Surgical Pathology of the Gastrointestinal System: Bacterial, Fungal, Viral, and Parasitic Infections

*For Drs. George F. Gray, Jr.; Rodger C. Haggitt;
and William A. Webb; they taught me most of what
I know, but only a small portion of what they know.*

Preface

Each organism's environment, for the most part, consists of other organisms.
– Kevin Kelly

Enteric infections are the second most common cause of death in the world, among all ages, preceded only by cardiovascular disease. The amount of anatomic pathology training that most of us receive pertaining to infectious disease pathology is at odds with these statistics. Most infectious disease pathology training is provided in the microbiology laboratory and is divorced from the examination of tissue sections. There are many situations, however, in which the histologic findings as well as microbiological data are critical to both the diagnosis and the management of an infectious disease.

This book is designed to serve as a practical reference for the pathologic diagnosis of infectious diseases of the gastrointestinal tract. In addition to discussing the morphologic features of the various infections, I have tried to emphasize how infectious diseases mimic other entities that we frequently encounter in gastrointestinal pathology, such as chronic idiopathic inflammatory bowel disease and ischemic enterocolitis. Much of the book is obviously devoted to illustrations, and the text is not intended as an exhaustive review but rather to provide pertinent clinical, diagnostic, and epidemiologic information that will be valuable to the practicing pathologist.

I have been fortunate in my career to train and work with many pathologists who loved infectious diseases of the gastrointestinal tract, and several of them have contributed large numbers of photographs to my collection over the years. It is my hope that the reader will benefit, as I have, from these wonderful materials that have been entrusted to me.

Little Rock, Arkansas   Laura Webb Lamps

Acknowledgments

I am indebted to so many friends and colleagues who have contributed photographs, slides, and tissue to me over the years; most of you are listed individually throughout the book in association with the material that you so generously contributed.

I particularly wish to thank my chairman, Dr. Bruce Smoller, for giving me the gift of time to write this book. I would also like to thank my colleagues in the pathology department for graciously supporting my time off service, and our fabulous secretarial and AV team, Victoria Hart, Mandy Trantham, Paula Lee, Donald Sandlin, and Sara Thompson.

Finally, I wish to thank my family for their support and encouragement: my father and stepmother, Dr. William A. and Ouida Webb; my brother Allen Webb; my dear husband and volunteer grammar editor Paul Ward; and my sister-equivalent and talented colleague, Dr. Amy Hudson.

Contents

Chapter 1

General Approach to the Diagnosis of Gastrointestinal Infections

Keywords Infection • Enteric • Colitis • Enterocolitis • Bacteria • Fungus • Virus • Parasite • Diarrhea

Gastrointestinal infections are one of the most important causes of morbidity and mortality worldwide. Enteric pathogens are the leading cause of childhood death in the world and are the second leading cause of death among all ages. Many enteric infections are transmitted to humans through contaminated food and water, and improvements in water quality, sanitation, and food hygiene practice have decreased food- and water-borne transmission of disease in many areas of the world. Conversely, problems associated with the modern practice of mass production and widespread distribution of food products most likely have contributed to the transmission of food-borne gastrointestinal illness, because food may be improperly stored at any point in the process, and food contaminated at one location may be shipped to many regions of a country and even to other nations.

Other aspects of modern living that contribute to the transmission of enteric pathogens include camping and water sports involving untreated water sources, poor swimming pool hygiene, more frequent consumption of restaurant and prepackaged foods, more widespread consumption of raw or poorly cooked meats and seafood, and travel, particularly from an area of good sanitation to one of poor sanitation.

The number of bone marrow and solid organ transplant patients is also increasing, as well as the population of patients with other immunocompromising conditions. For all of the above reasons, and as global urbanization, immigration, and transcontinental travel become more frequent, infectious diseases that were once limited to certain regions of the world, or relegated to the realm of textbook esoterica, could easily traverse the microscope stage of any anatomic pathologist, anywhere.

In many instances, diagnosing infectious diseases is a task for the clinician and the microbiologist. There are many situations, however, in which the histologic findings as interpreted by a skilled anatomic pathologist are critical to both diagnosis and management of infectious diseases. Examples include raising the possibility of an infectious disease when evaluating a tissue section, when it has not been previously considered in the differential diagnosis, and recommending useful ancillary tests such as microbiological cultures and serologic studies; the ability to perform special stains, molecular studies, or immunohistochemistry to diagnose an infection when cultures were not performed; and the ability to identify pathogens in tissue sections that cannot be cultured or identified by other means. In addition, many morphologic methods used for tissue diagnosis can be performed much quicker than microbiological culture, particularly when fungal or mycobacterial infections are considered.

The goals of the surgical pathologist in evaluating gastrointestinal specimens for infection are generally twofold. First, acute self-limited and/or infectious processes should be distinguished from chronic idiopathic inflammatory bowel disease (ulcerative colitis and Crohn's disease), ischemia, and other chronic atypical colitides such as lymphocytic colitis. Second, dedicated attempts must be made to identify the specific infectious organism(s). In recent years, the surgical pathologist's ability to diagnose infectious processes in tissue sections has grown exponentially with the advent of new histochemical stains, immunohistochemistry, and molecular assays. As these techniques have developed, our knowledge of the morphologic changes caused by various organisms also has increased.

Many enteric infections are self-limited, particularly in immunocompetent patients. Those who undergo endoscopic evaluation generally have chronic or debilitating diarrhea and systemic symptoms or are immunocompromised. A discussion with the gastroenterologist regarding symptoms and macroscopic findings, as well as knowledge of travel history, food intake (such as sushi or poorly cooked meat), sexual practices, and immune status, can be invaluable in evaluating specimens for infectious diseases.

Morphological approach to diagnosis of infections of the gastrointestinal tract. Despite the long list of pathogens that affect the GI tract, most produce morphologic changes that can be broadly categorized into one of a few histologic patterns (see also Tables 1.1 and 14.1):

L.W. Lamps, *Surgical Pathology of the Gastrointestinal System: Bacterial, Fungal, Viral, and Parasitic Infections,*
DOI 10.1007/978-1-4419-0861-2_1, © Springer Science+Business Media, LLC 2009

Table 1.1 Classification of bacterial infections of the gastrointestinal tract by histologic pattern

Minimal or no inflammatory change	Acute self-limited colitis pattern	Pseudo-membranous pattern	Predominantly granulomatous	Diffuse histiocytic	Predominantly lympho-histiocytic	Architectural distortion	Ischemic pattern
Toxigenic *Vibrio cholerae* O1	*Shigella*	Entero-hemorrhagic	*Yersinia*	*Rhodococcus equi*	LGV	Marked	Enterohemorrhagic *E. coli*
	Campylobacter	*E. coli*	*M. tuberculosis*		*Salmonella typhimurium*	*Salmonella typhimurium*	*C. difficile*
Enteropathogenic *E. coli*	*Aeromonas*	*C. difficile*	*Actinomycosis*	Whipple's disease		*Shigella*	
Enteroadherent *E. coli*	Occasionally *Salmonella* (especially non-typhoid)	Occasionally *Shigella*	*MAI* (immuno-competent patients)	*MAI* (immuno-compromised patients)		Focal or mild: *Aeromonas*	
Spirochetosis						*Campylobacter*	
Neisseria species	Other *Vibrio* species						
	Occasionally *C. difficile*						
	Syphilis (+/− increased plasma cells)						

1. Organisms that produce mild or no histologic changes (such as toxigenic *Vibrio cholerae* O1, *Neisseria gonorrhea,* and many enteric viruses).
2. Organisms that produce histologic features of acute infectious-type or acute self-limited colitis (AITC/ASLC) or focal active colitis (FAC); many bacterial infections fall into this category, including *Campylobacter, Aeromonas,* and some *Salmonella* species (see Table 1.1).
3. Organisms that can be specifically identified in tissue sections, or that produce specific or characteristic histologic features, such as *Strongyloides, Clostridium difficile*-related pseudomembranous colitis, necrotizing granulomatous infection associated with *Mycobacterium tuberculosis*, or viral inclusions.

Surgical pathologists should also be aware of the infections that are most likely to mimic other inflammatory bowel diseases, particularly Crohn's disease, ulcerative colitis, and ischemic colitis (see Table 1.2).

Acute self-limited or acute infectious-type colitis patterns. The "acute self-limited colitis (ASLC)" pattern is one of the patterns most commonly seen in enteric infections. This process usually resolves within several weeks, without residual histologic findings or recurrent symptoms. Many infectious agents can produce the ASLC pattern, including numerous bacteria, viruses, and parasites. In some cases, however, the infection may not be self-limited and even can be fatal; for this reason, many pathologists and clinicians prefer the essentially synonymous term "acute infectious-type colitis (AITC)."

The characteristic findings in ASLC/AITC can be summarized as cryptitis in a background of preserved crypt architecture (Fig. 1.1). Other characteristic findings include neutrophils in the lamina propria, crypt abscesses, crypt rup-

Table 1.2 Infectious mimics of chronic idiopathic inflammatory bowel disease and ischemic colitis

Mimics of Crohn's disease	Mimics of ulcerative colitis	Mimics of ischemic colitis
Cytomegalovirus	*Shigella* species	Cytomegalovirus
Salmonella typhimurium	Non-typhoid *Salmonella* species	*Aspergillus*
Shigella species	*Entamoeba histolytica*	Zygomycetes
Yersinia	*Aeromonas* species	Enterohemorrhagic *E. coli*
M. tuberculosis	*Campylobacter* (rarely)	*C. difficile* (pseudomembranous colitis)
Aeromonas species	Lymphogranuloma venereum	*C. perfringens*
Campylobacter (rarely)		
Lymphogranuloma venereum		
Entamoeba histolytica		

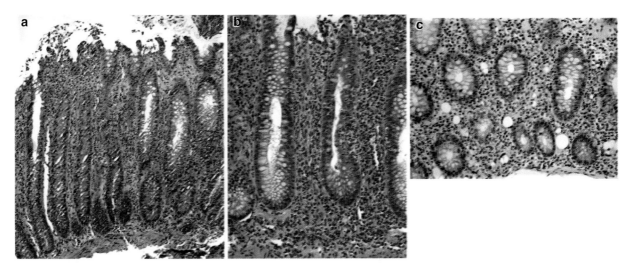

Fig. 1.1 Diffuse cryptitis in a background of preserved crypt architecture is typical of acute infectious-type colitis (**a–c**). Note surface epithelial damage and superficial mucosal erosion (**a** and **b**), as well as a neutrophilic infiltrate in the lamina propria (**b** and **c**)

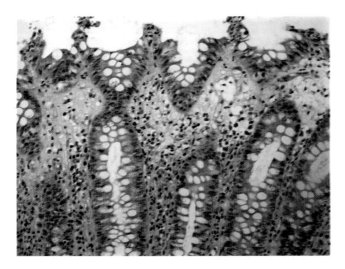

Fig. 1.2 Mucosal edema and neutrophils in the upper third of the mucosa, as well as surface injury and neutrophilic inflammation, in a case of AITC

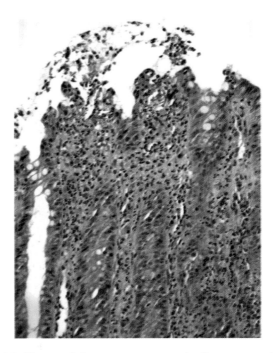

Fig. 1.3 The acute inflammatory component is often most prominent in the mid- to upper levels of the crypts

ture, edema, and surface epithelial damage with superficial mucosal erosion (Fig. 1.2). The acute inflammatory component is often most prominent in the mid- to upper levels of the crypts (Fig. 1.3). The inflammatory changes may be focal or diffuse. The lamina propria may contain increased mononuclear cells as well as neutrophils, but basal plasma cells should not be present.

Histological changes of chronicity are usually present even in the initial biopsy specimen in patients with chronic idiopathic inflammatory bowel disease, and the lack of features of chronicity (crypt distortion, Paneth cell metaplasia, and basal lymphoplasmacytosis) helps to distinguish ASLC from chronic idiopathic inflammatory bowel disease. It is important to realize, however, that many infectious agents can produce changes that closely mimic other inflammatory

bowel diseases, and the surgical pathologist should be aware of these entities as he or she considers differential diagnoses (see Tables 1.1 and 1.2). Further complicating this issue is that many enteric pathogens may cause exacerbations or relapses of chronic idiopathic inflammatory bowel disease, producing a histologically confusing picture; this reinforces the necessity of a diligent search for pathogens (including stool cultures) even in patients with the established diagnosis of chronic idiopathic inflammatory bowel disease.

Focal active colitis. Focal active colitis (FAC) is the term that should be used to describe focal neutrophilic crypt injury

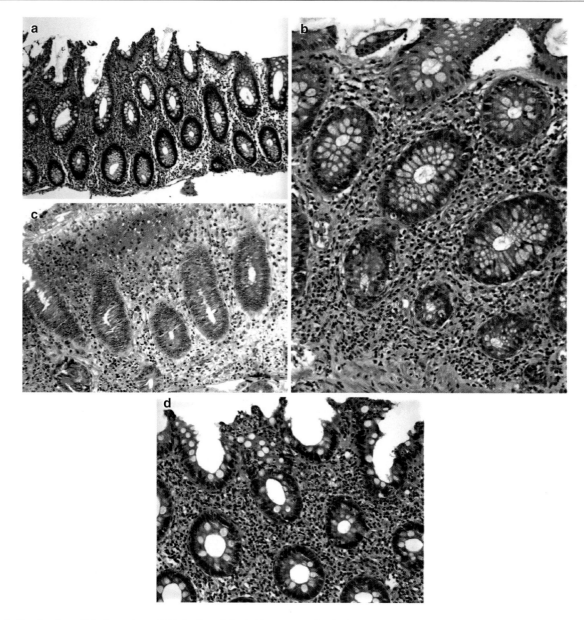

Fig. 1.4 Focal active colitis due to bacterial infection. Colonic biopsy shows focal cryptitis and increased inflammatory cells in the lamina propria. Note more normal epithelium to the right (**a**). High-power view shows very focal cryptitis in a background of increased mixed inflam- mation in the lamina propria and preserved crypt architecture (**b**). Focal increase in neutrophils in the lamina propria, with mucosal edema and reactive epithelial changes (**c**). Focal cryptitis with surface mucosal injury and infiltration by neutrophils (**d**)

(Fig. 1.4). The spectrum of morphologic changes encom- passed by the term FAC ranges from a single crypt abscess or focus of cryptitis to multiple foci of neutrophilic crypti- tis or crypt abscesses within one or more large bowel biop- sies. Infection, particularly resolving infection, is the most common underlying cause of FAC, although adverse drug reaction, bowel prep injury, and Crohn's disease (particularly in children) also can produce this spectrum of morphologic changes.

Resolving infectious colitis. Since most patients do not present for endoscopy until several weeks after the onset of symptoms, pathologists are less and less frequently exposed to the classic histologic features of AITC as described above. This is important, because the resolving phase of infectious colitis is more challenging to diagnose. At this stage, one may find only occasional foci of neutrophilic cryptitis (focal active colitis) and a patchy increase in lamina propria inflam- mation, which may, in fact, contain abundant plasma cells and increased intraepithelial lymphocytes (Fig. 1.5). Since these features are also seen in Crohn's disease and in lym- phocytic colitis, it is important to be aware of the patient's symptoms (particularly acute versus chronic onset) and, ide- ally, the culture results, because the exact diagnosis may be difficult to resolve on histologic grounds alone.

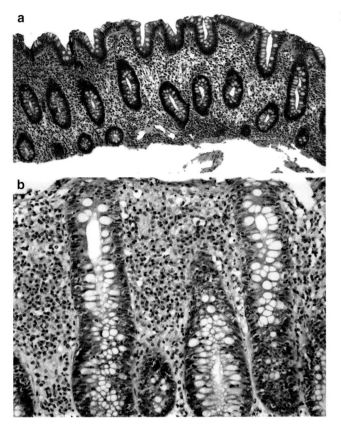

Fig. 1.5 Resolving infectious colitis. At low power, the lymphoplasmacytic infiltrate in the lamina propria can mimic lymphocytic colitis (**a**). High-power view shows increased plasma cells in the lamina propria, along with numerous intraepithelial lymphocytes and only rare intraepithelial neutrophils (**b**)

Selected References

1. Abrams GD. Surgical pathology of the infected gut. Am J Surg Pathol 11 Suppl 1:16–24, 1987.
2. Greenson JK, Stern RA, Carpenter SL, Barnett JL. The clinical significance of focal active colitis. Hum Pathol 28:729–33, 1997.
3. Hibbs RG. Diarrhoeal disease: current concepts and future challenges. Introduction. Trans Roy Soc Trop Med Hyg 87 Suppl 3:1–2, 1993.
4. Kumar NB, Nostrant TT, Appelman HD. The histopathologic spectrum of acute self-limited colitis (acute infectious-type colitis). Am J Surg Pathol 6:523–9, 1982.
5. Mylonaki M, Langmead L, Pantes A, et al. Enteric infection in relapse of inflammatory bowel disease: importance of microbiological examination of stool. Eur J Gastroenterol Hepatol 16: 775–8, 2004.
6. Savarino SJ, Bourgeois AL. Diarrhoeal disease: current concepts and future challenges. Epidemiology of diarrhoeal diseases in developed countries. Trans Roy Soc Trop Med Hyg 87 Suppl 3:7–11, 1993.
7. Surawicz CM. The role of rectal biopsy in infectious colitis. Am J Surg Path 12 Supp 1:82–8, 1988.
8. Surawicz CM, Haggitt RC, Husseman M, McFarland LV. Mucosal biopsy diagnosis of colitis: acute self-limited colitis and idiopathic inflammatory bowel disease. Gastroenterol 107:755–63, 1994.
9. Volk EE, Shapiro BD, Easley KA, Goldblum JR. The clinical significance of a biopsy-based diagnosis of focal active colitis: a clinicopathologic study of 31 cases. Mod Pathol 11:789–94, 1998.
10. Watts JC. Surgical pathology and the diagnosis of infectious diseases (editorial). Am J Clin Pathol 102:711–12, 1994.
11. Xin W, Brown PI, Greenson JK. The clinical significance of focal active colitis in pediatric patients. Am J Surg Pathol 27:1134–8, 2003.

Part I
Bacterial Infections of the Gastrointestinal Tract

Abstract Bacterial infections of the gastrointestinal tract are an important cause of morbidity and mortality worldwide, and can mimic other gastrointestinal diseases including ischemic colitis and chronic idiopathic inflammatory bowel disease. Although many bacterial infections of the gastrointestinal tract are diagnosed using microbiological cultures, tissue biopsy is an important diagnostic tool, especially as stool cultures are often not obtained prior to beginning antibiotic therapy. This section addresses common and uncommon bacterial infections affecting the gastrointestinal tract, including clinical setting, important associations with food and water, macroscopic and histologic features, differential diagnoses, and useful laboratory tests that can aid in diagnosis.

Chapter 2

Aeromonas, Vibrio cholerae, and Related Bacteria

Keywords *Aeromonas* sp • *Vibrio* sp • *Plesiomonas* sp • *Edwardsiella* sp • Colitis • Bacteria

Aeromonas species are ubiquitous in soil and water sources throughout the world. Infection commonly results from exposure to untreated water, but also may result from consuming contaminated foods such as produce, meat, and dairy products. Aeromonads are not part of the normal human intestinal flora. They were initially believed to be nonpathogenic, as they are occasionally isolated from the stool of asymptomatic persons. They are increasingly recognized as a cause of gastroenteritis in both healthy and immunocompromised adults and children, based on the recovery of the organism from the stool of symptomatic patients in the absence of other pathogens, and subsequent complete response to antibiotic therapy. The motile *Aeromonas hydrophila* and *Aeromonas sobria* most often cause gastrointestinal disease in humans, although other species may as well.

Gastrointestinal *Aeromonas* infections most frequently present in the late spring, summer, and early fall. Children are most commonly affected. A mild, self-limited diarrheal illness is most frequently described, sometimes accompanied by nausea, vomiting, and cramping abdominal pain. A more severe, dysentery-like illness occurs in 15–25% of patients, featuring bloody or mucoid diarrhea and fecal leukocytes. This variant is most likely to mimic chronic idiopathic inflammatory bowel disease endoscopically. A minority of patients experiences a subacute, chronic diarrhea lasting months to years, and the chronic nature of the symptoms may mimic chronic idiopathic inflammatory bowel disease clinically.

Pathologic features. Endoscopically, findings include mucosal edema, friability, erosions, exudates, and loss of vascular pattern (Fig. 2.1). The distribution is often segmental, either right- or left-sided, and may mimic ischemic colitis, Crohn's disease, or ulcerative colitis macroscopically. A severe pancolitis mimicking fulminant ulcerative colitis has been described as well. The histologic features are usually those of acute self-limited colitis, including cryptitis,

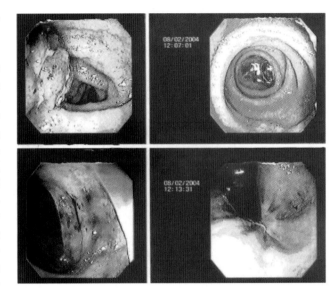

Fig. 2.1 Both *Aeromonas* and *Plesiomonas* colitis can show mucosal erythema, erosions, and friability (courtesy Dr. Karl Landberg)

crypt abscesses, and a neutrophilic infiltrate in the lamina propria (Fig. 2.2). However, ulceration (Fig. 2.3) and focal architectural distortion may be seen in some cases (Fig. 2.4).

Differential diagnosis. The differential diagnosis includes other infectious colitides, ischemic colitis, and chronic idiopathic inflammatory bowel disease. Stool cultures are critical to diagnosis, and certain selective media may be required.

When architectural distortion is present in a patient with chronic symptoms or macroscopic features mimicking chronic idiopathic inflammatory bowel disease, it may be difficult to resolve the issue of *Aeromonas* infection versus Crohn's disease or ulcerative colitis. *Aeromonas* has been reported as a cause of exacerbations in idiopathic inflammatory bowel disease as well. For these reasons, some authorities recommend culturing for *Aeromonas* in all patients with refractory chronic inflammatory bowel disease, as well as patients (particularly children) with a presumed initial presentation of chronic idiopathic inflammatory bowel

L.W. Lamps, *Surgical Pathology of the Gastrointestinal System: Bacterial, Fungal, Viral, and Parasitic Infections,*
DOI 10.1007/978-1-4419-0861-2_2, © Springer Science+Business Media, LLC 2009

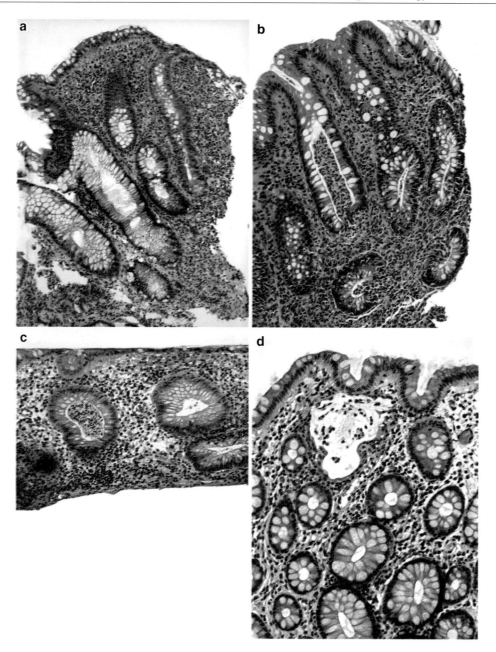

Fig. 2.2 *Aeromonas* colitis. Low-power view shows cryptitis and a mixed inflammatory infiltrate in the lamina propria (**a**). Well-developed neutrophilic cryptitis and crypt abscesses are common features (**b–d**)

disease. Although there are no histologic features specific for *Aeromonas* infection (as with many infections of the gastrointestinal tract), it is important for the surgical pathologist to realize that this is one of the bacteria that can most closely mimic chronic idiopathic inflammatory bowel disease.

Plesiomonas shigelloides and *Edwardsiella tarda* are similar freshwater bacteria. Although less commonly isolated than *Aeromonas* species, they are believed to cause a similar clinical, macroscopic, and histologic spectrum of disease (Fig. 2.5).

Vibrio cholerae, specifically the toxigenic O1 strain, is the causative agent of cholera, an important worldwide cause of watery diarrhea and dysentery that may lead to significant dehydration, electrolyte imbalance, and death within hours. In the United States, most cases occur in patients who have traveled to or emigrated from endemic or epidemic areas. Most infections are due to consumption of raw or undercooked seafood, especially shellfish. Other *Vibrios*, including non-O1 strains of *V. cholerae*, *V. hollisae,* and *V. parahaemolyticus*, also can cause severe gastroenteritis.

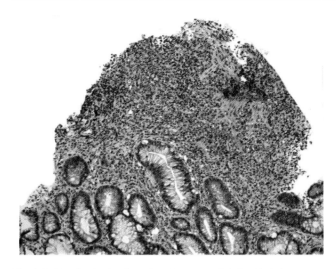

Fig. 2.3 Focal colonic ulcerations in a case of right-sided *Aeromonas* colitis, proven by culture and PCR assay, which mimicked Crohn's disease clinically

Symptoms of cholera include abrupt onset of diarrhea, usually profusely watery and rarely bloody, accompanied by abdominal pain, vomiting, muscle cramps, and fever. Strains other than toxigenic O1 *V. cholerae* are more likely to cause bloody diarrhea, fecal leukocytes, and dissemination to extraintestinal sites; however, the clinical scenarios produced by toxigenic *V. cholerae* O1 and other *Vibrios* may be indistinguishable. Disseminated infection is a particularly important risk with immunocompromised patients; patients with underlying liver disease, partial or total gastrectomy, and diseases of iron metabolism are also at risk for more serious *Vibrio* infections.

Despite the severity of the illness, toxigenic *V. cholerae* O1 is a non-invasive organism that causes minimal or no histologic changes in the gut. Rare non-specific findings such as small bowel mucin depletion, degenerative surface epithelial changes, and a mild increase in lamina propria mononuclear cells have been reported rarely.

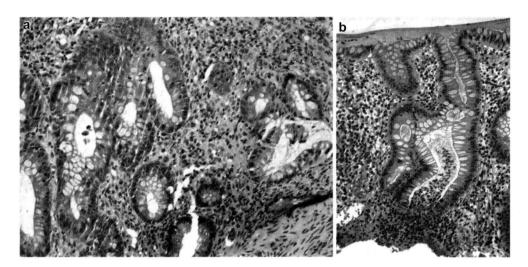

Fig. 2.4 Architectural distortion in *Aeromonas* infection may mimic chronic idiopathic inflammatory bowel disease (**a** and **b**)

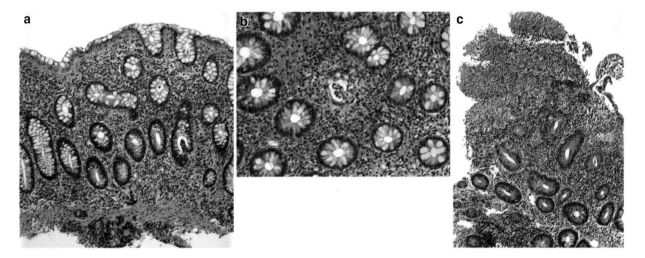

Fig. 2.5 Culture-proven *Plesiomonas* colitis showing patchy architectural distortion (**a**), cryptitis, and crypt abscesses (**b**). An ulcerative ileitis was also present (**c**)

Non-toxigenic O1 and other non-cholerae *Vibrio* species may show an erosive enterocolitis with active neutrophilic inflammation and associated hemorrhage. Useful ancillary diagnostic tests include culture, darkfield examination of stool, and serologic studies. A history of travel to or emigration from an endemic or epidemic area also can be invaluable.

Selected References

Aeromonas, Plesiomonas, *and* Edwardsiella

1. Champsaur H, Andremont A, Mathieu D, et al. Cholera-like illness due to *Aeromonas sobria*. J Inf Dis 145:248–54, 1982.
2. Deutsch SF, Wedzina W. *Aeromonas sobria* associated left sided segmental colitis. Am J Gastro 92:2104–6, 1997.
3. Doman DB, Golding MI, Goldberg HJ, Doyle RB. *Aeromonas hydrophila* colitis presenting as medically refractory inflammatory bowel disease. Am J Gastroenterol 84:83–5, 1989.
4. Farraye FA, Peppercorn MA, Ciano PS, Kavesh WN. Segmental colitis associated with *Aeromonas hydrophila*. Am J Gastroenterol 84:436–8, 1989.
5. George WL, Nakata MM, Thompson J, White ML. *Aeromonas*-related diarrhea in adults. Arch Int Med 145:2207–11, 1985.
6. Gluskin I, Batash D, Shoseyov D, et al. A 15-year study of the role of *Aeromonas* spp. In gastroenteritis in hospitalized children. J Med Microbiol 37:315–8, 1992.
7. Goldsweig CD, Pacheco PA. Infectious colitis excluding *E. coli* O157:H7 and *C. difficile*. Gastroenterol Clin North Am 30(3):709–33, 2001.
8. Gracey M, Burke V, Robinson I. *Aeromonas*-associated gastroenteritis. Lancet 2(8311):1304–6, 1982.
9. Janda JM, Abbott SL, Morris JG Jr. *Aeromonas, Plesiomonas,* and *Edwardsiella*. In: Blaser MJ, Smith PD, Ravdin JI, et al. Infections of the Gastrointestinal Tract. New York: Raven Press, 1995, pp. 905–17.
10. Kain KC, Kelly MT. Clinical features, epidemiology, and treatment of *Plesiomonas shigelloides* diarrhea. J Clin Microbiol 27:998–1001, 1989.
11. Kourany M, Vasquez MA, Saenz R. Edwardsiellosis in man and animals in Panama: clinical and epidemiological characteristics. Am J Trop Med Hyg 26:1183–90, 1977.
12. Lindberg MR, Havens JM, Lauwers GY, et al. *Aeromonas*: an emerging food-borne cause of infectious colitis. Mod Pathol 21:127A, 2008.
13. Marsik F, Werlin SL. *Aeromonas hydrophila* colitis in a child. J Pediatr Gastroenterol Nutr 3:808–11,1984.
14. Merino S, Rubires X, Knochel S, Tomas JM. Emerging pathogens: *Aeromonas* spp. Int J Food Microbiol 28:157–68, 1995.
15. Roberts IM, Parenti DM, Albert MB. *Aeromonas hydrophila*-associated colitis in a male homosexual. Arch Int Med 147:1502–3, 1987.
16. Travis LB, Washington JA. The clinical significance of stool isolates of *Aeromonas*. Am J Clin Path 85: 330–6, 1986.
17. von Graevenitz A, Mensch AH. The genus *Aeromonas* in human bacteriology: report of 30 cases and review of the literature. N Engl J Med 278:245–9, 1968.

Vibrio *Species*

18. Abbott SL, Janda JM. Severe gastroenteritis associated with *Vibrio hollisae* infection: report of two cases and review. Clin Inf Dis 18:310–12, 1994.
19. Besser RE, Feikin DR, Eberhart-Phillips JE, et al. Diagnosis and treatment of cholera in the United States: are we prepared? JAMA 272:1203–5, 1994.
20. Carpenter CCJ, Mahmoud AAF, Warren KS. Algorithms in the diagnosis and management of exotic diseases. XXVI. Cholera. J Infect Dis 136:461–4, 1977.
21. Goldsweig CD, Pacheco PA. Infectious colitis excluding *E. coli* O157:H7 and *C. difficile*. Gastroenterol Clin North Am 30(3):709–33, 2001.
22. Hughes JM, Hollis DG, Gangarosa EJ, Weaver Re. Non-cholera *Vibrio* infections in the United States. Ann Intern Med 88:602–6, 1978.
23. Hughes JM, Boyce JM, Aleem ARMA, et al. *Vibrio parahaemolyticus* enterocolitis in Bangladesh: report of an outbreak. Am J Trop Med Hyg 27:106–12, 1978.
24. Pastore G, Schiraldi G, Fera G, et al. A biopsy study of gastrointestinal mucosa in cholera patients during an epidemic in southern Italy. Am J Dig Dis 21:613–7, 1976.
25. Seas C, Miranda J, Gil AI, et al. New insights on the emergence of cholera in Latin American during 1991: the Peruvian experience. Am J Trop Med Hyg 62:513–17, 2000.
26. Shuangshoti S, Reinprayoon S. Pathologic changes of gut in non-O1 *Vibrio cholerae* infection. J Med Assoc Thai 78:204–9, 1995.

Chapter 3

Campylobacter Species

Keywords *Campylobacter* sp. • Colitis • Guillain–Barre syndrome

These Gram-negative bacteria are the most common stool isolate in the United States and are a major cause of diarrhea worldwide. *Campylobacter* (derived from the Greek for "curved rod") is most commonly associated with consuming undercooked poultry, raw milk, or untreated water. It is a common veterinary pathogen, and human infection may be contracted from sick animals. *Campylobacter jejuni* is most commonly associated with food-borne gastroenteritis, along with *C. coli* and *C. laridis*, whereas *C. fetus* and other less common species are more often seen in immunosuppressed patients and homosexual men.

Campylobacter infects patients of all ages, but infants, children, and young adults are most often affected. The incidence in HIV-positive patients is higher than the general population, and severe, chronic, recurrent, or disseminated infections are more common in this group. Most infections are self-limited, especially in immunocompetent patients; antibiotics and supportive care may be required in patients with lengthy, severe, or disseminated infections, as well as in immunocompromised patients. *Campylobacter* infection is associated with the subsequent development of several autoimmune disorders, including Guillain–Barre syndrome (which is associated with *Campylobacter* in up to 40% of cases), Henoch-Schonlein purpura, and reactive arthropathy. *Campylobacter* infection may also cause exacerbations of underlying chronic idiopathic inflammatory bowel disease.

Signs and symptoms typically include fever, malaise, cramping abdominal pain (often severe), and watery diarrhea, which often contains blood and leukocytes. Abdominal pain may be the dominant symptom in many patients. Nausea, vomiting, tenesmus, headache, and myalgias are variably present. Symptoms generally resolve within 1–2 weeks, but relapse is common.

Pathologic features. Endoscopic findings include friable colonic mucosa with associated erythema and hemorrhage. Ulceration and inflammatory exudates may be present. Segmental colitis or a pancolitis macroscopically mimicking ulcerative colitis has been reported rarely. Colonoscopy may be unremarkable, however.

Histologic examination most frequently shows features of acute infectious or self-limited colitis, including cryptitis

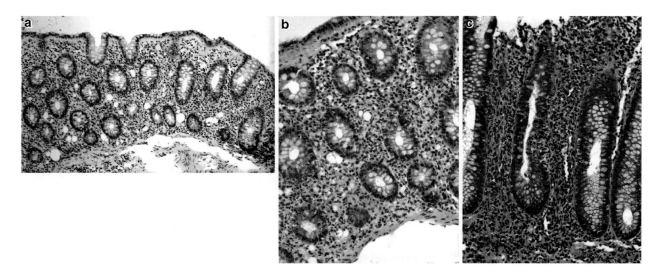

Fig. 3.1 Preservation of crypt architecture (**a**), cryptitis, and a neutrophilic infiltrate in the lamina propria in culture-proven *Campylobacter* colitis (**b** and **c**)

L.W. Lamps, *Surgical Pathology of the Gastrointestinal System: Bacterial, Fungal, Viral, and Parasitic Infections*,
DOI 10.1007/978-1-4419-0861-2_3, © Springer Science+Business Media, LLC 2009

(Fig. 3.1), crypt abscesses (Fig. 3.2), surface epithelial damage (Fig. 3.3), and a neutrophilic infiltrate in the lamina propria. Marked edema and superficial mucosal erosion with associated hemorrhage may be seen as well (Fig. 3.4). Findings may be patchy or focal. Of note, *C. jejuni* has been detected by molecular methods in almost 20% of patients who have the "focal active colitis" pattern of inflammation on colon biopsy. Mild crypt distortion, crypt epithelial damage, and crypt loss are occasionally present (Fig. 3.5), although crypt architecture is usually well preserved. Similar morphologic findings may be seen in the small bowel.

Differential diagnosis. The differential diagnosis predominantly includes other infections that produce the acute infectious or self-limited colitis pattern, such as *Salmonella*, *Shigella*, and *Aeromonas*. Occasionally, when crypt distortion is seen, *Campylobacter* colitis can mimic chronic idio-

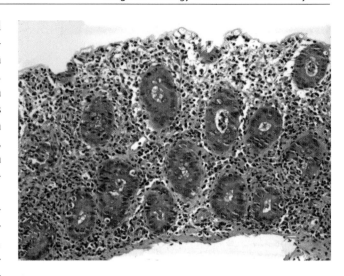

Fig. 3.3 Surface epithelial damage in *Campylobacter* colitis. The underlying mucosa shows cryptitis, crypt abscesses, and preservation of crypt architecture

pathic inflammatory bowel disease. Stool culture is an invaluable aid to diagnosis; serologic studies, darkfield examination of stool, and molecular assays are also available.

Selected References

1. Arguilles BF, Martin IH, Fernandez MJ, Vivas JJP. Recurrence of Henoch-Schonlein purpura in association with *Campylobacter jejuni* colitis. J Clin Gastroenterol 34:492–3, 2002.
2. Blaser MJ, Parsons RB, Wang WLL. Acute colitis caused by *Campylobacter fetus* ss. *jejuni*. Gastroenterol 78:448–53, 1980.
3. Blaser MJ, Berkowitz ID, LaForce FM, et al. *Campylobacter* enteritis: clinical and epidemiological features. Ann Intern Med 91:179–85, 1979.
4. Goldsweig CD, Pacheco PA. Infectious colitis excluding *E. coli* 0157:H7 and *C. difficile*. Gastroenterol Clin North Am 30(3):709–33, 2001.

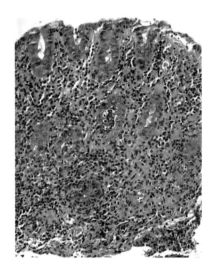

Fig. 3.2 Crypt abscesses, cryptitis, and reactive epithelial changes in *Campylobacter* colitis

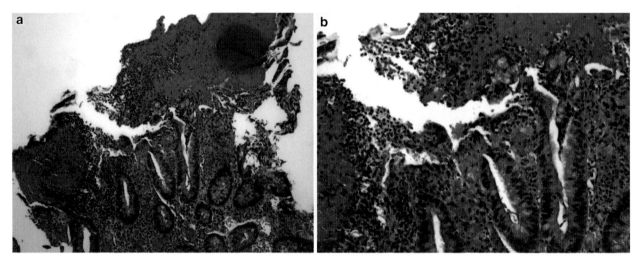

Fig. 3.4 Surface mucosal erosion with associated hemorrhage and acute inflammatory exudates in *Campylobacter* colitis (**a** and **b**)

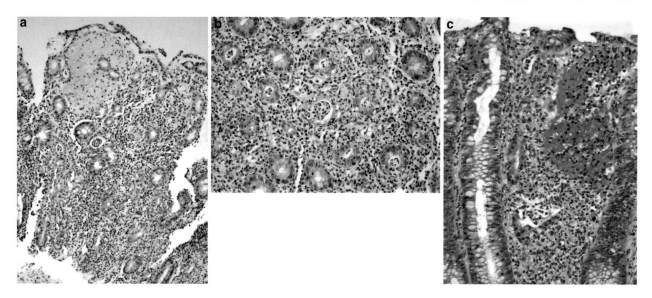

Fig. 3.5 Patchy crypt distortion (**a**), crypt epithelial damage (**b**), and crypt destruction (**c**) are occasionally seen in *Campylobacter* colitis, mimicking chronic idiopathic inflammatory bowel disease

5. Fields PI, Swerdlow DL. *Campylobacter jejuni*. Clin Lab Med 19:489–503, 1999.
6. Lambert ME, Schofield PF, Ironside AG, Mandal BK. *Campylobacter* colitis. Br Med J 1:857–9, 1979.
7. Price AB, Jewkes J, Sanderson PJ. Acute diarrhoea: *Campylobacter* colitis and the role of rectal biopsy. J Clin Pathol 32:990–7, 1979.
8. Schneider ES, Havens JM, Scott MA, et al. Molecular diagnosis of *C. jejuni* infection in cases of focal active colitis. Am J Surg Pathol 30:782–5, 2006.
9. Siegal D, Syed F, Hamid N, Cunha BA. *Campylobacter jejuni* pancolitis mimicking idiopathic ulcerative colitis. Heart Lung 34:288–90, 2005.
10. Skirrow MB. *Campylobacter* enteritis: a "new" disease. Br Med J 2:9–11, 1977.
11. Tee W, Anderson BN, Ross BC, Dwyer B. Atypical *Campylobacters* associated with gastroenteritis. J Clin Microbiol 25:1248–52, 1987.
12. Turgeon DK, Fritsche TR. Laboratory approaches to infectious diarrhea. Gastroenterol Clin North Am 30(3):693–707, 2001.

Chapter 4

Helicobacter pylori and Related Species

Keywords *Helicobacter* sp • Gastritis • Special stain

Helicobacter pylori, originally classified as *Campylobacter pyloridis*, is a spirillar or coccoid Gram-negative bacterium that infects the stomach. The incidence of *H. pylori* (HP) infection is decreasing, in part due to eradication, but it remains one of the most common bacterial infections worldwide and reportedly infects over half of the entire human race. Person-to-person transmission via fecal–oral, oral–oral, and gastric–oral routes accounts for most cases, but the possibility of acquisition from zoonotic or environmental sources cannot be excluded. Risk factors include young age and low socioeconomic status.

H. pylori infection is associated with many gastrointestinal diseases, including chronic gastritis, atrophic gastritis, peptic ulcers, gastric adenocarcinoma, and lymphomas of the mucosa-associated lymphoid tissue (MALT) type. However, the exact mechanisms by which HP causes disease remain unclear. Patients with *H. pylori*-associated gastritis may present with dyspepsia, epigastric pain, nausea, vomiting, and GI bleeding. Many infected patients are asymptomatic, however.

Pathologic features. There is generally poor correlation between endoscopic findings and the presence or severity of histologic findings. Mucosal changes are very non-specific and include erythema, mucosal granularity, and abnormal vascular pattern. Nodularity of the mucosa may be seen, especially in children, and may correlate with lymphoid hyperplasia.

The antrum is most commonly affected, although the fundic and cardiac mucosa also are commonly involved. The inflammatory pattern most commonly associated with HP infection is chronic, active gastritis, featuring a mononuclear cell infiltrate in the lamina propria that is rich in plasma cells (Fig. 4.1), along with neutrophils that may infiltrate the glandular epithelium (Fig. 4.2). Scattered eosinophils are also

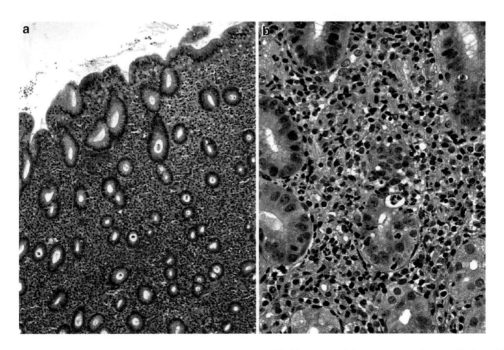

Fig. 4.1 The lamina propria of the antrum is expanded by a mononuclear cell infiltrate containing numerous plasma cells (**a** and **b**)

L.W. Lamps, *Surgical Pathology of the Gastrointestinal System: Bacterial, Fungal, Viral, and Parasitic Infections,*
DOI 10.1007/978-1-4419-0861-2_4, © Springer Science+Business Media, LLC 2009

Fig. 4.2 In chronic, active gastritis due to *H. pylori*, neutrophils may be present in the lamina propria as well and may infiltrate the glandular epithelium (**a** and **b**; **b** – courtesy Dr. Rodger C. Haggitt)

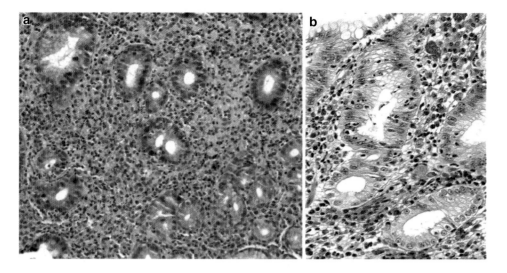

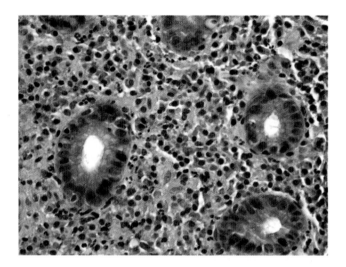

Fig. 4.3 Scattered eosinophils may be present within the inflammatory milieu

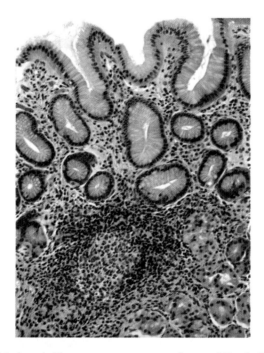

Fig. 4.4 Lymphoid aggregates are a common feature of *H. pylori* infection, which may contain prominent germinal centers

common within the inflammatory infiltrate (Fig. 4.3). Lymphoid aggregates are a frequent feature (Fig. 4.4), with variably present germinal centers, and a significant intraepithelial lymphocytosis may be seen as well (Fig. 4.5). Although mucosal architecture is usually well preserved, the epithelium may show mucus depletion, reactive nuclear changes, or a serrated appearance. The severity of the inflammation does not usually correlate with the number of organisms found. Although intestinal metaplasia may be seen in association with HP infection (most commonly in the context of multifocal atrophic gastritis), HP is rarely seen overlying areas of intestinal metaplasia.

Proton pump inhibitors and medications used to eradicate HP may result in a migration of the bacteria proximally toward the corpus, as well as a decrease in inflammatory activity. The absence of active inflammation does

not necessarily imply an absence of *H. pylori*, however. The chronic inflammatory infiltrate and presence of lymphoid follicles abate more slowly, and these changes are usually present a year or more after eradication of the organism.

H. pylori are tiny (2–5 μm), slightly basophilic, spirillar, "comma," or "seagull" shaped organisms (Fig. 4.6) that are present in the mucus layer at the surface of the epithelium. They reside both at the luminal surface and within the pits (Fig. 4.7); invasive organisms are seldom seen. The distribution of HP may be very focal and patchy (Fig. 4.8). Further-

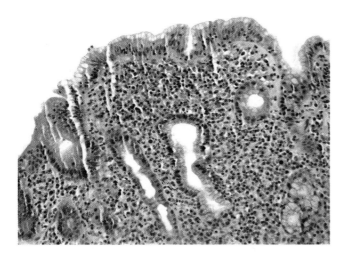

Fig. 4.5 Helicobacter infection may cause a notable intraepithelial lymphocytosis, seen here in both surface and glandular epithelium

more, under suboptimal conditions, the usually spirillar bacteria may undergo transformation to coccoid forms (Fig. 4.9) that closely resemble mucus droplets, non-pathogenic bacteria, or other organisms such as fungal spores or coccidians. Although the precise clinical significance of coccoid forms is uncertain, they are usually associated with spirillar forms, and the diagnosis of HP infection when only coccoid forms are present should be entertained with caution.

Many authorities recommend two biopsies from the antrum (one from the lesser and one from the greater curvature) and one or more from the gastric corpus to adequately evaluate the status of HP infection. Although the need for special stains in the diagnosis of HP remains controversial,

most agree that some form of stain is necessary, particularly if infection is patchy, intestinal metaplasia is present, or the patient has been treated previously. Useful stains include Giemsa, Diff-quick (Fig. 4.10), and silver impregnation stains such as the Warthin-Starry or Steiner. The latter may be combined with H&E and Alcian blue (pH 2.5) to produce the popular "triple" or "Genta" stain that also allows for evaluation of gastric morphology (Fig. 4.11). Silver impregnation stains are expensive and technically more difficult, but the bacteria are easy to identify using this method as they stain dark black, and appear fatter. Gram stain and the fluorescent acridine orange stain also will detect HP, although these are not routinely used. The more recently introduced immunostain has gained popularity due to the ease of identification and specificity (Fig. 4.12). However, the immunostain may cross-react with other *Helicobacter* species (see below).

Differential diagnosis. The differential diagnosis primarily includes other causes of non-erosive, non-specific gastritis, including autoimmune gastritis, Crohn's disease, infectious gastroenteritis, adverse drug reaction, and the lymphocytic gastritis associated with celiac disease. If there is a particularly dense inflammatory infiltrate, *H. pylori*-related gastritis must be distinguished from MALT lymphoma. Architectural destruction (Fig. 4.13), infiltration of lymphocytes into the submucosa (Fig. 4.14), and numerous lymphoepithelial lesions (Fig. 4.15) favor a neoplastic process, but gene rearrangement studies may be required to confirm the diagnosis.

H. pylori must be distinguished from contaminating oropharyngeal flora, which also may stain on non-specific histochemical stains, by the morphology of the organism. It must also be distinguished from other less common *Helicobacter* species (see below).

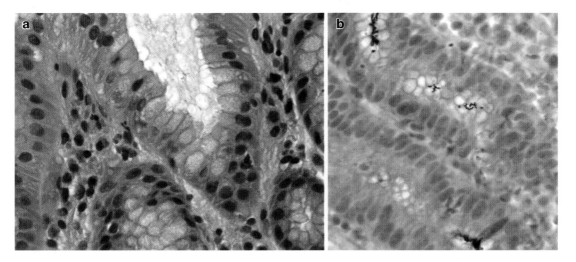

Fig. 4.6 *H. pylori* are tiny (2–5 μm) organisms that may appear slightly basophilic within the mucus layer on H&E staining (**a**). Their characteristic spirillar, "comma," or "seagull" shapes can be seen easily on immunostaining (**b**)

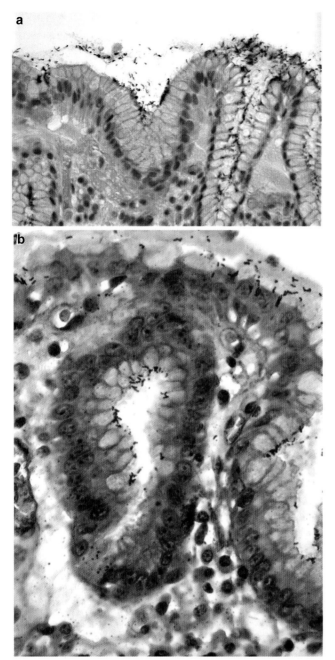

Fig. 4.7 *H. pylori* can be present within the surface mucus layer of both luminal surface epithelium and deeper glandular epithelium (**a**, *H. pylori* immunostain; **b**, Genta stain, courtesy Dr. Rodger C. Haggitt)

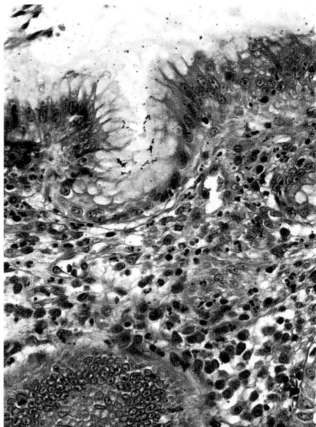

Fig. 4.8 The distribution of bacteria may be very patchy or focal (Genta stain, courtesy Dr. Rodger C. Haggitt)

Numerous ancillary studies exist for diagnosing HP. Culture of the organism is extremely difficult and is most commonly used today when antibiotic susceptibility testing is needed. The CLO and other urease tests are rapid, inexpensive, and have sensitivity and specificity comparable to histology. Breath tests measuring excretion of carbon isotopes are quick, accurate (as a positive result indicates active infection), and non-invasive, but they are expensive, not widely available, and there is a slight radiation

exposure with some methods. Serologic studies have excellent sensitivity and specificity and are inexpensive. A positive result in the absence of treatment implies current infection; however, positive serologic studies may persist for quite some time following eradication of the bacteria. Molecular detection assays also exist but are not widely available.

Helicobacter heilmannii and other species. *H. heilmannii* (HH), a less commonly encountered *Helicobacter* species formerly known as *Gastrospirillum hominis*, is associated with animal contact, particularly dogs, cats, cattle, and pigs. It causes symptoms similar to HP and may infect both children and adults. *H. heilmannii* infection has been associated rarely with ulcer formation, particularly in the context of non-steroidal anti-inflammatory drug use. Co-infection with HP and HH has also been well-documented.

Although the gastritis caused by HH is morphologically indistinguishable from that caused by HP, it is often more focal, less severe, and associated with fewer organisms. HH infection is also usually restricted to the antrum. Some authors have also reported foveolar hyperplasia, vascular dilatation, edema, and increased intracytoplasmic mucin in

Fig. 4.9   *H. pylori* may undergo transformation to coccoid forms (**a** and **b**, *H. pylori* immunostain)

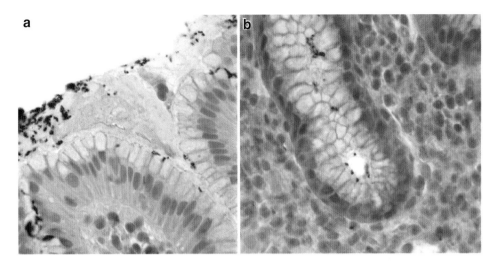

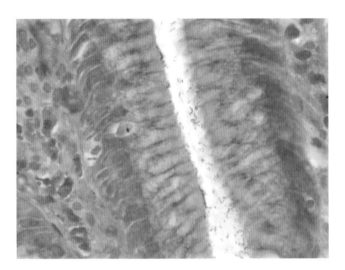

Fig. 4.10   Modified Diff-Quik stain shows blue *H. pylori* against a lighter blue background in a gastric cardia biopsy

Fig. 4.11   The Genta or triple stain combines a Steiner silver impregnation stain, H&E, and Alcian blue pH 2.5 (courtesy Dr. Rodger C. Haggitt)

association with HH. Intestinal metaplasia, gastric adenocarcinoma, and MALT lymphoma are less commonly associated with HH.

   H. heilmannii is longer (4–10 μm in length) and more tightly spiraled than HP (Fig. 4.16). *H. heilmannii* is detectable by the same histochemical stains used for HP detection (Fig. 4.17), and they are also immunopositive for the anti-*H. pylori* immunohistochemical stains (Fig. 4.18). *H. felis* is also known to infect humans rarely, but its ability to cause gastritis remains unclear.

   Other rarely encountered *Helicobacter* species include (but are not limited to) *H. cinaedi*, *H. pullorum*, *H. canadensis*, and *H. fennelliae*, which are believed to cause

Campylobacter-like lower GI symptoms in immunocompromised patients; *H. canis* and *H. winghamensis*, which cause gastroenteritis; and *H. rappini*, which also causes diarrhea. Virtually all of these species have one or more animal hosts. As special microbiological techniques are required to isolate these organisms, the prevalence of infection in humans, and their relationship with their animal reservoirs, remains poorly understood.

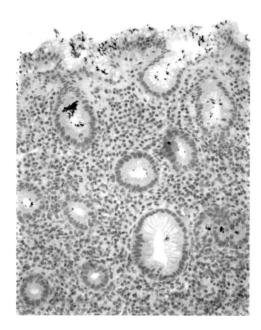

Fig. 4.12 The *H. pylori* immunostain allows for easy screening at low power

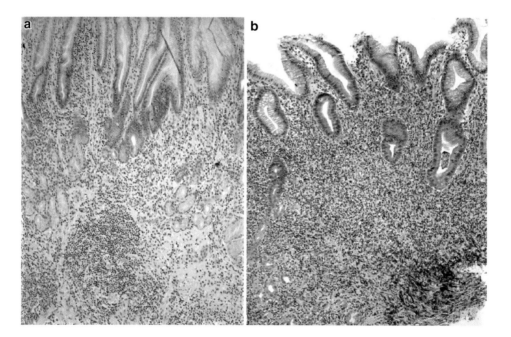

Fig. 4.13 Gastric antral MALT lymphoma, showing numerous intraepithelial lesions (**a**) as well as a small lymphocytic infiltrate that separates the glands, effaces normal architecture, and extends into the submucosa (**a** and **b**)

Fig. 4.14 A dense small lymphocytic infiltrate extends through the muscularis mucosa and into the submucosa in a gastric MALT lymphoma

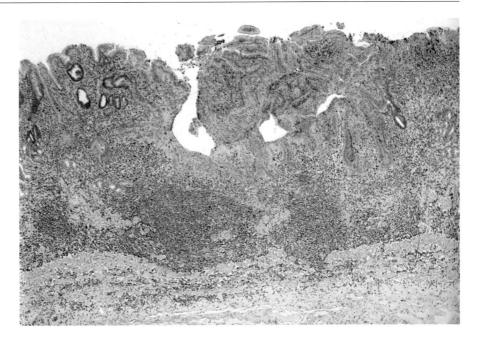

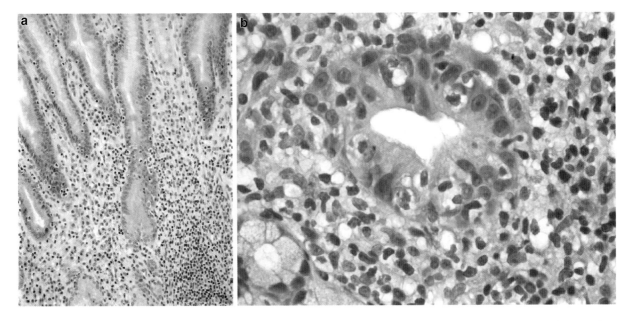

Fig. 4.15 Lymphoepithelial lesions are common in MALT lymphoma (**a**); lymphocytes may virtually overrun the glandular epithelium (**b**)

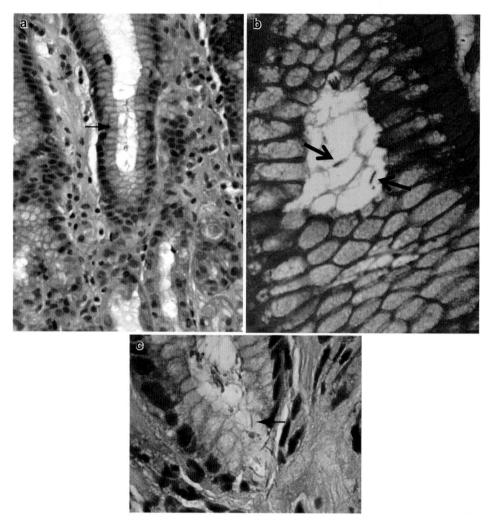

Fig. 4.16 *H. heilmannii* is longer (4–10 μm in length) and more tightly spiraled than HP (**a**, courtesy Dr. Joel Greenson; **b** and **c**, courtesy Dr. Brian West)

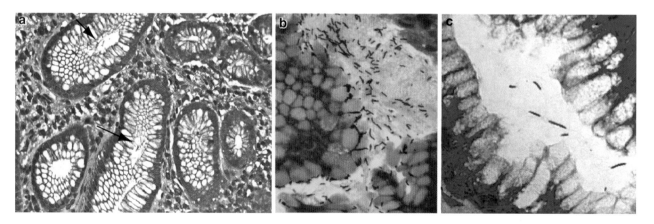

Fig. 4.17 *H. heilmannii* are detectable by the same histochemical stains used for HP detection (**a**, Giemsa stain, courtesy Dr. Joel Greenson; **b**, modified triple stain, courtesy Dr. Dhanpat Jain; **c**, Giemsa stain, courtesy Dr. Brian West). Note the longer, more tightly spiraled bacterial morphology (**b** and **c**)

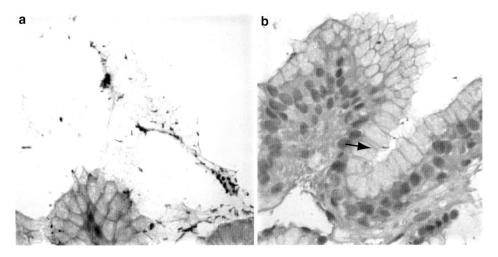

Fig. 4.18 *H. heilmannii* are immunoreactive with the anti-*H. pylori* immunohistochemical stains (**a** and **b**)

Selected References

Helicobacter pylori

1. Ashton-Key M, Diss TC, Isaacson PG. Detection of *Helicobacter pylori* in gastric biopsy and resection specimens. J Clin Pathol 49:107–11, 1996.
2. Brown KE, Peura DA. Diagnosis of *Helicobacter pylori* infection. Gastroenterol Clin North Am 22(1):105–15, 1993.
3. El-Zimaity HMT, Segura AM, Genta RM, Graham DY. Histologic assessment of *Helicobacter pylori* status after therapy: comparison of Giemsa, Diff-Quick, and Genta stains. Mod Pathol 11:288–91, 1998.
4. Farinha P, Gascoyne RD. *Helicobacter pylori* and MALT lymphoma. Gastroenterol 128:1579–1605, 2005.
5. Genta RM, Robason GO, Graham DY. Simultaneous visualization of *Helicobacter pylori* and gastric morphology: a new stain. Hum Pathol 25:221–6, 1994.
6. Genta RM, Graham DY. Comparison of biopsy sites for the histopathologic diagnosis of *Helicobacter pylori*: a topographic study of *H. pylori* density and distribution. Gastrointest Endosc 40:342–5, 1994.
7. Genta RM, Huberman RM, Graham DY. The gastric cardia in *Helicobacter pylori* infection. Hum Pathol 25:915–9, 1994.
8. Genta RM, Hamner HW, Graham DY. Gastric lymphoid follicles in *Helicobacter pylori* infection: frequency, distribution, and response to triple therapy. Hum Pathol 24:577–83, 1993.
9. Genta RM, Graham DY. *Helicobacter pylori*: the new bug on the (paraffin) block. Virch Arch 425:339–47, 1994.
10. Goldstein NS. Chronic inactive gastritis and coccoid *Helicobacter pylori* in patients treated for gastroesophageal reflux disease or with *H. pylori* eradication therapy. Am J Clin Pathol 118:719–26, 2002.
11. Laine L, Lewin DN, Naritoku W, Cohen H. Prospective comparison of H&E, Giemsa, and Genta stains for the diagnosis of *Helicobacter pylori*. Gastrointest Endosc 45:463–7, 1997.
12. Ota H, Katsuyama T, Nakajima S, et al. Intestinal metaplasia with adherent *Helicobacter pylori*: a hybrid epithelium with both gastric and intestinal features. Hum Pathol 29:846–50, 1998.
13. Owen DA. Gastritis and carditis. Mod Pathol 16:325–41, 2003.
14. Parsonnet J. *Helicobacter pylori* and gastric cancer. Gastroenterol Clin North Am 22(1):89–104, 1993.
15. Robert ME, Weinstein WM. *Helicobacter pylori*-associated gastric pathology. Gastroenterol Clin North Am 22(1):60–73, 1993.
16. Uemura N, Okamoto S, Yamamoto S, et al. *Helicobacter pylori* infection and the development of gastric cancer. N Engl J Med 345:784–9, 2001.
17. Wotherspoon AC, Ortiz-Hidalgo C, Falzon MR, Isaacson PG. *H. pylori*-associated gastritis and primary B-cell gastric lymphoma. Lancet 338:1175–6, 1991.
18. Wu ML, Lewin KJ. Understanding *Helicobacter pylori*. Hum Pathol 32:247–9, 2001.

Helicobacter heilmannii *and Other Species*

19. Debongnie JC, Donnay M, Mairesse J. *Gastrospirillum hominis* ("*Helicobacter heilmannii*"): a cause of gastritis, sometimes transient, better diagnosed by touch cytology? Am J Gastroenterol 90:411–16, 1995.
20. Fritz EL, Slavik T, Delport W, et al. Incidence of *Helicobacter felis* and the effect of coinfection with *Helicobacter pylori* on the gastric mucosa in the African population. J Clin Microbiol 44:1692–6, 2006.
21. Ierardi E, Monno RA, Gentile A, et al. *Helicobacter heilmannii* gastritis: a histological and immunohistochemical trait. J Clin Pathol 54:774–7, 2001.
22. Jhala D, Jhala N, Lechago J, Haber M. *Helicobacter heilmannii* gastritis: associated with acid peptic diseases and comparison with *Helicobacter pylori* gastritis. Mod Pathol 12:534–8, 1999.
23. Kaklikkaya N, Ozgur O, Aydin F, Cobanoglu U. *Helicobacter heilmannii* as causative agent of chronic active gastritis. Scand J Infect Dis 34:768–70, 2002.
24. Lee A, O'Rourke J. Gastric bacteria other than *Helicobacter pylori*. Gastroenterol Clin North Am 22(1):21–42, 1993.
25. Mention K, Michaud L, Duimber D, et al. Characteristics and prevalence e of *Helicobacter heilmanii* infection in children undergoing upper gastrointestinal endoscopy. J Pediatr Gastroenterol Nutr 29:533–9, 1999.

26. Singhal AV, Sepulveda AR. *Helicobacter heilmannii* gastritis: A case study with review of the literature. Am J Surg Pathol 29:1537–9, 2005.

27. Solnick JV. Clinical significance of *Helicobacter* species other than *Helicobacter pylori*. Clin Infect Dis 36:349–54, 2003.

28. Stolte M, Kroher G, Meining A, et al. A comparison of *Helicobacter pylori* and *H. heilmannii* gastritis. A matched control study involving 404 patients. Scand J Gastroenterol 32:28–33, 1997.

29. Sykora J, Hejda V, Varvarovska J, et al. *Helicobacter heilmannii* gastroduodenal disease and clinical aspects in children with dyspeptic symptoms. Acta Paediatr 93:707–9, 2004.

Chapter 5

Salmonella Species

Keywords *Salmonella* sp. • Typhoid • Non-typhoid species • Enteric fever • Colitis • Enterocolitis

These Gram-negative bacilli are transmitted through contaminated food and water and are prevalent where sanitation is poor. They also are an important cause of both sporadic food poisoning in developed countries and traveler's diarrhea. *Salmonella* is present in meat, dairy products, eggs and egg products, and occasionally vegetables and fruits; they may survive partial cooking, freezing, and drying. Food handlers can be a reservoir for transmission, and infection can be acquired from animals.

Patients with low gastric acidity are at increased risk of salmonellosis, and AIDS patients have a greater risk of *Salmonella* infection as well. Although most *Salmonella* infections in developed countries resolve with antibiotics and supportive care, intestinal infection may progress to septicemia and death, particularly in the elderly, the very young, or patients with immune compromise or co-morbid conditions. Delayed treatment is associated with higher mortality, and antibiotics are particularly important for neonates, older patients, the immunocompromised, and patients with cardiac valve abnormalities or indwelling prostheses. A chronic carrier state rarely develops in the gallbladder. Interestingly, patients with schistosomiasis are at increased risk for salmonellosis, as the bacteria penetrate and multiply within the parasites, which then serve as a nidus for recurrent infection.

The discussion of *Salmonella* infection may be divided generally into typhoid and non-typhoid serotypes (commonly referred to as species). *S. typhi* is the most common causative agent of typhoid fever, although *S. paratyphi* occasionally causes a similar clinicopathologic spectrum. Non-typhoid species (including *S. enteritidis*, *S. typhimurium*, *S. muenchen*, *S. anatum*, *S. newport*, *S. paratyphi*, and *S. give*) generally cause a more self-limited gastroenteritis.

Typhoid (enteric) fever. Patients with typhoid fever typically present with fever (which generally rises over several days), abdominal pain, headache, and occasionally initial constipation. Abdominal rash ("rose spots"), delirium, hep-atosplenomegaly, and leukopenia are fairly common. Diarrhea, which begins in the second or third week of infection, is initially watery but may progress to severe gastrointestinal bleeding and perforation.

Pathologic features. Any level of the alimentary tract may be involved, but the characteristic pathology is most prominent in the ileum, appendix, and right colon. Grossly, the bowel wall is thickened, and raised nodules may be seen corresponding to hyperplastic Peyer's patches (Fig. 5.1). Apthoid ulcers overlying Peyer's patches (Fig. 5.2), linear ulcers, ovoid ulcers, or full thickness ulceration and necrosis are common as the disease progresses. Perforation and toxic megacolon may complicate typhoid fever, and suppurative mesenteric lymphadenitis is variably present. Occasionally, the mucosa is grossly normal or only mildly inflamed and edematous.

The inflammatory infiltrate in typhoid fever is typically mononuclear (Fig. 5.3). Following hyperplasia of Peyer's patches (Fig. 5.4), acute inflammation of the overlying

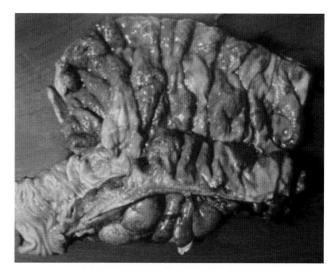

Fig. 5.1 Ileocolonic resection specimen in typhoid fever. The bowel wall is thickened and nodular, with ulcers corresponding to hyperplastic Peyer's patches. The necrosis and hyperemia are transmural, extending into the mesenteric fat. (Courtesy Dr. A. Brian West)

L.W. Lamps, *Surgical Pathology of the Gastrointestinal System: Bacterial, Fungal, Viral, and Parasitic Infections,*
DOI 10.1007/978-1-4419-0861-2_5, © Springer Science+Business Media, LLC 2009

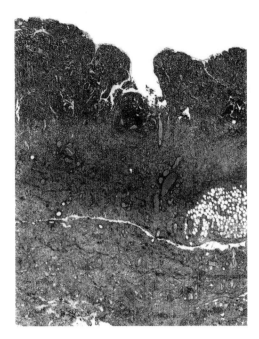

Fig. 5.2 Ileal ulcer overlying a Peyer's patch in typhoid fever. Necrosis and hemorrhage extend deeply into the submucosa. (Courtesy Dr. A. Brian West)

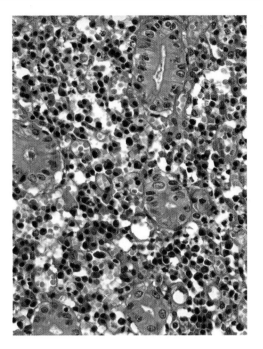

Fig. 5.3 The inflammatory infiltrate in typhoid fever is predominantly mononuclear, composed of plasma cells, lymphocytes, and histiocytes; neutrophils are usually inconspicuous. (Courtesy Dr. A. Brian West)

epithelium develops. Eventually macrophages, mixed with occasional lymphocytes and plasma cells, infiltrate and obliterate the lymphoid follicles; neutrophils are usually inconspicuous. Necrosis then begins in the Peyer's patch and spreads to the surrounding mucosa, which eventually ulcerates (Fig. 5.5). The ulcers are typically very deep, with the base at the level of the muscularis propria, and occasionally penetrating through it. Granulomas are rarely seen. Architectural distortion that may mimic ulcerative colitis or Crohn's disease can be seen as well (Fig. 5.6).

Non-typhoid Salmonella species. These species generally cause a less severe gastroenteritis with vomiting, nausea, fever, and watery diarrhea, presenting within 8–48 hours of ingesting contaminated food or water. Non-typhoid species rarely cause severe bloody diarrhea or toxic megacolon. Non-typhoid *Salmonellae* most commonly infect children less than 1 year of age and are one of the more common infectious causes of colon perforation in this population.

The gross findings are often milder, including mucosal erythema, hemorrhage, ulceration, and exudates. Lesions can be focal, and occasionally the mucosa is grossly normal or only mildly hyperemic and edematous. The histologic features are typically those of non-specific acute infectious-type colitis or enterocolitis (Fig. 5.7) (see also Chapter 1). Severe cases may have mucus depletion, cryptitis, fibrinous exudates, and small microthrombi, and occasionally significant crypt distortion may be seen (Fig. 5.8).

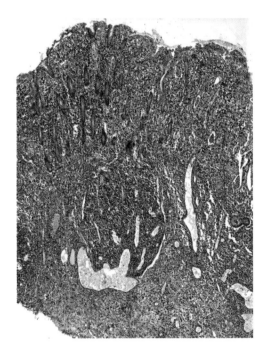

Fig. 5.4 Hyperplastic Peyer's patch with overlying mucosal inflammation and surrounding edema. (Courtesy Dr. A. Brian West)

More recent descriptions of the pathology of *Salmonella* infection have reported a fair amount of histological overlap in the features of typhoid and non-typhoid species (Fig. 5.9). It is important to note that patients with typhoid fever may lack the classic ulcer overlying a Peyer's patch and may have

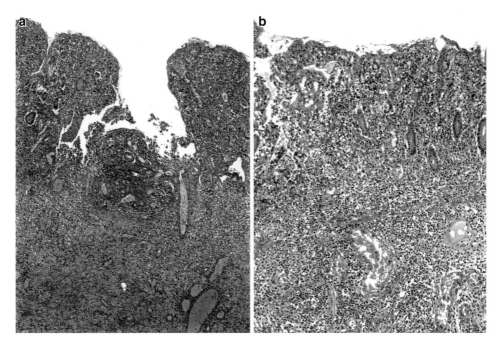

Fig. 5.5 Ulceration overlying a hyperplastic Peyer's patch, the hallmark lesion of typhoid fever (**a**). In the adjacent right colon, a lymphoid follicle is infiltrated by mononuclear cells, with overlying mucosal ulceration (**b**). (Courtesy Dr. A. Brian West)

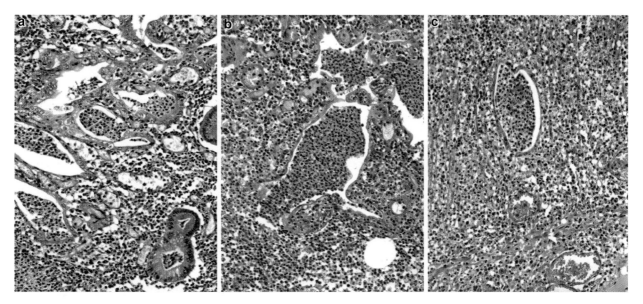

Fig. 5.6 Typhoid fever commonly shows marked architectural distortion that can mimic chronic idiopathic inflammatory bowel disease (**a–c**, courtesy Dr. A. Brian West)

histologic features more consistent with acute self-limited colitis (similar to non-typhoid species). Conversely, patients with non-typhoid salmonellosis may have severe colitis with ulceration and transmural involvement.

Differential diagnosis. The differential diagnosis of typhoid fever includes yersiniosis and other enteric bacterial pathogens, as well as ulcerative colitis and Crohn's dis-

ease. There may be significant histologic overlap between salmonellosis and chronic idiopathic inflammatory bowel disease, especially when architectural distortion is present. Clinically, the incubation period of *S. typhi* infection is longer (10–15 days) than with other similar enteric pathogens. Typhoid fever often lacks neutrophils in comparison to other enteric pathogens as well as idiopathic

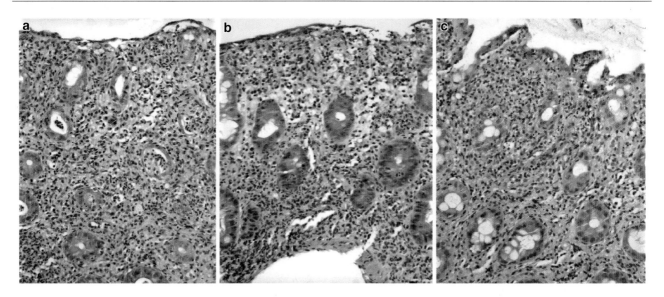

Fig. 5.7 The histologic features of non-typhoid salmonellosis are most often those of acute infectious-type colitis. A colon biopsy shows cryptitis and crypt abscess formation, along with a mixed inflammatory infiltrate in the lamina propria (**a**). The mucosa is edematous, but crypt architecture is preserved overall (**b**). Neutrophils are most prominent in the upper half of the mucosa, with surface epithelial injury (**c**)

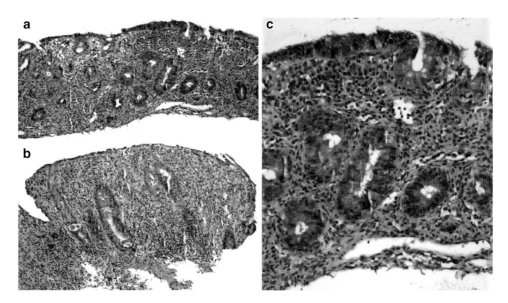

Fig. 5.8 Mild or focal architectural distortion is occasionally seen in non-typhoid *Salmonella* infection, mimicking chronic idiopathic inflammatory bowel disease (**a** and **b**). Higher power view shows mild crypt disorganization and basal plasmacytosis (**c**)

inflammatory bowel disease, and granulomas are unusual in salmonellosis. Although significant crypt distortion has been reported in some cases of typhoid fever, it is generally more pronounced in ulcerative colitis.

The differential diagnosis of non-typhoid *Salmonella* includes other causes of acute self-limited infectious colitis, as well as chronic idiopathic inflammatory bowel disease.

In addition, *Salmonella* infection may complicate pre-existing chronic idiopathic inflammatory bowel disease. Stool and/or blood cultures with appropriate biochemical tests for species identification may be invaluable in resolving the differential diagnosis in both typhoid fever and non-typhoid *Salmonella* infection.

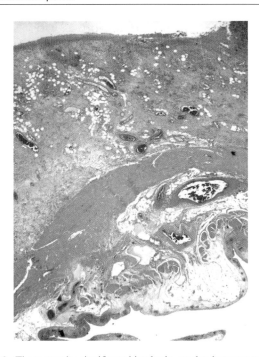

Fig. 5.9 There may be significant histologic overlap between typhoid fever and non-typhoid salmonellosis. This case of *S. newport* infection shows severe morphologic features including extensive ulceration and transmural inflammation and edema. (Courtesy Dr. Fiona Graeme-Cook)

Selected References

1. Azad AK, Islam R, Salam MA, et al. Comparison of clinical features and pathologic findings in fatal cases of typhoid fever during the initial and later stages of the disease. Am J Trop Med Hyg 56:490–3, 1997.
2. Boyd JF. Pathology of the alimentary tract in *Salmonella typhimurium* food poisoning. Gut 26:935–44, 1985.
3. Chang YJ, Yan DC, Kong MS, et al. Non-traumatic colon perforation in children: a 10-year review. Pediatr Surg Int 22:665–9, 2006.
4. Edwards BH. *Salmonella* and *Shigella* species. Clin Lab Med 19(3): 469–87, 1999.
5. Goldsweig CD, Pacheco PA. Infectious colitis excluding *E. coli* 0157:H7 and *C. difficile.* Gastroenterol Clin North Am 30(3): 709–33, 2001.
6. Kazlow PG, Freed J, Rosh JR, et al. *Salmonella typhimurium* appendicitis. J Pediatr Gastroenterol Nutr 13:101–3, 1991.
7. Kelly JK, Owen DA. Bacterial diarrheas and dysenteries. In Connor DH, Chandler FW et al. (eds): Pathology of Infectious Diseases, Stamford, CT: Appleton and Lange, 1997, pp. 421–9.
8. Kraus MD, Amatya B, Kimula Y. Histopathology of typhoid enteritis: morphologic and immunophenotypic findings. Mod Pathol 12:949–55, 1999.
9. Mallory FB. A histological study of typhoid fever. J Exp Med 3:611–38, 1898.
10. McGovern VJ, Slavutin LJ. Pathology of *Salmonella* colitis. Am J Surg Pathol 3:483–90, 1979.
11. Pegues DA, Hohmann EL, Miller SI. *Salmonella* including *S. typhi*. In Blaser MJ, Smith PD et al. (eds): Infections of the Gastrointestinal Tract, New York: Raven Press, 1995, pp. 785–809.
12. Sachdev HPS, Chadha V, Malhotra V, et al. Rectal histopathology in endemic *Shigella* and *Salmonella* diarrhea. J Pediatr Gastroenterol Nutr 13:33–8, 1993.

Chapter 6

Shigella Species

Keywords *Shigella* sp. • Dysentery • Colitis

Shigellae are virulent, invasive Gram-negative bacilli that are a major cause of infectious diarrhea worldwide. Shigellosis is most common in developing countries where sanitation is poor, and it is endemic in tropical and subtropical parts of Africa, Southern Asia, and Central America. The *Shigellae* include four species: *S. dysenteriae*, *S. flexneri*, *S. boydii*, and *S. sonnei*. *Shigella dysenteriae* is the most virulent and the most common species isolated, although *S. sonnei* and *S. flexneri* are increasingly reported in the United States. Transmission is either food- or water-borne, although person-to-person transmission is also possible through the fecal–oral route. It has the highest infectivity rate among all of the enteric Gram-negative bacteria, and symptoms may result from ingestion of only 10–100 organisms.

Children under 6 years of age are commonly affected, as are homosexual males and malnourished or debilitated patients. Outbreaks of shigellosis are associated with crowded living conditions and poor hygiene and often are seen in nursing homes, day-care centers, and prisons. *Shigella* can be sexually transmitted as well, and there is an increase in sexually transmitted shigellosis in the male homosexual population in the United States. Similar to salmonellosis, the gross and microscopic features of shigellosis may closely mimic chronic idiopathic inflammatory bowel disease.

The onset of symptoms is usually within 12–50 h of consumption of contaminated food or water. Constitutional symptoms are the earliest manifestation, including abdominal pain, malaise, and fever. Diarrhea is often watery initially, followed by the onset of bloody diarrhea containing mucus or pus, and accompanied by tenesmus. Complications include severe dehydration, sepsis, perforation, toxic megacolon, reactive arthritis, Reiter's syndrome, and hemolytic–uremic syndrome. *S. dysenteriae* is most likely to cause dysentery and serious complications. *S. flexneri* and *S. sonnei* are usually moderately severe and self-limited, although the illness may take a week or more to resolve.

Pathologic features. Grossly, the large bowel is typically affected (the distal left side usually more severely), but the ileum may be involved as well. Initially, distribution is often continuous and can mimic ulcerative colitis; patchy involvement is more common as the disease resolves. The mucosa is edematous and hemorrhagic, with exudates that may form pseudomembranes. Ulcerations are variably present.

Morphologic changes are usually most severe in the rectum. Early changes are generally those of acute infectious-type colitis, including a superficial neutrophilic infiltrate (Fig. 6.1), edema, mucin depletion, cryptitis (Fig. 6.2), crypt abscesses (often superficial) (Fig. 6.3), and ulceration. Apthoid ulcers similar to Crohn's disease are variably present. Pseudomembranes similar to *Clostridium difficile* infection are fairly common (Fig. 6.4), and microthrombi can be seen. As the disease continues, there is increased mucosal destruction with many neutrophils and mononuclear inflammatory cells in the lamina propria. Architectural changes mimicking idiopathic inflammatory bowel disease are well described in shigellosis, including crypt branching, crypt disorganization, crypt dilatation, and marked crypt distortion (Fig. 6.5).

Differential diagnosis. The differential diagnosis of early shigellosis is primarily that of other infections, particularly enteroinvasive *Escherichia coli* and non-typhoid *Salmonella*. Pseudomembranous shigellosis may closely resemble the colitis caused by *C. difficile*; the *C. difficile* antigen test can be very helpful in this instance. Later in the course of the disease, it may be extremely difficult to distinguish shigellosis from Crohn's disease or ulcerative colitis both endoscopically and histologically. Clinical presentation (e.g., rapid onset of symptoms) may be very helpful in resolving the differential diagnosis. Stool cultures are essential, and specimens should be rapidly inoculated onto appropriate culture plates, since *Shigella* is fastidious and dies quickly. Multiple cultures may be necessary. Molecular assays for the diagnosis of shigellosis are also available.

L.W. Lamps, *Surgical Pathology of the Gastrointestinal System: Bacterial, Fungal, Viral, and Parasitic Infections*,
DOI 10.1007/978-1-4419-0861-2_6, © Springer Science+Business Media, LLC 2009

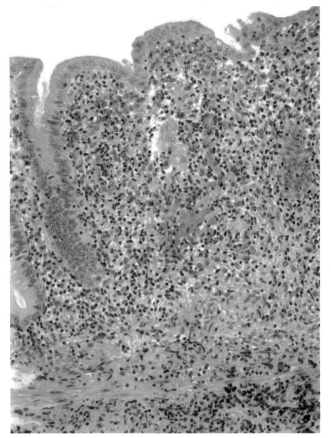

Fig. 6.1 Colon biopsy from a culture-proven case of shigellosis, featuring a neutrophilic infiltrate in the lamina propria with focal crypt destruction (courtesy Dr. Mary Bronner)

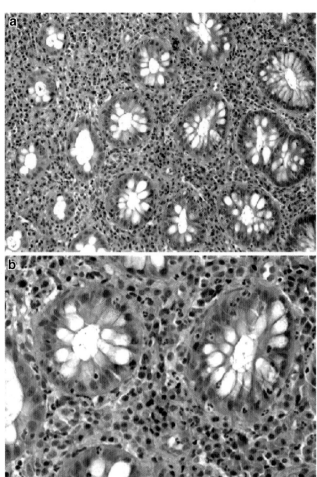

Fig. 6.2 Cryptitis with a mixed inflammatory infiltrate in the lamina propria (**a** and **b**)

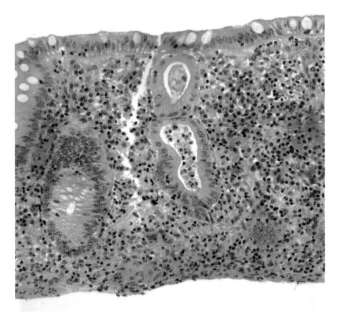

Fig. 6.3 Crypt abscess in a case of *S. sonnei* infection (courtesy Dr. Mary Bronner)

Fig. 6.4 Pseudomembranes similar to *C. difficile* infection are fairly common in shigellosis (**a** and **b**, courtesy Dr. John Hart)

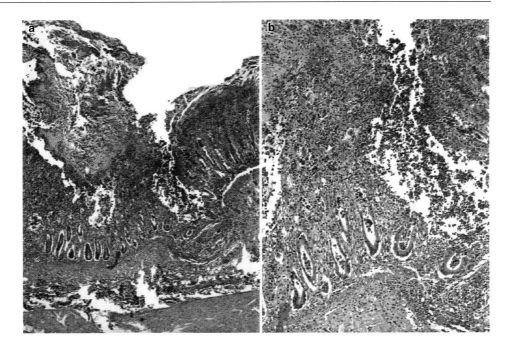

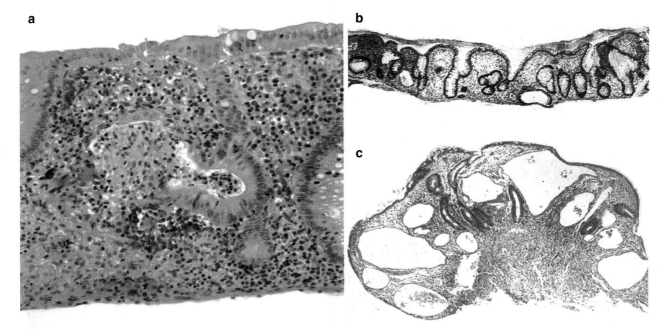

Fig. 6.5 Focal architectural distortion with crypt destruction and a mucin granuloma (**a**, case courtesy Dr. Mary Bronner). Severe architectural changes in resolving shigellosis that mimic chronic idiopathic inflammatory bowel disease (courtesy Lippincott Williams and Wilkins, Fig. 22.5, from Riddell, Lewin, and Weinstein, Gastrointestinal Pathology and Its Clinical Implications, 1992)

Selected References

1. Acheson DWK, Keusch GT. *Shigella* and enteroinvasive *E. coli*. In Blaser MJ, Smith PD et al. (eds): Infections of the Gastrointestinal Tract, New York, NY: Raven Press, 1995, pp. 763–84.

2. Edwards BH. *Salmonella* and *Shigella* species. Clin Lab Med 19(3):469–87, 1999.

3. Goldsweig CD, Pacheco PA. Infectious colitis excluding *E. coli* 0157:H7 and *C. difficile*. Gastroenterol Clin North Am 30(3):709–33, 2001.

4. Gracey M. Bacterial diarrhoea. Clin Gastroenterol 15(1):21–37, 1986.

5. Islam MM, Azad Ak, Bardhan PK, et al. Pathology of shigellosis and its complications. Histopathol 24:65–71, 1994.

6. Kelber M, Ament ME. *Shigella dysenteriae* I: a forgotten cause of pseudomembranous colitis. J Pediatr 89:595–6, 1976.

7. Kelly JK, Owen DA. Bacterial diarrheas and dysenteries. In Connor DH, Chandler FW et al. (eds): Pathology of Infectious Diseases, Stamford, CT: Appleton and Lange, 1997, pp. 421–9.

8. Khuroo MS, Mahajan R, Zargar SA, et al. The colon in shigellosis: serial colonoscopic appearances in *Shigella dysenteriae* I. Endoscopy 22: 35–8, 1990.

9. Mathan MM, Mathan VI. Morphology of rectal mucosa of patients with shigellosis. Rev Inf Dis 13(Suppl 4): S314–8, 1991.

10. Sachdev HPS, Chadha V, Malhotra V, et al. Rectal histopathology in endemic *Shigella* and *Salmonella* diarrhea. J Pediatr Gastroenterol Nutr 13:33–8, 1993.

11. Speelman P, Kabir I, Islam M. Distribution and spread of colonic lesions in shigellosis: a colonoscopic study. J Infect Dis 1984;150:899–903.

Chapter 7

Escherichia coli Species

Keywords *E. coli* sp • Enteroinvasive • Enteroadherent • Enterotoxigenic • Enteropathogenic • Enterohemorrahgic • Colitis • Ischemia • Diarrhea • O157:H7

Escherichia coli is the most common Gram-negative human pathogen. The diarrheagenic *E. coli* are generally classified into five groups, as discussed below (see also Table 7.1). Virtually all are transmitted through contaminated food or water. These infections are probably markedly underdiagnosed, since routine stool cultures will not distinguish pathogenic strains from normal intestinal flora. If pathogenic *E. coli* stains are suspected, then the clinical laboratory should be notified to search for them specifically, so that specific culture techniques on specialized agars and serotyping may be instituted. Pathogenic *E. coli* strains are often cleared rapidly from stool, often within 4–7 days; thus cultures should be taken as early as possible.

Enterotoxigenic E. coli (*ETEC*). ETEC are a major cause of traveler's diarrhea, as well as infantile diarrhea in develop-ing countries. Although infection most frequently occurs in areas with poor sanitation, major food-borne outbreaks also have been described in industrialized countries. ETEC are transmitted by contaminated food and water; the most serious outbreaks in the United States have involved semisoft cheese, during which multiple lots of cheese were affected by contaminated water used in processing, as well as contaminated processing machinery, and several states were involved. Transmission also has been associated with fresh produce and seafood.

These non-invasive *E. coli* produce enterotoxins that cause secretory diarrhea. Symptoms include watery diarrhea similar to cholera, sometimes accompanied by nausea, vomiting, low-grade fever, diarrhea, headache, and abdominal cramping. Symptoms usually present within 1–2 days of consumption. The gross and microscopic pathology of ETEC has not been described in humans. Animal studies show very mild histopathologic changes that are similar to those seen in cholera.

Table 7.1 General features of the major diarrheagenic *E. coli*

Group	Abbreviation	Pathogenesis/phenotype	Clinical features	Pathology
Enterotoxigenic *E. coli*	ETEC	Elaborate secretory toxins that do not damage mucosa	Traveler's diarrhea: profuse watery diarrhea +/– cramps, vomiting; similar to cholera; food-borne outbreaks in developed countries	Not well described in humans; presumed similar to minimal histologic changes seen in cholera
Enteropathogenic *E. coli*	EPEC	Adhere to epithelial cells	Usually infants; low-grade fever, vomiting, mucoid diarrhea; chronic diarrhea in AIDS patients	Not well described, but similar to EAEC
Enteroinvasive *E. coli*	EIEC	Invade epithelial cells	Dysentery-like illness with fever, urgency and tenesmus. Blood, mucus, WBC in stool; similar to *Shigella*	Not described in humans; presumably similar to shigellosis
Enterohemorrhagic *E. coli*	EHEC	Elaborate cytotoxins	Bloody diarrhea, often no fever; associated with HUS	Features similar to ischemia; often right colon
Enteroadherent *E. coli* (including enteroaggregative *E. coli*)	EAEC	Adhere to epithelial cells	Watery diarrhea, often chronic; vomiting, abdominal pain; chronic diarrhea in AIDS patients	Adherent Gram-negative bacteria with little inflammatory reaction

L.W. Lamps, *Surgical Pathology of the Gastrointestinal System: Bacterial, Fungal, Viral, and Parasitic Infections*, DOI 10.1007/978-1-4419-0861-2_7, © Springer Science+Business Media, LLC 2009

Enteropathogenic E. coli (EPEC). EPEC are predominantly an infection of infants and neonates. Infection is clinically similar to EAEC, although the O:H serotypes are different. These non-invasive *E. coli* cause mucoid, non-bloody diarrhea, accompanied by fever, malaise, and vomiting. The diarrhea can be chronic, and EPEC has been increasingly recognized as a cause of chronic diarrhea and wasting in AIDS patients. The gross and microscopic pathology of EPEC has not been well described in humans.

Enteroadherent E. coli (EAEC). EAEC are an important cause of traveler's diarrhea and pediatric diarrhea worldwide, and these non-invasive *E. coli* are increasingly recognized as a cause of chronic diarrhea and wasting in AIDS patients. Typically, these organisms produce non-bloody, non-mucoid, watery diarrhea with vomiting and low-grade fever. As they are non-invasive, dissemination with sepsis is not thought to occur.

Endoscopic findings are usually unremarkable. Histologic examination shows degenerative surface epithelial cell changes, including epithelial disarray, cytoplasmic vacuolization, nuclear pyknosis, and sloughing (Fig. 7.1). There are variably present intraepithelial inflammatory cells, but there is no associated cryptitis or architectural distortion. A coating of adherent Gram-negative bacteria at the surface epithelium is the most prominent feature. The bacteria may be tightly or loosely adherent (Fig. 7.2). As the histologic findings can be patchy and resemble an exaggerated brush border, they may be easily missed at low power. In addition, biopsies of infected patients may be entirely normal microscopically. The main entities in the differential diagnosis are normal mucosa and spirochetosis; the bacteria in EPEC and EAEC are not spirillar, in contrast to spirochetosis, and generally stain Gram negative.

Enteroinvasive E. coli. The EIEC are relatively recently recognized as pathogens, probably because they were previously confused with other *E. coli* strains or *Shigella*. They are very similar to *Shigella* genetically and in their clinical presentation and pathogenesis. In fact, there is some cross-reactivity with *Shigella* antigens in serologic tests. These organisms can be transmitted via contaminated cheese, water, and person-to-person contact; they are also a cause of traveler's diarrhea.

Symptoms include diarrhea, tenesmus, fever, malaise, and abdominal cramps. Diarrhea is generally watery and may contain mucus or blood. Fecal leukocytes are common. Since they are able to invade the colonic epithelium, EIEC can produce severe colitis as well as systemic bacteremia; this can be a particular problem in AIDS patients. The pathology of EIEC has not been well described in humans. Since these organisms are similar to *Shigella*, the pathology could be anticipated to resemble shigellosis.

Enterohemorrhagic E. coli (EHEC). This pathogen gained national attention in 1993 when a massive outbreak in the western United States was linked to contaminated hamburger patties served at a fast-food restaurant. Although contaminated meat is the most frequent mode of transmission, infection also may occur through contaminated water, milk, produce, and person-to-person contact. The most common strain of enterohemorrhagic *E. coli* is O157:H7, although there are others. EHEC adheres to intestinal epithelial cells and produces a cytotoxin similar to that of *Shigella dysenteriae*; however, there is no tissue invasion.

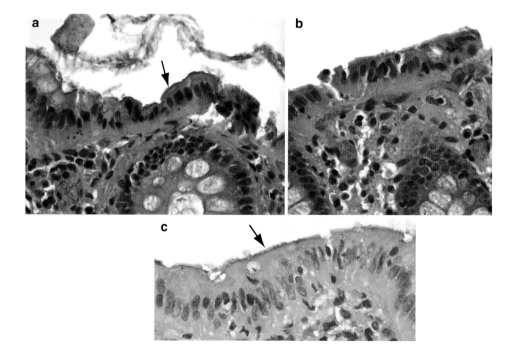

Fig. 7.1 Enteroadherent *E. coli* with associated surface epithelial disarray, along with occasional intraepithelial inflammatory cells (**a** and **b**). The coating of adherent bacteria may resemble an exaggerated brush border (**c**)

Fig. 7.2 Tissue Gram stain highlights the bacteria at the mucosal surface (**a**, courtesy Dr. Mary Bronner) which may be tightly (**b**) or loosely (**c**) adherent

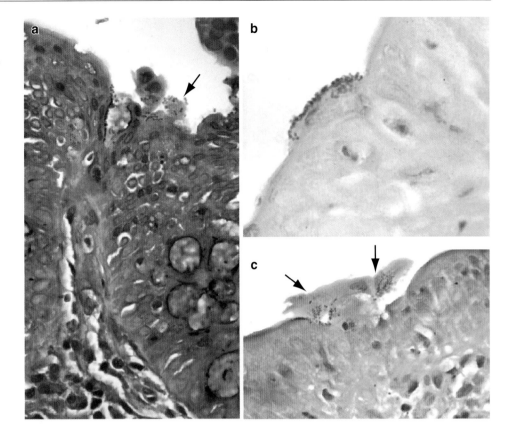

Gastrointestinal symptoms usually consist of bloody diarrhea with severe abdominal cramps. Unlike most infectious diseases, fever is mild or absent. Non-bloody, watery diarrhea may occur in some cases, or precede the development of bloody diarrhea. Only one-third of patients have fecal leukocytes. The most serious complication of EHEC is the development of the hemolytic–uremic syndrome, and children and the elderly are at particular risk for grave illness. Ironically, the use of antibiotics to treat EHEC appears to increase the risk of development of HUS in some studies.

Pathologic features. Patients typically have severe mural edema, with associated hemorrhage. Mucosa is eroded and ulcerated, and ulcers often have an overlying purulent exudate. Edema may be so marked as to cause obstruction, and surgical resection may be required to relieve this or to control bleeding (Fig. 7.3). The right colon is usually most severely affected.

The histologic features closely resemble ischemic colitis due to other causes, and include marked edema and hemorrhage in the lamina propria and submucosa, with associated mucosal acute inflammation (Fig. 7.4), crypt withering (Figs. 7.4 and 7.5), and lamina propria hyalinization (Fig. 7.6). Microthrombi may be present within small caliber blood vessels (Fig. 7.7), and pseudomembranes resembling antibiotic-associated pseudomembranous colitis are occasionally present as well (Fig. 7.8). Mucosal necrosis

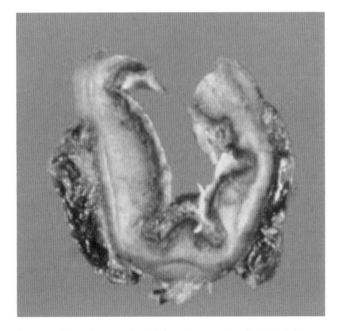

Fig. 7.3 Gross photograph of right colon resection for EHEC. Severe mural edema is present, with associated hemorrhage and overlying mucosal ulceration with purulent exudate. (Courtesy Dr. Robert D. Collins)

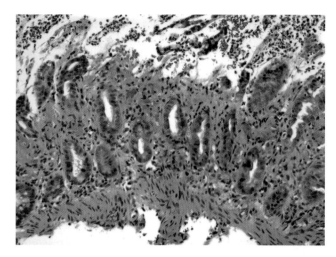

Fig. 7.4 Right colon biopsy of EHEC showing mucosal hemorrhage and lamina propria hyalinization, along with crypt withering, reactive epithelial changes, and an acute inflammatory exudate

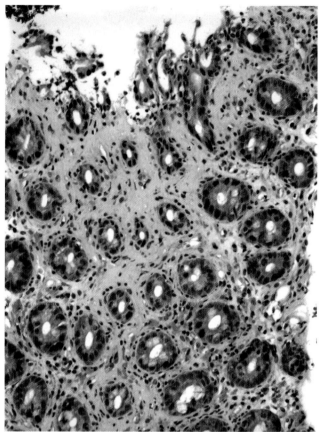

Fig. 7.6 Marked lamina propria hyalinization in EHEC, mimicking ischemia of other causes

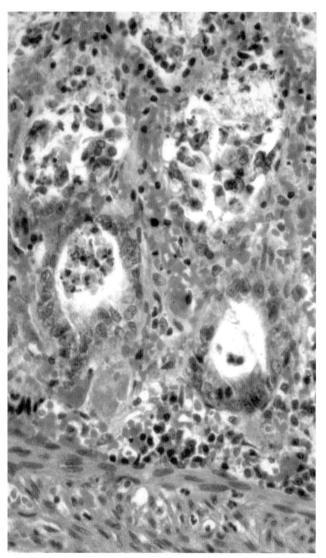

Fig. 7.5 Crypt withering in EHEC, with small fibrin thrombi in mucosal vessels

is frequently seen, often involving the upper portion of the mucosa but sparing the deeper crypts (Fig. 7.9).

Differential diagnosis. The differential diagnosis for EHEC primarily includes *C. difficile*-related pseudomembranous colitis and ischemic colitis of other causes, from which EHEC may be histologically indistinguishable. Clinical history, including the possibility of consumption of contaminated food, age of the patient, and macroscopic findings, may aid in distinguishing ischemia from *E. coli* infection. The *C. difficile* antigen test may be very helpful in distinguishing *C. difficile*-related colitis from EHEC. Recently, an antibiotic-associated hemorrhagic colitis has been reported in association with *Klebsiella oxytoca*. This colitis is hemorrhagic, segmental, most common in the right and transverse colon, and lacks pseudomembranes. A history of antibiotic usage, especially penicillins, may help distinguish this infection from EHEC.

Stool culture is invaluable in making the diagnosis; however, routine stool cultures cannot distinguish 0157:H7 from normal intestinal flora, since microbiologic diagnosis requires screening on selective agar. An immunohisto-

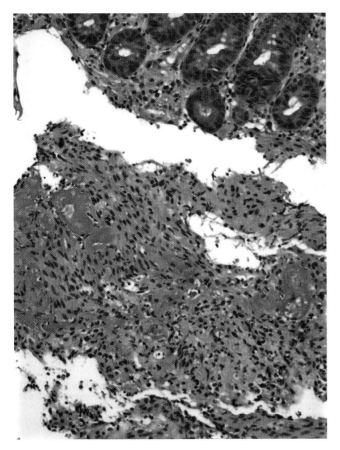

Fig. 7.7 Prominent fibrin thrombi in the superficial submucosa

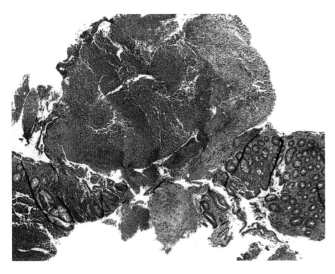

Fig. 7.8 Abundant necroinflammatory debris overlying the mucosa in a right colon biopsy from a case of EHEC

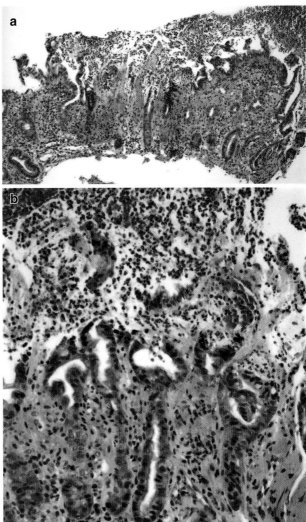

Fig. 7.9 Low-power view of a biopsy from a case of EHEC, showing lamina propria hemorrhage and fibrosis, along with crypt withering (**a**). Higher power view shows mucosal necrosis involving the upper portion of the mucosa but sparing the deeper crypts (**b**)

Selected References

General

chemical stain for this organism has recently been described as well, and molecular assays exist but are not widely available.

1. Clarke SC. Diarrhoeagenic *Escherichia coli*-an emerging problem? Diagn Microbiol Infect Dis 41:93–8, 2001.
2. Gilligan PH. *Escherichia coli*: EAEC, EHEC, EIEC, ETEC. Clin Lab Med 19(3):505–21, 1999.
3. Kelly JK, Owen DA. *Escherichia coli* diarrhea. In Connor DH, Chandler FW et al. (eds): Pathology of Infectious Diseases, Stamford, CT: Appleton and Lange, 1997, pp. 555–62.
4. Levine MM. *Escherichia coli* that cause diarrhea: enterotoxigenic, enteropathogenic, enteroinvasive, enterohemorrhagic, and enteroadherent. J Inf Dis 155:377–89, 1987.

Enterotoxigenic *E. coli*

5. Beatty ME, Adcock PM, Smith SW, et al. Epidemic diarrhea due to enterotoxigenic *E. coli*. Clin Infect Dis 42:329–34, 2006.
6. Devasia RA, Jones TF, Ward J, et al. Endemically acquired food-borne outbreak of enterotoxin-producing *Escherichia coli* serotype O169:H41. Am J Med 119(168):e7–10, 2006.
7. Gorbach SL, Kean BH, Evans DG, et al. Travelers' diarrhea and toxigenic *Escherichia coli*. NEJM 292:933–6, 1975.
8. Macdonald KL, Eidson M, Strohmeyer C, et al. A multistate outbreak of gastrointestinal illness caused by enterotoxigenic *E. coli* in imported semisoft cheese. J Inf Dis 151:716–20, 1985.
9. Qadri F, Svennerholm AM, Faruque AS, Sack RB. Enterotoxigenic *Escherichia coli* in developing countries: epidemiology, microbiology, clinical features, treatment, and prevention. Clin Micro Rev 18:465–83, 2005.
10. Rowe B, Gross RJ, Scotland SM, et al. Outbreak of infantile enteritis causes by enterotoxigenic *E. coli* 06.H16. J Clin Pathol 1978; 31:217–19.
11. Sack RB. Human diarrheal disease caused by enterotoxigenic *Escherichia coli*. Ann Rev Microbiol 29:333–53, 1975.
12. Yoder JS, Cesario S, Plotkin V. Outbreak of enterotoxigenic *Escherichia coli* infection with an unusually long duration of illness. Clin Inf Dis 42:1513–17, 2006.

Enteroadherent *E. coli*

13. Kotler DP, Giang TT, Thiim M, et al. Chronic bacterial enteropathy in a patient with AIDS. J Inf Dis 171:552–8, 1995.
14. Mathewson JJ, Johnson PC, DuPont HL, et al. A newly recognized cause of travelers' diarrhea: enteroadherent *Escherichia coli*. J Inf Dis 151:471–5, 1985.
15. Orenstein JM, Kotler DP. Diarrheogenic bacterial enteritis in acquired immune deficiency syndrome: a light and electron microscopic study of 52 cases. Hum Pathol 26:481–92, 1995.
16. Savarino SJ. Enteroadherent E. coli: a heterogeneous group of *E. coli* implicated as diarrhoeal pathogens. Trans Roy Soc Trop Med Hyg 87(Suppl 3):49–53, 1993.

Enteroinvasive *E. coli*

17. Bessesen MT, Wang E, Echeverria P, Blaser MJ. Enteroinvasive *Escherichia coli:* a cause of bacteremia in patients with AIDS. J Clin Microbiol 29:2675–77, 1991.
18. Tulloch EF, Ryan EJ, Formal SB, Franklin FA. Invasive enteropathic *E. coli* dysentery. Ann Intern Med 79:13–17, 1973.
19. Wanger AR, Murray BE, Echeverria P, et al. Enteroinvasive *E. coli* in travelers with diarrhea. J Inf Dis 158:640–2, 1988.

Enterohemorrhagic *E. coli*

20. Cobden I. Germs, arteries, or both? Differentiating *E. coli* O157:H7 from ischemic colitis. Am J Gastroenterol 93:1022–3, 1998.
21. Griffin PM, Olmstead LC, Petras RE. *Escherichia coli* 0157:H7-associated colitis: a clinical and histological study of 11 cases. Gastroenterol 99:142–49, 1990.
22. Griffin PM. E. coli 0157:H7 and other enterohemorrhagic *E. coli*. In Blaser MJ, Smith PD et al. (eds): Infections of the Gastrointestinal Tract, New York, NY: Raven Press, 1995, pp. 739–61.
23. Hogenauer C, Langner C, Beubler E, et al. Klebsiella oxytoca as a causative organisms of antibiotic-associated hemorrhagic colitis. N Eng J Med 355(23):2418–26, 2006.
24. Kelly J, Oryshak A, Wenetsek M, Grabiec J, Handy S. The colonic pathology of E. coli 0157:H7 infection. Am J Surg Pathol 14:87–92, 1990.
25. Su C, Brandt LJ, Sigal SH, et al. The immunohistological diagnosis of E. coli 0157:H7 colitis: possible association with colonic ischemia. Am J Gastroenterol 1998; 93:1055–9.
26. Tarr PI, Neill MA. *Escherichia coli* O157:H7. Gastroenterol Clin North Am 30(3):735–51, 2001.
27. Welinder-Olsson C, Kaijser B. Enterohemorrhagic *E. coli* (EHEC). Scand J Infect Dis 37:405–16, 2005.

Chapter 8

Yersinia enterocolitica and *Yersinia pseudotuberculosis*

Keywords *Yersinia enterocolitica* • *Yersinia pseudotuberculosis* • Granuloma • Colitis • Ileitis • Appendicitis • Crohn's disease • Lymphadenopathy

Yersinia is one of the most common causes of bacterial enteritis in Western and Northern Europe. It has a worldwide distribution; the incidence of infection is rising within both Europe and the United States, although this may be due to better methods of detection and wider recognition of *Yersinia* species as important enteric pathogens. *Y. enterocolitica* (*YE*) and *Y. pseudotuberculosis* (*YP*) are the species that cause human gastrointestinal disease. *Yersinia* infection can be transmitted by both food and water, and the bacteria is associated with meat, dairy products, chocolate, poultry, and produce. Pork-related infection has been particularly well documented. Infection also can be acquired from animals. *Yersinia* has a preference for cold temperatures; thus, there is a natural affinity for refrigerated food, and there is speculation that infection is more common in cooler months. Familial, hospital-acquired, transplacental, and transfusion-associated infections also have been well documented.

These Gram-negative coccobacilli cause appendicitis, ileitis, colitis, and mesenteric lymphadenitis. *Yersinia* infection is responsible for many cases of isolated granulomatous appendicitis as well. Although yersiniosis is usually a self-limited process, chronic infections (including chronic colitis) have been well documented. Risk factors for serious infection include immunocompromise or debilitation, diabetes mellitus, cirrhosis, and deferoxamine therapy or iron overload. Complications of gastrointestinal infection include sepsis, abscess formation, perforation, and obstruction from inflammatory masses.

Infants, children, and young adults are most commonly infected. Patients commonly present with diarrhea (variably bloody), abdominal pain (which may be diffuse, periumbilical, or right lower quadrant), nausea, vomiting, and weight loss. Fever, pharyngitis, and leukocytosis may be present as well. Symptoms often have been present for weeks to months, leading to misdiagnosis as chronic idiopathic inflammatory bowel disease. Reactive polyarthritis and erythema nodosum are also associated with *Yersinia* infection.

Patients with granulomatous appendicitis due to *Yersinia* often present with signs and symptoms indistinguishable from acute non-specific appendicitis. Some patients with yersiniosis, however, are initially believed to be suffering from appendicitis, but upon exploration are found to have inflammation of the terminal ileum and mesenteric nodes that clinically mimics appendicitis (the "pseudoappendicular syndrome").

Pathologic features. *Yersinia* preferentially involves the ileum, right colon, and appendix, although any area of the bowel can be affected. Involvement may be segmental or patchy. Grossly, involved bowel has a thickened, edematous wall with nodular inflammatory masses centered on Peyer's patches (Fig. 8.1). Aphthoid and linear ulcers may be seen, along with mucosal friability, edema, and loss of vascular pattern (Fig. 8.2). Exudates are variably present. The findings may macroscopically mimic either Crohn's disease or ulcerative colitis, depending on the distribution. Involved appendices are enlarged and hyperemic, similar to suppurative appendicitis, and perforation is common. Involved lymph nodes may show gross foci of necrosis.

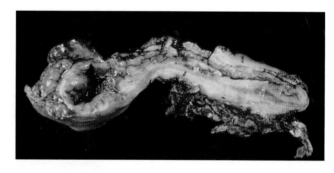

Fig. 8.1 Appendectomy specimen from a patient with *YE*-associated granulomatous appendicitis. The appendix has an edematous, thickened wall with nodular masses centered on Peyer's patches and ulcerated hemorrhagic mucosa

L.W. Lamps, *Surgical Pathology of the Gastrointestinal System: Bacterial, Fungal, Viral, and Parasitic Infections,*
DOI 10.1007/978-1-4419-0861-2_8, © Springer Science+Business Media, LLC 2009

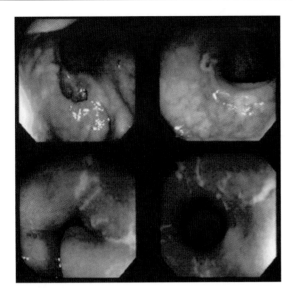

Fig. 8.2 Endoscopic photographs from a patient with *YE*-associated ileocolitis. Findings included patchy linear ulcerations with mucosal friability and hyperemia

Both suppurative and granulomatous patterns of inflammation are common and are often mixed. *YE* typically features epithelioid granulomas, along with hyperplastic Peyer's patches and overlying ulceration (Figs. 8.3 and 8.4). Gastrointestinal infection with *YP* has been described characteristically as a granulomatous process with central microabscesses (Fig. 8.5), almost always accompanied by mesenteric adenopathy. There is significant overlap between the histological features of *YE* and *YP* infection, however, and either species may show epithelioid granulomas with prominent lymphoid cuffing (Fig. 8.6), lymphoid hyperplasia, transmural lymphoid aggregates (Fig. 8.7), mucosal ulceration, and lymph node involvement. The transmural inflammation, fissuring and/or aphthoid ulcers (Fig. 8.8), focal architectural distortion (Fig. 8.9), skip lesions, and granulomas may closely mimic Crohn's disease.

Involved mesenteric lymph nodes often show follicular hyperplasia with scattered microabscesses and epithelioid granulomas (Fig. 8.10). Non-specific reactive lymphoid hyperplasia without microabscesses or granulomas is also a frequent finding in infected patients, however.

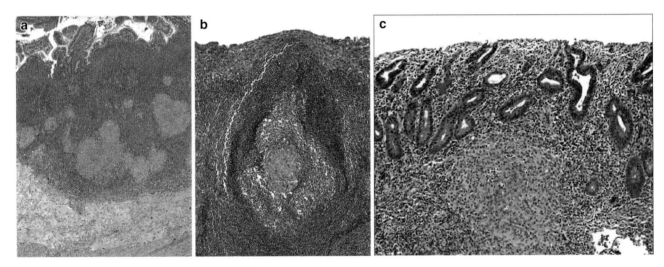

Fig. 8.3 *YE* infection is characterized by hyperplastic lymphoid tissue associated with granulomatous inflammation (**a**, ileum; **b**, appendix; **c**, colon). Higher power view shows overlying architectural distortion (**c**, courtesy Dr. Robert Odze)

Fig. 8.4 *YE* infection may feature deep ulcerations, accompanied by lymphoid hyperplasia, transmural lymphoid aggregates, and granulomatous inflammation (**a** and **b**; **a** courtesy Dr. Robert Odze)

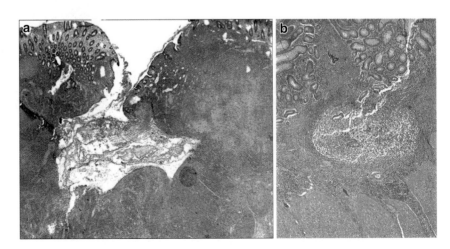

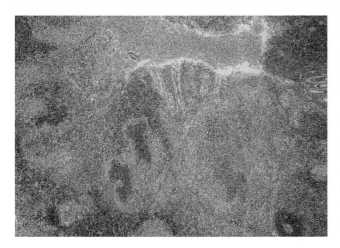

Fig. 8.5 *YP* appendicitis featuring irregular granulomas with central abscesses, lymphoid hyperplasia, and overlying mucosal ulceration

Differential diagnosis. The major differential diagnosis includes other infectious processes, particularly mycobacteria and *Salmonella*. Acid-fast stains and culture results help distinguish mycobacterial infection from yersiniosis. The specific clinical features, and the presence of greater numbers of neutrophils, microabscesses, and granulomas, may help to distinguish yersiniosis from salmonellosis. Gram stains are usually not helpful for the diagnosis of *Yersinia*, but cultures, serologic studies, and PCR assays may be very useful in confirming the diagnosis. Sarcoidosis, foreign body reaction to fecal material, and granulomatous inflammation secondary to delayed (interval) appendectomy with antibiotic therapy are also in the differential diagnosis of *Yersinia*-associated granulomatous appendicitis. Lymphogranuloma venereum and cat scratch disease also may affect the mesenteric lymph nodes and produce similar histologic features, but these organisms (especially cat scratch disease) only rarely involve the bowel itself (see Chapter 13).

Crohn's disease and yersiniosis may be very difficult to distinguish from one another. In addition to the gross and microscopic similarities, *Yersinia* DNA has been detected in many cases of longstanding Crohn's disease; however, the significance of this remains unclear. Features

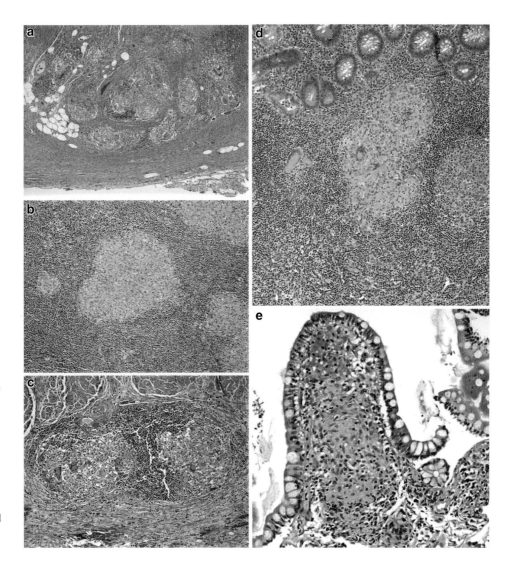

Fig. 8.6 Epithelioid granulomas, often with prominent lymphoid cuffs or an associated lymphoid infiltrate, may be a feature of infection with either species (**a–c**). Giant cells are variably present. Granulomatous appendicitis with lymphoid hyperplasia surrounding epithelioid granulomas (**d**). Epithelioid granulomas in an ileal biopsy from a patient with yersiniosis (**e**)

Fig. 8.7 Transmural lymphoid aggregates in a linear array with associated fibrosis can closely mimic Crohn's disease (**a** and **b**)

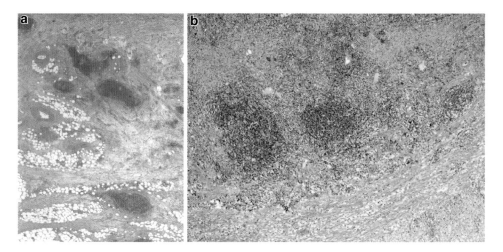

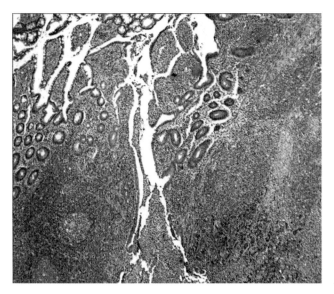

Fig. 8.8 Fissuring ulcer with surrounding lymphoid hyperplasia and granulomatous inflammation in a case of *Yersinia* infection of the ileum. (Courtesy Dr. Robert Odze)

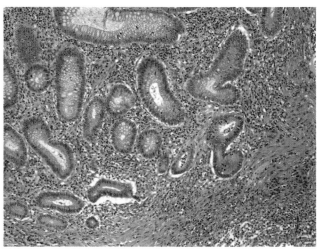

Fig. 8.9 Focal mucosal architectural distortion with associated neutrophilic infiltrate in a case of *Yersinia*-associated granulomatous appendicitis

favoring Crohn's disease include fistula formation, cobblestoning of mucosa, presence of creeping fat, and histologic changes of chronicity including crypt distortion, thickening

of the muscularis mucosa, and prominent neural hyperplasia. However, some cases are simply indistinguishable on histologic grounds alone.

Isolated granulomatous appendicitis, in the past, frequently has been interpreted as representing primary Crohn's

Fig. 8.10 Multiple epithelioid granulomas characterize *Yersinia*-related mesenteric adenitis (**a–b**)

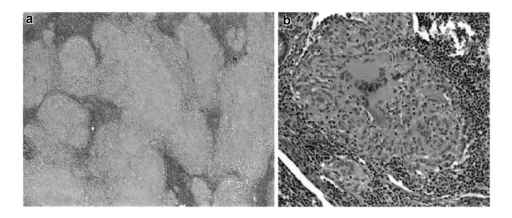

disease of the appendix. However, patients with granulomatous inflammation confined to the appendix rarely (less than 10%) develop generalized inflammatory bowel disease.

Selected References

1. Attwood SEA, Cafferkey MT, Keane FBV. *Yersinia* infections in surgical practice. Br J Surg 76:499–504, 1989.
2. Attwood SEA, Cafferkey MT, West AB, et al. *Yersinia* infection and acute abdominal pain. Lancet 1(8532): 529–33, 1987.
3. Bronner MP. Granulomatous appendicitis and the appendix in idiopathic inflammatory bowel disease. Semin Diagn Pathol 21:98–107, 2004.
4. Dudley TH, Dean PJ. Idiopathic granulomatous appendicitis, or Crohn's disease of the appendix revisited. Hum Pathol 24:595–601, 1993.
5. El-Maraghi NRH, Mair N. The histopathology of enteric infection with *Yersinia pseudotuberculosis*. Am J Clin Pathol 71:631–639, 1979.
6. Fredriksson-Ahomaa M, Stolle A, Korkeala H. Molecular epidemiology of *Yersinia enterocolitica* infections. FEMS Immunol Med Microbiol 47:315–29, 2006.
7. Gleason TH, Patterson SD. The pathology of *Yersinia enterocolitica* ileocolitis. Am J Surg Pathol 6:347–355, 1982.
8. Lamps LW, Madhusudhan KT, Greenson JK, et al. The role of *Y. enterocolitica* and *Y. pseudotuberculosis* in granulomatous appendicitis: a histologic and molecular study. Am J Surg Pathol 25:508–15, 2001.
9. Lamps LW, Madhusudhan KT, Havens JM, et al. Pathogenic *Yersinia enterocolitica* and *Yersinia pseudotuberculosis* DNA is detected in bowel and mesenteric nodes from Crohn's disease patients. Am J Surg Pathol 27(2):220–7, 2003.
10. Lamps LW. Beyond acute inflammation: a review of appendicitis and infections of the appendix. Diagn Histopathol 14:68–77, 2008.
11. Mazzoleni G, deSa D, Gately J, Riddell RH. *Yersinia enterocolitica* infection with ileal perforation associated with iron overload and deferoxamine therapy. Dig Dis Sci 36:1154–60, 1991.
12. Natkin J, Beavis KG. *Yersinia enterocolitica* and *Yersinia pseudotuberculosis*. Clin Lab Med 19:523–36, 1999.
13. Paff JR, Triplett DA, Saari TN. Clinical and laboratory aspects of *Yersinia pseudotuberculosis* infections, with a report of two cases. Am J Clin Pathol 66:101–10, 1976.
14. Saebo A, Lassen J. Acute and chronic gastrointestinal manifestations associated with *Yersinia enterocolitica* infection: a Norwegian 10-year follow-up study on 458 hospitalized patients. Ann Surg 215:250–5, 1992.
15. Simmonds SD, Noble MA, Freeman HJ. Gastrointestinal features of culture-positive *Yersinia enterocolitica* infection. Gastroenterol 92:112–7, 1987.
16. Van Noyen R, Selderslaghs R, Bekaert J, et al. Causative role of *Yersinia* and other enteric pathogens in the appendicular syndrome. Eur J Clin Microbiol Infect Dis 10:735–41, 1991.
17. Vantrappen G, Agg HO, Ponette E, et al. *Yersinia* enteritis and enterocolitis: gastroenterological aspects. Gastroenterol 72:220–7, 1977.
18. Winblad S, Nilehn B, Sternby NH. *Yersinia enterocolitica* (*Pasteurella* X) in human enteric infections. Brit Med J 2:1363–6, 1966.

Chapter 9

Mycobacterial Infections

Keywords Mycobacterial sp. • Tuberculosis • Granuloma • Histiocytic • Acid-fast • Crohn's disease

Mycobacterium tuberculosis. There has been a remarkable resurgence of tuberculosis in Western countries, due in large part to the AIDS population, but also to institutional overcrowding and immigrant populations. Tuberculosis also remains common in developing countries. Gastrointestinal tuberculosis may be acquired through several mechanisms, including the swallowing of infected sputum in pulmonary tuberculosis, ingestion of contaminated milk (rare where pasteurization is common), via hematogenous spread from pulmonary or military disease, and direct extension from adjacent organs.

Gastrointestinal symptoms (rather than pulmonary) may be the initial presentation of disease, and extrapulmonary manifestations of tuberculosis are more common in AIDS patients than immunocompetent persons. In addition, primary gastrointestinal tuberculosis in the absence of pulmonary infection has been well documented.

Symptoms and signs of gastrointestinal tuberculosis vary with the site(s) of involvement. The ileocecal and jejuno-ileal areas are most commonly involved, probably due to the abundance of lymphoid tissue. Associated mesenteric adenopathy is very common. Involvement of the ascending colon, duodenum, and rectum is less frequent. Gastroesophageal, appendiceal, and anal/perianal involvement are rare, but merit special mention due to the clinicopathologic implications (below). Peritoneal tuberculosis is slightly more common than gastrointestinal involvement, and may cause ascites as well as clinically significant adhesions.

Regardless of site of involvement, patients often have non-specific symptoms including weight loss, fever, abdominal pain, diarrhea, or a palpable abdominal mass. Other symptoms include night sweats, malaise, anorexia, GI bleeding, and signs of malabsorption. Symptoms have often been present for months. Laboratory abnormalities include an elevated erythrocyte sedimentation rate and mild anemia.

Gastroesophageal tuberculosis. Esophageal tuberculosis is most often due to extension from adjacent involved organs such as lung or mediastinal lymph nodes. Common clinical symptoms include dysphagia, odynophagia, aspiration due to tracheo-esophageal fistula, and hematemesis. Ulcers are the most common finding, but strictures also have been reported. Gastric tuberculosis is slightly more common than esophageal involvement, and patients usually present with abdominal pain, nausea, and vomiting, most often due to either ulcerative lesions or gastric outlet obstruction.

Anal/perianal tuberculosis. Anal tuberculosis is rare in Western countries, but fairly common in nations in which tuberculosis is endemic. Patients with anal/perianal tuberculosis often do not have pulmonary disease, and present with anal ulceration, fissures, fistulas, abscesses, and mass lesions that can mimic malignancy, Crohn's disease, or other sexually transmitted diseases.

Appendiceal tuberculosis. Tuberculosis of the appendix is most often associated with ileocecal infection, although it is much rarer than ileocecal infection. Periappendicular tuberculosis also has been well described, and may be associated with peritoneal tuberculosis.

Pathologic features. Strictures and ulcers (often occurring together) (Fig. 9.1) are the most common endoscopic findings, along with thickened mucosal folds and inflammatory nodules. The ulcers are often circumferential and transverse.

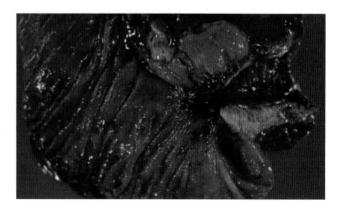

Fig. 9.1 Ulcerated stricture in a patient with ileal tuberculosis. (Courtesy Dr. George Gray, Jr)

L.W. Lamps, *Surgical Pathology of the Gastrointestinal System: Bacterial, Fungal, Viral, and Parasitic Infections,*
DOI 10.1007/978-1-4419-0861-2_9, © Springer Science+Business Media, LLC 2009

Multiple and segmental lesions with skip areas are common, which can easily mimic Crohn's disease. The ileocecal valve is often deformed and gaping when this segment of the bowel is involved. Large inflammatory masses ("tuberculomas") may be seen, most often involving the ileocecum, and well described complications include obstruction, perforation, and hemorrhage. Mesenteric lymphadenopathy is very common; mesenteric lymph nodes are enlarged and may be matted. Foci of necrosis can be seen grossly in some cases (Fig. 9.2).

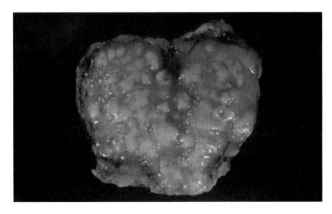

Fig. 9.2 Mesenteric lymph node with tuberculous lymphadenitis. The lymph node is enlarged, with multiple grossly visible foci of caseous necrosis. (Courtesy Dr. George Gray)

The wall of the bowel is often thickened and edematous, with transmural inflammation (Fig. 9.3), lymphoid hyperplasia, and fibrosis in later stages of disease. Ulcers may be superficial or deep (Fig. 9.4), and may overlie hyperplastic Peyer's patches (aphthoid ulcers). The characteristic histologic lesion consists of caseating, often confluent, granulomas (Fig. 9.5), present at any level of the gut wall, but most common in the submucosa (Fig. 9.6). A rim of lymphocytes is often present at the periphery of the granulomas (Fig. 9.7), and giant cells are variably present (Fig. 9.8). Older lesions

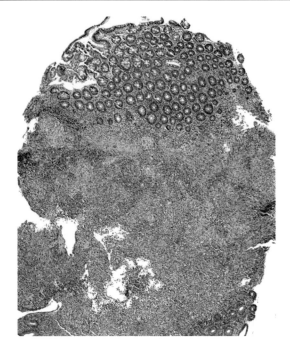

Fig. 9.3 Marked submucosal granulomatous inflammation and inflammation extending deeply into the bowel wall are seen in this biopsy from the right colon of a patient with tuberculosis

are frequently hyalinized and calcified, and well-formed granulomas may be rare and difficult to find. Inflammation of submucosal vessels is common (Fig. 9.9), and architectural distortion that mimics chronic idiopathic inflammatory bowel disease is frequently seen overlying areas of granulomatous inflammation (Fig. 9.10). Characteristic granulomas are often present within involved lymph nodes as well, with confluence and caseation (Figs. 9.8c and 9.11).

Acid-fast stains sometimes demonstrate organisms, preferentially within necrotic areas or macrophages (Fig. 9.12), but culture is usually required for definitive diagnosis. The acid-fast bacilli of *M. tuberculosis* are typically rod-shaped

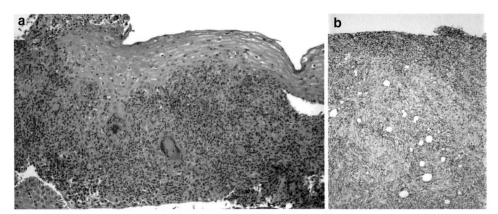

Fig. 9.4 Superficial ulceration in a patient with esophageal tuberculosis, with underlying submucosal granulomatous inflammation (**a**, courtesy Dr. Philip Ferguson). Broad areas of ulceration with underlying granulomatous inflammation and fibrosis in the right colon of a patient with *M. tuberculosis* infection (**b**)

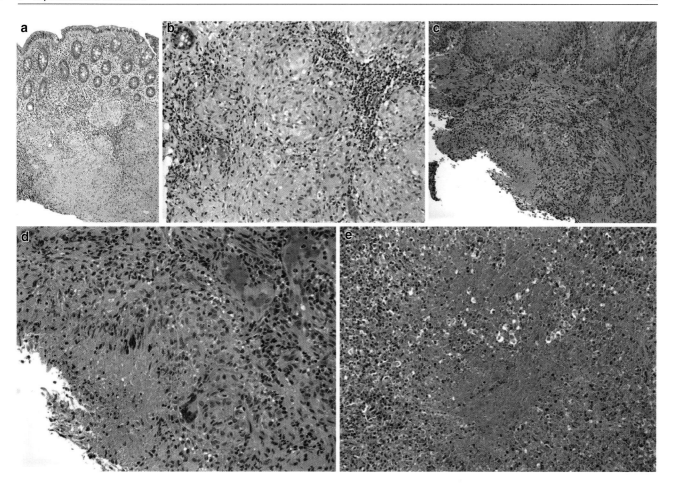

Fig. 9.5 Numerous epithelioid, confluent granulomas characterize gastrointestinal tuberculosis (**a** and **b**). Well-formed epithelioid submucosal granuloma with central caseation from an esophageal biopsy (**c** and **d**, courtesy Dr. Philip Ferguson). High-power view of abundant necrotic debris at the center of a tuberculoid granuloma (**e**)

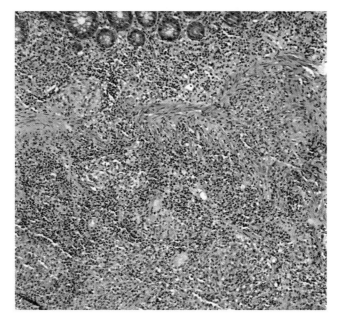

Fig. 9.6 Tuberculoid granulomas and/or granulomatous inflammation are often most prominent in the submucosa

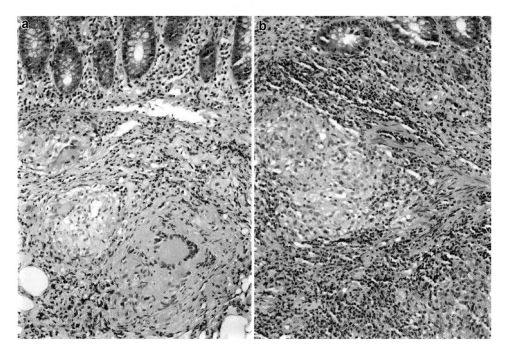

Fig. 9.7 A rim of lymphocytes or a lymphocytic infiltrate is often associated with the granulomas in tuberculosis (**a** and **b**)

Fig. 9.8 Prominent giant cells
within granulomatous
inflammation in an esophageal
biopsy from a patient with
tuberculosis (**a**, courtesy Dr.
Philip Ferguson). Granuloma
with necrosis and prominent
giant cells in a mesenteric lymph
node from a patient with
abdominal tuberculosis (**b**,
courtesy Dr. Margie Scott)

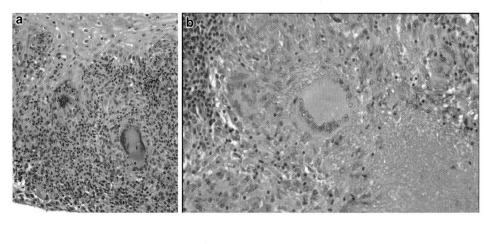

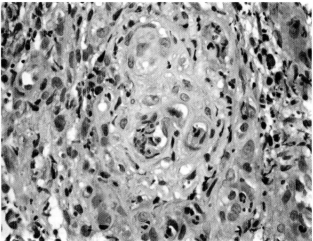

Fig. 9.9 Inflammation of small vessels in the submucosa of the right colon from a patient with colonic tuberculosis

Fig. 9.10 Cryptitis, crypt abscesses, and architectural distortion overlying areas of granulomatous inflammation from a patient with colonic tuberculosis (**a** and **b**)

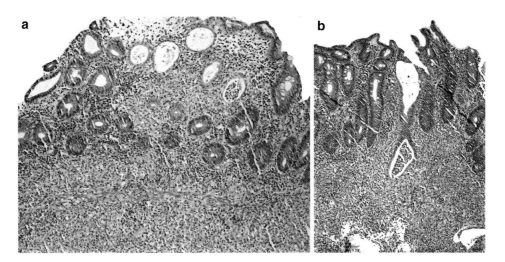

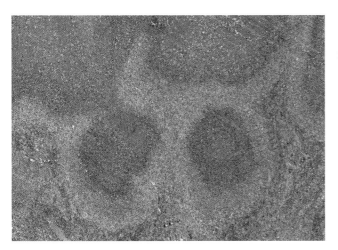

Fig. 9.11 Confluent, caseating granulomas from a mesenteric lymph node in a patient with abdominal tuberculosis (courtesy Dr. Margie Scott)

and have a "beaded" morphology. Organisms may be abundant in immunocompromised patients (Fig. 9.13), yet rare and difficult to detect in immunocompetent persons (Fig. 9.14), and the number of organisms may vary with the age of the lesion and previous anti-tubercular therapy. PCR assays are becoming more widely available, but sensitivity suffers with this methodology as well if the number of organisms is very low. PPD tests may be helpful, but are unreliable in immunocompromised or debilitated patients. Some atypical mycobacteria, such as *M. kansasii* and *M. bovis,* may cause similar pathologic findings.

Differential diagnosis. The differential diagnosis includes other granulomatous infectious processes, especially yersiniosis and fungal disease (Table 9.1), as well as sarcoidosis, granulomatous drug reactions, and unusual autoimmune diseases such as Behcet's disease. The granulomas of yersiniosis are typically non-caseating, with striking lymphoid

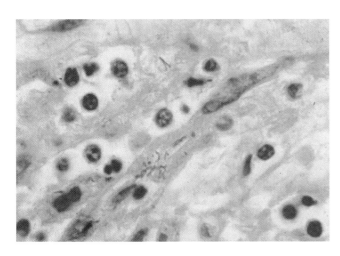

Fig. 9.12 Acid-fast stains highlight intracellular bacilli (*stained red*) within macrophages

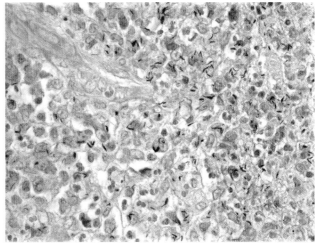

Fig. 9.13 Innumerable mycobacteria in a mesenteric lymph node from an immunocompromised patient with tuberculosis (courtesy Dr. Margie Scott)

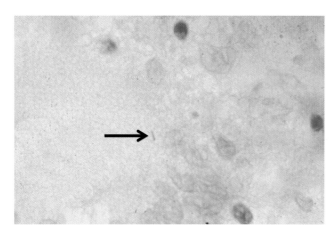

Fig. 9.14 Mycobacteria may be rare and very difficult to find in immunocompetent patients

Table 9.1 A comparison of histologic features useful in the differential diagnosis of *M. tuberculosis*, *Yersinia*, and Crohn's disease

	M. tuberculosis	*Yersinia*	Crohn's disease
Caseating granulomas	Frequent	Rare	Absent
Confluent granulomas	Frequent	Frequent	Absent
Numerous granulomas	Common	Common	Rare
Prominent lymphoid cuff	Frequent	Frequent	Uncommon
Lymphoid hyperplasia	Common	Very common	Uncommon
Ulcers (both aphthous and deep)	Common	Common	Common
Architectural distortion	Common	Common	Common
Changes of chronicity unassociated with sites of granulomatous inflammation	Absent	Absent	Common
Multiple sites of involvement	Common	Rare	Common
Mucosal cobblestoning	Uncommon	Uncommon	Common
Fistula formation	Uncommon	Rare	Common
Anal/perianal disease	Rare	Absent	Common

cuffs, but there may be considerable histologic overlap. Culture, AFB and fungal stains, and PCR assays may be invaluable in resolving the differential diagnosis.

Patients with sarcoidosis usually have coexistent mediastinal or pulmonary lesions, as well as an elevated serum angiotensin converting enzyme. Patients with Behcet's disease typically have a skin rash and/or oral ulcerations. Granulomatous drug reactions must be excluded based on the evaluation of the patient's medication history, as well as a temporal association between symptoms and use of the offending drug. In the appendix, granulomatous reaction to foreign material and granulomatous changes in the context of a delayed or interval appendectomy may also mimic mycobacterial infection.

Crohn's disease may be very difficult to distinguish from tuberculosis, particularly in countries where tuberculosis is common (Table 9.1). Features favoring Crohn's disease are the presence of linear rather than circumferential ulcers, transmural lymphoid aggregates, deep fistulas and fissures, and mucosal changes of chronicity that are present away from areas of granulomatous inflammation. Tuberculosis also commonly lacks mucosal cobblestoning.

A further confounding factor is that tuberculosis has recently been associated with the use of infliximab, a tumor necrosis factor alpha neutralizing agent used in treating Crohn's disease and rheumatoid arthritis. The pattern of involvement in these patients is somewhat unusual, with a majority of patients exhibiting extrapulmonary tuberculosis. The emergence of infection is often associated with initiation of treatment.

Mycobacterium avium-intracellulare complex. This is the most common mycobacterium isolated from the GI tract. It is usually found in patients with AIDS and other immune-compromising conditions, although it is rarely seen in immunocompetent persons. It is often a late manifestation of AIDS, reflecting low CD4 counts.

Disseminated MAI infection remains the most common systemic bacterial infection among AIDS patients. Gastrointestinal involvement is usually a feature of disseminated infection, and the lungs, liver, spleen, bone marrow, and lymph nodes are frequently involved in addition to the gastrointestinal tract. Symptoms include diarrhea (usually chronic and non-bloody), nausea, vomiting, and weight loss; fever and night sweats are often present as well. Abdominal pain is a less-frequent symptom.

Pathologic features. The small bowel is preferentially involved, but colonic and gastroesophageal involvement may be present, as well as mesenteric adenopathy. Appendiceal involvement has been rarely described.

Endoscopy is often normal. When macroscopic findings are present, MAI infection most often manifests as 2–4-mm raised, granular white mucosal nodules with surrounding erythema. Small ulcers and mucosal hemorrhages have been described as well. Involved mesenteric lymph nodes are enlarged, solid, and firm, with variably present foci of necrosis.

Histologic manifestations vary with site and immune status of the patient. Immunocompetent patients typically have well formed, often epithelioid granulomas either with or without necrosis (Fig. 9.15). Small bowel biopsies from immunocompromised patients generally show villi distended by a diffuse infiltration of histiocytes containing bacilli (Fig. 9.16), with little inflammatory response (Fig. 9.17) other than occasional poorly formed granulomas (Fig. 9.18). Similar histiocytic infiltrates may be seen in the colon and other areas of the GI tract (Fig. 9.19).

Fig. 9.15 Multiple well-delineated, epithelioid granulomas in the ileum of an immunocompetent patient with MAI infection (**a** and **b**)

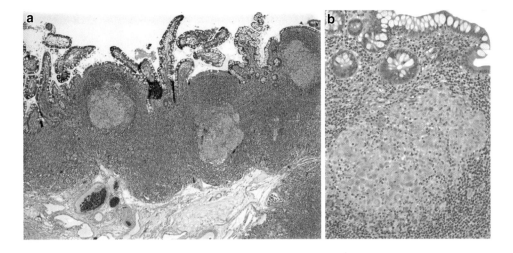

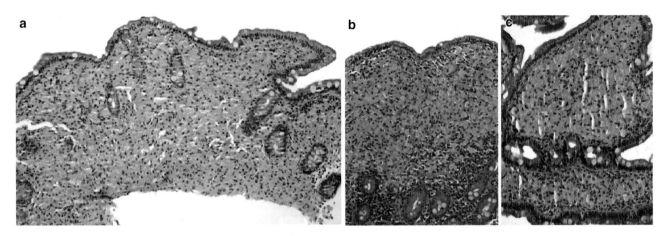

Fig. 9.16 Small bowel biopsies from AIDS patients with MAI infection show the characteristic diffuse histiocytic infiltrate leading to marked villous blunting (**a–c**)

Bacilli stain with acid-fast stains (Fig. 9.20), as well as PAS and GMS (Fig. 9.21) (any rapidly dividing bacteria may stain positively on GMS stain, and this should not dissuade the pathologist from an erroneous diagnosis of fungal infection). Mycobacteria (including *M. tuberculosis* and *M. leprae*) may also stain for desmin, actin, and keratin. Culture and PCR assays may be extremely helpful in diagnosis. Organisms are generally abundant in the immunocompromised host (Fig. 9.20), but may be harder to detect in healthy patients.

Differential diagnosis. The differential diagnosis primarily includes other infectious processes. It is particularly important to distinguish atypical mycobacterial infection from *M. tuberculosis*, because the anti-tubercular drug regimen varies. MAI more often features diffuse histiocytic infiltrates and poorly formed granulomas with abundant organisms, rather than the well-formed granulomas typical of tuberculosis. Rarely, other atypical mycobacteria, including *M. fortuitum*, *M. chelonei*, and *M. sulgai*, may infect the gastrointestinal tract and cause histologic findings similar to MAI infection. Culture and molecular assays are invaluable tools for distinguishing between mycobacterial species.

Both MAI and the Whipple bacillus are PAS positive, but the Whipple bacillus is not acid-fast, and PCR assays will also distinguish the two bacteria. *Rhodococcus equi*, a rare infection found in immunocompromised patients (see Chapter 13), produces a similar histiocytic infiltrate. These intracellular coccobacillary organisms are Gram and PAS positive and also stain with modified acid-fast stains. *Rhodococcus* is more granular on PAS than the bacilli of MAI, however, and is negative with routine Ziehl–Neelsen stain. Culture and molecular assays also may differentiate these two organisms. Although, as mentioned above, MAI stain with both PAS and GMS, fungal organisms appear morphologically different than MAI.

Fig. 9.17 Other than scattered mononuclear cells, few other inflammatory cells are typically associated with the histiocytic infiltrate of MAI infection (**a**–**c**). (**a**, courtesy Dr. Lucas Campbell)

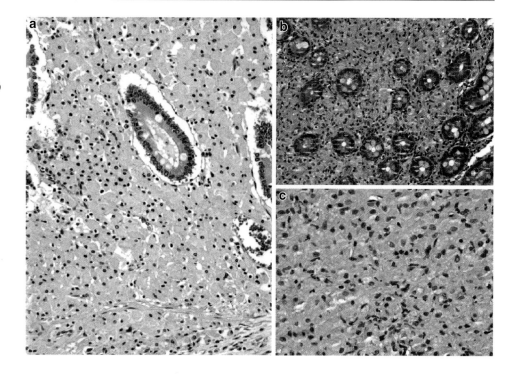

Fig. 9.18 Some immunocompromised patients with atypical mycobacterial infection may show small, poorly formed granulomas (**a** and **b**). (Courtesy Drs. Rebecca Wilcox and John Hart)

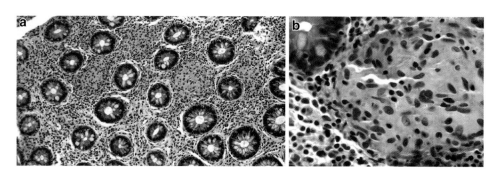

Fig. 9.19 When the colon is involved by MAI infection, a similar histiocytic infiltrate is seen filling the lamina propria (**a** and **b**)

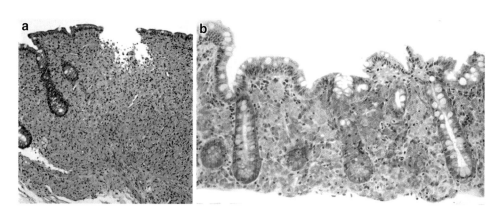

In addition to involvement of mesenteric nodes by histiocytic infiltrates similar to those found in the gut, atypical mycobacteria can cause histiocytic spindle-cell nodules (Fig. 9.22). These lesions mimic sarcomas or other malignancies, particularly, as described above, if they are immunopositive for cytokeratin, actin, or desmin. However, AFB stains reveal innumerable bacteria in the spindled cells.

Fig. 9.20 Ziehl–Neelsen stain shows innumerable acid-fast bacilli filling histiocytes within the lamina propria, leading to marked villous blunting (**a–c**)

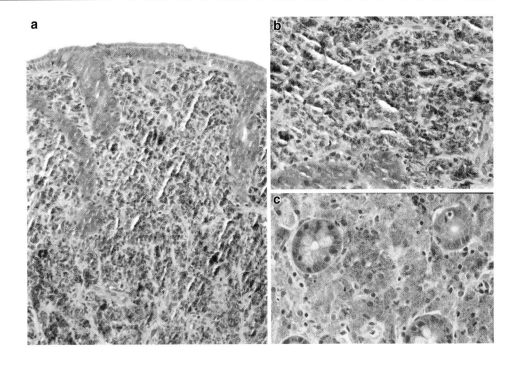

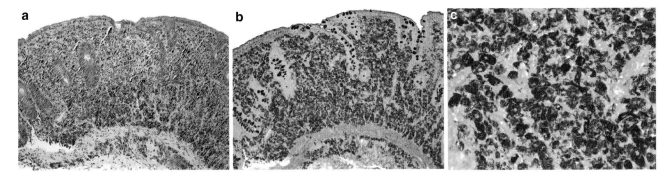

Fig. 9.21 MAI may be GMS positive as well, but should not be confused with fungi (**a**, Ziehl-Neelsen stain; **b** and **c**, GMS stain on same case)

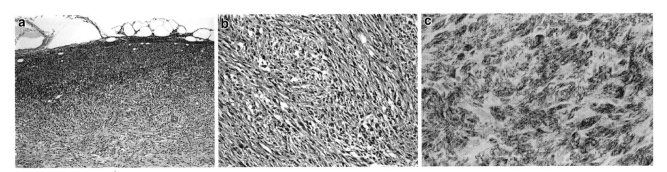

Fig. 9.22 Atypical mycobacterial spindle-cell nodule in mesenteric lymph node. The periphery of the lymph node shows a granulomatous response adjacent to the spindle-cell nodule (**a**). The marked spindle-cell proliferation can mimic a malignancy (**b**). AFB stain highlights numerous mycobacteria within the spindle cells (**c**). (**a** and **b**, courtesy Drs. Rebecca Wilcox and John Hart)

Selected References

M. tuberculosis

1. Ani AN, Solanke TF. Anal fistula: a review of 82 cases. Dis Colon Rectum 19:51–5, 1976.
2. Chung CC, Choi CL, Kwok SP, et al. Anal and perianal tuberculosis: a report of three cases in 10 years. J R Coll Surg Edinb 42:189–90, 1997.
3. Gordon AH, Marshall JB. Esophageal tuberculosis: definitive diagnosis by endoscopy. Am J Gastroenterol 85:174–7, 1990.
4. Horvath KD, Whelan RL. Intestinal tuberculosis: return of an old disease. Am J Gastroenterol 93:692–6, 1998.
5. Iochim HL. Granulomatous lesions of lymph nodes. In Iochim HL (ed): Pathology of Granulomas, New York, NY: Raven Press, 1983, pp. 151–8.
6. Keane J, Gershon S, Wise RP, et al. Tuberculosis associated with infliximab, a tumor necrosis factor alpha-neutralizing agent. N Eng J Med 345:1098–104, 2001.
7. Lamps LW. Beyond acute inflammation: a review of appendicitis and infections of the appendix. Diagn Histopathol 14:68–77, 2008.
8. Marshall JB. Tuberculosis of the gastrointestinal tract and peritoneum. Am J Gastroenterol 88:989–99, 1993.
9. Pulimood AB, Peter S, Ramakrishna BS, et al. Segmental colonoscopic biopsies in the differentiation of ileocolonic tuberculosis from Crohn's disease. J Gastroenterol Hepatol 20:688–96, 2005.
10. Pulimood AB, Ramakrishna BS, Kurian G, et al. Endoscopic mucosal biopsies are useful in distinguishing granulomatous colitis due to Crohn's disease from tuberculosis. Gut 45:537–41, 1999.
11. Sharma MP, Bhatia V. Abdominal tuberculosis. Indian J Med Res 120:305–15, 2004.
12. Singh MK, Arunabh, Kapoor VK. Tuberculosis of the appendix-a report of 17 cases and a suggested aetiopathological classification. Post Med J 63:855–7, 1987.

MAI (Mycobacterium avium-intracellulare) and Other Atypical Mycobacteria

13. Armstrong D. Opportunistic infections in the acquired immune deficiency syndrome. Sem Oncol 14(2)Suppl 3:40–7, 1987.
14. Benson CA, Ellner JJ. *Mycobacterium avium* complex infection and AIDS: advances in theory and practice. Clin Infect Dis 17:7–20, 1993.
15. Chen KTK. Mycobacterial spindle cell pseudotumor of lymph nodes. Am J Surg Pathol 16:276–81, 1992.
16. Hellyer TJ, Brown IN, Taylor MB, et al. Gastro-intestinal involvement in *Mycobacterium avium-intracellulare* infection of patients with HIV. J Inf 26:55–66, 1993.
17. Farhi DC, Mason UG, Horsburgh CR. Pathologic findings in disseminated *Mycobacterium avium-intracellulare* infection: a report of 11 cases. Am J Clin Pathol 85:67–72, 1986.
18. Lamps LW. Infectious disorders of the upper gastrointestinal tract, excluding *H. pylori*. Diagn Histopathol 14:427–36, 2008.
19. Monsour HP, Quigley EMM, Markin RS, et al. Endoscopy in the diagnosis of gastrointestinal *Mycobacterium avium-intracellulare* infection. J Clin Gastroenterol 13 (1): 20–4, 1991.
20. Pere D, Ris J, Lopez-Contreras J, et al. Appendicitis due to *Mycobacterium avium* complex in a patient with AIDS. Arch Intern Med 156:1114.
21. Roth RI, Owen RL, Keren DF, et al. Intestinal infection with *Mycobacterium avium-intracellulare* in acquired immune deficiency syndrome (AIDS): histological and clinical comparison with Whipple's disease. Dig Dis Sci 5:497–504, 1985.
22. Umlas J, Federman M, Crawford C, et al. Spindle cell pseudotumor due to *Mycobacterium avium-intracellulare* in patients with acquired immunodeficiency syndrome (AIDS). Am J Surg Pathol 15:1181–7, 1991.

Chapter 10

Clostridial Infections

Keywords *Clostridium* sp. • Pseudomembranous colitis • Pig-bel • Neutropenic enterocolitis • Enteritis necroticans

Clostridia are some of the most potent toxigenic bacteria in existence. This group of bacteria is responsible for important gastrointestinal diseases including pseudomembranous/antibiotic-associated colitis (usually *Clostridium difficile*), enteritis necroticans or pig-bel (usually *C. perfringens* [*welchii*]), and neutropenic enterocolitis (frequently *C. septicum*).

Clostridium difficile. *C. difficile* is the most common nosocomial gastrointestinal pathogen. Infection is usually related to prior antibiotic exposure (especially orally administered antibiotics), since the organisms cannot infect in the presence of normal colonic flora. The association between *C. difficile* and antibiotic-associated diarrhea was initially described in the 1970s, and the incidence has dramatically increased since that time. Pathogenic strains produce two enterotoxins: toxin A, the activation of which leads to fluid secretion and mucosal permeability, and toxin B, which has little enterotoxic activity in vivo.

The majority of patients are elderly, although infection is certainly not limited to this group. Other risk factors (in addition to prior antibiotic use) include severe co-morbid conditions, indwelling nasogastric tubes, gastrointestinal procedures, antacids, admission to an intensive care unit, and duration of hospitalization. In addition, the incidence of *C. difficile* infection has increased in patients with chronic idiopathic inflammatory bowel disease and negatively affects clinical outcome in terms of both hospitalization and need for colectomy.

Recurrent disease is common despite successful treatment and is seen in up to 50% of cases; the incidence of recurrent disease appears to be increasing. Risk factors include new exposure to antibiotics, especially multiple antibiotics, age greater than 65 years, severe underlying illness, and a lengthy hospital stay. Furthermore, the incidence of severe or life-threatening *C. difficile* colitis in North America has increased recently. This increase has been linked to an epidemic strain of *C. difficile* known as strain BI/NAP1; this strain is hyper-

virulent, with increased production of both toxins A and B, and is resistant to fluoroquinolones.

Some patients are asymptomatic despite the presence of toxigenic strains in stool. Presentation in symptomatic patients is very variable, ranging from mild diarrhea to pseudomembranous colitis (PMC) to fulminant colitis with perforation or toxic megacolon. Watery diarrhea is most common initially, and may be accompanied by abdominal pain, cramping, fever, and leukocytosis (sometimes marked). Bloody diarrhea is variably seen. Symptoms can occur up to several weeks after discontinuation of antibiotic therapy. Patients with more severe disease may not have diarrhea, and the only clues to diagnosis may be fever, marked leukocytosis, and a markedly tender, distended abdomen. Complications of severe infection include toxic megacolon, perforation, and death. An associated reactive polyarthritis also has been described.

Pathologic features. Endoscopically, classic PMC features yellow–white pseudomembranes that bleed when scraped (Fig. 10.1). The entire colon is often involved, but the disease may be patchy or segmental, and any segment of the bowel can be affected including the small bowel and the appendix. Pseudomembranes are most common in the distal left colon. In patients with ulcerative colitis, *C. difficile* infection of the ileal pouch–anal anastomosis has been well described. Atypical findings include mucosal erythema and friability without pseudomembranes, and typical histologic findings may be seen in the absence of macroscopically evident pseudomembranes.

Histologically, classic PMC features "volcano" or "mushroom" lesions (Fig. 10.2) with intercrypt necrosis (Fig. 10.3) and ballooned crypts (Fig. 10.4), giving rise to the laminated pseudomembrane composed of fibrin, mucin, and neutrophils (Fig. 10.5). The ballooned glands are filled with neutrophils and mucin, and the superficial epithelial cells are often lost (Fig. 10.6). The degenerated goblet cells may slough and spill into the lumen of degenerated and necrotic crypts (Fig. 10.7); this feature may mimic signet ring cell adenocarcinoma, and it is important to be aware of this reactive morphologic change in the context of PMC. More severe

L.W. Lamps, *Surgical Pathology of the Gastrointestinal System: Bacterial, Fungal, Viral, and Parasitic Infections,*
DOI 10.1007/978-1-4419-0861-2_10, © Springer Science+Business Media, LLC 2009

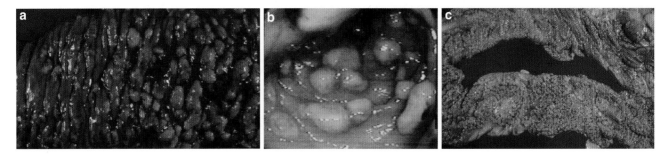

Fig. 10.1 Pseudomembranous colitis typically features yellow–white pseudomembranes (**a**, courtesy Dr. George F. Gray; **b**, courtesy Dr. William A. Webb) that bleed when scraped. The entire colon is often involved (**c**, courtesy Dr. Rodger C. Haggitt), but findings may be patchy

Fig. 10.2 The classic histologic feature of pseudomembranous colitis is the "volcano" or "mushroom" lesion. "Volcano"-like pseudomembrane overlies the mucosa (**a**). A smaller "mushroom" pseudomembrane is seen in a colonic biopsy (**b**)

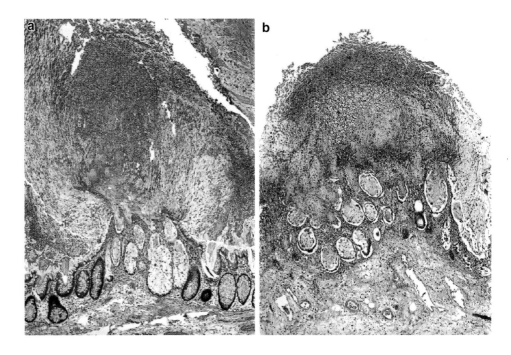

and prolonged PMC may lead to full thickness mucosal necrosis (Fig. 10.8). Non-specific, less characteristic lesions, usually focal active colitis with occasional crypt abscesses but lacking pseudomembranous features (Fig. 10.9), has been well described in association with a positive *C. difficile* toxin assay.

Differential diagnosis. It is important to note that "pseudomembranous colitis" is a descriptive phrase, not a specific diagnosis. Although most cases of PMC are related to *C. difficile*, other infectious entities (particularly enterohemorrhagic *Escherichia coli, Shigella*, and *Salmonella*), as well as ischemic colitis, may have a similar endoscopic and histologic appearance. A hyalinized lamina propria favors the diagnosis of ischemia. Other features, such as crypt withering, pseudomembranes, and mucosal necrosis, may be seen in either entity (Fig. 10.10). Endoscopically, pseudomembrane formation is more frequent in PMC, although it can be seen in ischemia as well; the presence of a polypoid or mass lesion is indicative of ischemia,

and is not seen in PMC. Recently, an antibiotic-associated hemorrhagic colitis has been reported in association with *Klebsiella oxytoca*. This colitis is hemorrhagic, segmental, most common in the right and transverse colon, and lacks pseudomembranes.

History of antibiotic use and stool assay for *C. difficile* toxin (either toxin A or B) may be invaluable in resolving the differential diagnosis. It is important to note, however, that the enzyme-linked immunoassay tests usually used in clinical practice have a high specificity (75–100%) but a limited sensitivity (63–99%). Therefore, a negative assay does not exclude *C. difficile* infection.

Clostridium perfringens (welchii). *C. perfringens* (formerly known as *C. welchii*) causes segmental necrotizing enteritis (also known as enteritis necroticans) related to food poisoning. This bacterium is also a cause of diarrhea unrelated to food poisoning, often associated with antibiotic use and hospitalization in elderly patients.

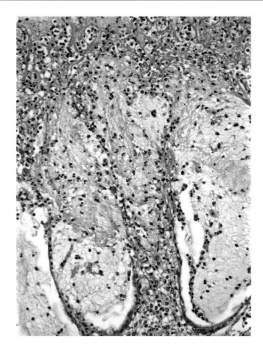

Fig. 10.3 Intercrypt necrosis is often present between dilated, ballooned crypts

Food-related infection, most commonly caused by *C. perfringens/welchii* type C, is most common in Southeast Asia and New Guinea, where it is known as "pig-bel." It was observed in Germany and Scandinavia during and following World War II, where it was known as "Darmbrand."

This organism is a normal commensal in both humans and swine. It has been hypothesized that persons with low-protein diets or chronic malnutrition have reduced digestive proteases, particularly if their regular diets are high in foods with abundant protease inhibitors, such as sweet potatoes. When

these individuals consume a meal high in animal protein that contains *C. welchii* type C and its toxin, there is an excess of toxin that persons with low protease activity are incapable of neutralizing, leading to disease. This hypothesis has been supported by animal experiments and supports observations regarding human disease as well. The onset of pig-bel usually follows a meal rich in infected meat and occurs in persons in endemic areas who routinely eat very low-protein diets and foods that are high in protease inhibitors. Cases in Europe during and after WWII were usually in patients who ate meat after a long period of protein malnutrition. Modern cases in Western countries usually follow eating binges or a meal rich in animal protein ingested by patients with malnutrition or malabsorption. Rare cases also have been reported after eating meals heavy in beans or raw peanuts, which also contain large amounts of trypsin inhibitors. Infection also has been associated with diabetes, possibly due to the delayed gastric emptying and reduced intestinal motility seen in these patients.

Symptoms include abdominal pain, bloody diarrhea, and vomiting, often with abdominal distension. Complications include perforation, obstruction, bowel gangrene, and septicemia with shock and rapid death. Mild or subacute forms have been reported, but the pathologic features have not been well described.

Pathologic features. Involvement is predominantly seen in, but not limited to, the jejunum. The bowel is often dusky gray-green, dilated, and edematous, similar to ischemia. The necrotic areas may be segmental and focal, with intervening areas of normal mucosa. The mucosal exudate may be similar to PMC, but inflammation and necrosis often become transmural and lead to perforation.

Histologically, the mucosa is edematous, necrotic, and ulcerated, with a heavy acute inflammatory infiltrate at

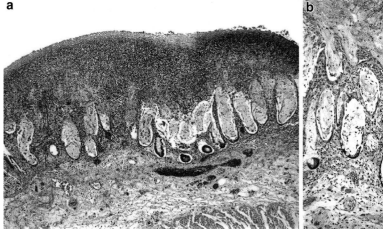
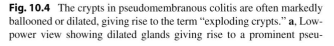
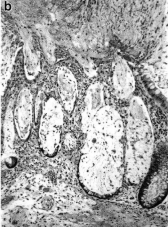

Fig. 10.4 The crypts in pseudomembranous colitis are often markedly ballooned or dilated, giving rise to the term "exploding crypts." **a**, Low-power view showing dilated glands giving rise to a prominent pseu-

domembrane. **b**, Higher power view of markedly dilated crypts giving rise to the pseudomembrane

Fig. 10.5 The pseudomembrane is characteristically laminated, and composed of mucin, fibrin, and neutrophils (**a** and **b**)

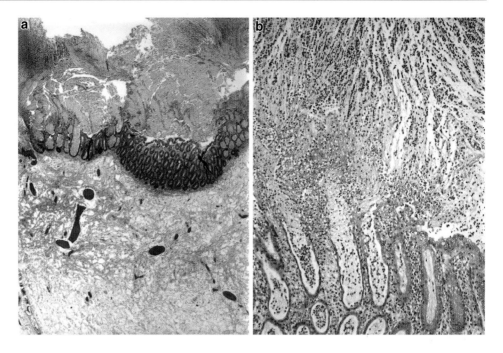

Fig. 10.6 The ballooned glands are filled with inspissated neutrophils and mucin, often accompanied by ulceration of surface epithelial cells (**a** and **b**)

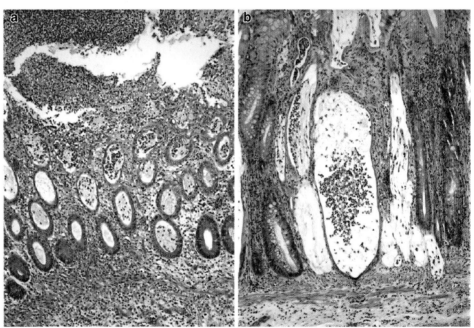

the edges of ulcers (Fig. 10.11). Small vessel vasculitis and microthrombi may be seen, as well as mucosal hemorrhage and crypt withering (Fig. 10.12). Pneumatosis may be present in severe cases (Fig. 10.13), particularly in the mucosa and submucosa. Gram-positive bacilli typical of *Clostridia* sometimes can be found in the necrotic exudate.

Differential diagnosis. The major entities in the differential diagnosis include ischemia and other infections that cause an ischemic-type injury, such as enterohemorrhagic *E.*

coli, which also commonly affects the right colon. The clinical history of consumption of large quantities of meat (especially pork or pork products) may be helpful, along with exclusion of other possible causes of ischemia. Cultures can help to distinguish *C. perfringens* from other bacteria; PCR and immunohistochemical assays exist but are not widely available.

Clostridium septicum. This organism was the first pathologic anaerobe identified by Pasteur in 1877, and it is a cause of gas gangrene in humans and animals. In the

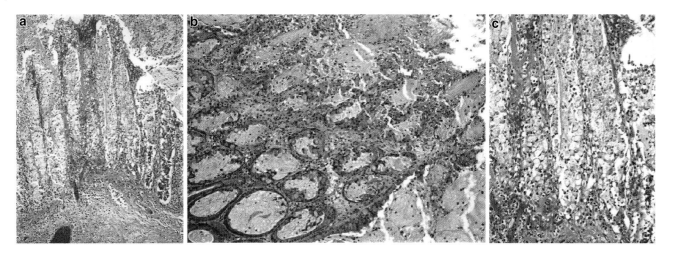

Fig. 10.7 The degenerated goblet cells may slough and spill into the lumens of degenerated crypts, known as "signet ring cell change (**a–c**)"

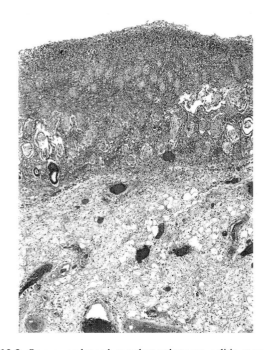

Fig. 10.8 Severe, prolonged pseudomembranous colitis may cause full-thickness mucosal necrosis, along with marked submucosal edema and inflammation

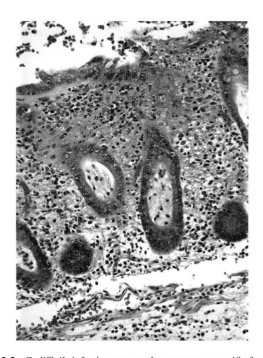

Fig. 10.9 *C. difficile* infection may produce very non-specific features, such as cryptitis, crypt abscesses, and a mucosal neutrophilic infiltrate, but lacks pseudomembranes

gastrointestinal tract, *C. septicum* is associated with neutropenic enterocolitis (typhlitis), a serious complication of both chemotherapy-related and primary neutropenia. Most patients have received chemotherapy within the previous month before the onset of colitis, and the incidence of typhlitis is believed to be related to the intensity of chemotherapy and degree of immunosuppression. *C. septicum* frequently has been reported as a causative agent, especially in adults; other commonly implicated bacteria include other *Clostridial* species, *E. coli*, *Pseudomonas*, and *Enterococci*.

An association with CMV also has been noted. *C. septicum* infection is also associated with malignancies (particularly adenocarcinoma) in the colon and distal ileum, and clostridial infection may be the first indication of such a tumor. It has been postulated that mucosal ulceration, perhaps secondary to injury from chemotherapy or an ulcerating malignancy, leads to invasion by these toxin-producing organisms, and that the pH and electrolyte balance in the distal ileum and right colon might be conducive to the organism's growth.

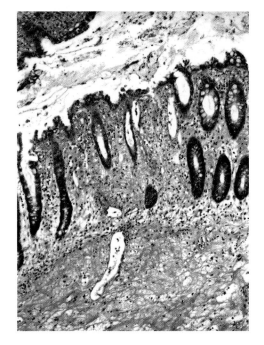

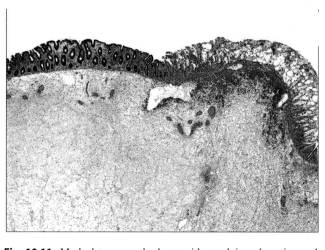

Fig. 10.11 Marked transmural edema with overlying ulceration and hemorrhage in a case of *C. perfringens* infection (courtesy Dr. Robert Odze)

Fig. 10.10 Crypt withering, mimicking ischemic colitis, can be seen in *C. difficile*-related pseudomembranous colitis

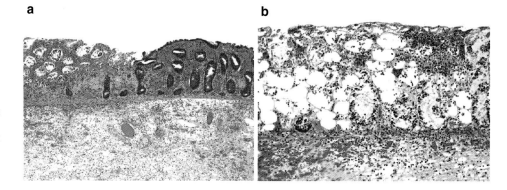

Fig. 10.12 Mucosal hemorrhage, necrosis, ulceration, and crypt withering are present in *C. perfringens* infection, with a heavy inflammatory infiltrate that extends into the submucosa (**a** and **b**, courtesy Dr. Robert Odze)

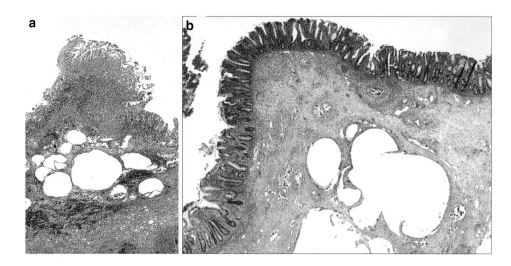

Fig. 10.13 Pneumatosis, particularly in the mucosa and submucosa, may be seen in *C. perfringens* infection. (**a**, courtesy Dr. David Owen; **b**, courtesy Dr. Robert Odze)

Fig. 10.14 Markedly dilated, dusky ileum and right colon in a case of chemotherapy-related neutropenic enterocolitis

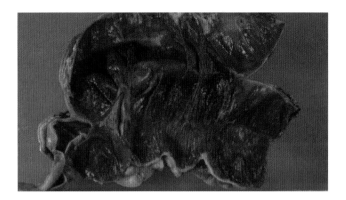

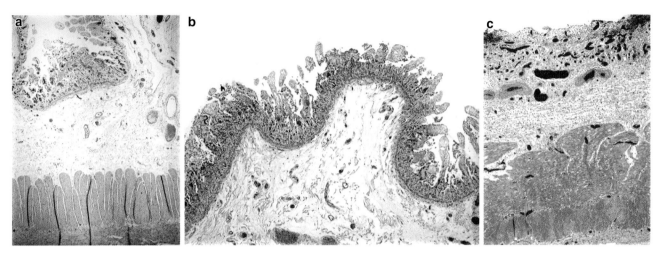

Fig. 10.15 Marked mural edema, with overlying mucosal hemorrhage and necrosis, are seen in the ileum (**a** and **b**) and right colon (**c**) of a patient with neutropenic enterocolitis

Patients usually present with the abrupt onset of gastrointestinal hemorrhage, fever, abdominal pain and distension, and diarrhea. The pain often initially localizes to the right lower quadrant, but quickly progresses to peritonitis, shock, and sepsis. Perforation is a well-described complication, and infection is often fatal.

Pathologic findings. The right colon (especially the cecum) is preferentially involved, although the ileum and other sites in the colon may be affected as well. Gross findings include diffuse dilatation, dusky discoloration, and marked edema of the bowel, with varying severity of ulceration and hemorrhage (Fig. 10.14). Exudates and pseudomembranes resembling *C. difficile* colitis are common.

Microscopically, changes range from mild hemorrhage to prominent submucosal edema (Fig. 10.15), ulceration (Fig. 10.16), marked hemorrhage, and necrosis, typically with a striking absence of inflammatory cells (Fig. 10.17). A few neutrophils may sometimes be found, however, despite peripheral neutropenia. Pneumatosis may occur rarely if the inciting organism is gas producing. Occasionally, organisms can be detected in the wall of the bowel or in mucosal or submucosal blood vessels, particularly on Gram stain.

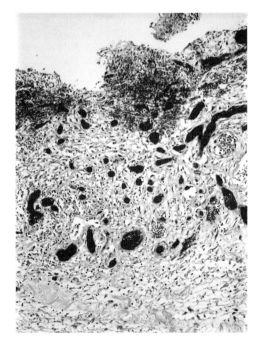

Fig. 10.16 Mucosal hemorrhage and ulceration in the right colon in a case of typhlitis

Fig. 10.17 Neutrophils are typically rare or absent (**a** and **b**). Only rare immature granulocytes are seen in the submucosal vessels (**c**)

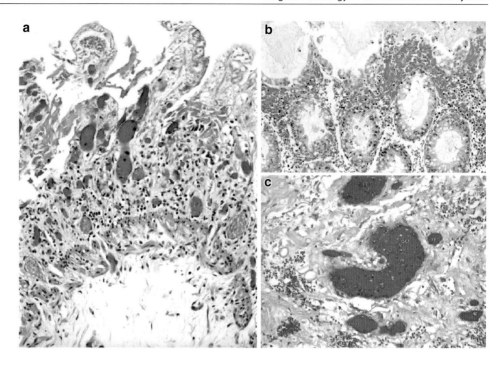

Differential diagnosis. The differential diagnosis includes ischemic colitis and pseudomembranous colitis. The appropriate clinical setting and dearth of inflammatory cells favor necrotizing enterocolitis. Isolation of the organism from blood cultures may be helpful in septic patients.

Selected References

General

1. Borriello SP. Clostridial disease of the gut. Clin Infect Dis 20(Suppl 2):S242–50, 1995.

C. difficile

2. Aslam S, Musher DM. An update on the diagnosis, treatment, and prevention of *Clostridium-difficile* associated disease. Gastroenterol Clin North Am 35(2):315–35, 2006.
3. Bartlett J. Narrative review: the new epidemic of *Clostridium difficile*-associated enteric disease. Ann Intern Med 145:758–64, 2006.
4. Beck A, McNeil C, Abdelsayed G, et al. *Salmonella* pseudomembranous colitis. Conn Med 71:339–42, 2007
5. Brown TA, Rajappannair L, Dalton AB, et al. Acute appendicitis in the setting of *Clostridium difficile* colitis: case report and review of the literature. Clin Gastroenterol Hepatol 5:969–71, 2007.
6. Coyne JD, Dervan PA, Haboubi NY. Involvement of the appendix in pseudomembranous colitis. J Clin Pathol 50:70–1, 1997.
7. Dignan CR, Greenson JK. Can ischemic colitis be differentiated from *C. difficile* colitis in biopsy specimens? Am J Surg Path 21:706–10, 1997.
8. Hogenauer C, Langner C, Beubler E, et al. *Klebsiella oxytoca* as a causative organism of antibiotic associated hemorrhagic colitis. N Eng J Med 355(23):418–26, 2006.
9. Issa M, Vijayapal A, Graham MB, et al. Impact of *C. difficile* on inflammatory bowel disease. Clin Gastroenterol Hepatol 5:345–51, 2007.
10. Kyne L, Farrell RJ, Kelly CP. *Clostridium difficile*. Gastroenterol Clin North Am 30(3):753–7, 2001.
11. Lundeen SJ, Otterson MF, Binion DG, et al. *Clostridium difficile* enteritis: an early postoperative complication in inflammatory bowel disease patients after colectomy. J Gastro Surg 11:138–42, 2007.
12. Mylonaki M, Langmead L, Pantes A, et al. Enteric infection in relapse of inflammatory bowel disease: importance of microbiological examination of stool. Eur J Gastroenterol Hepatol 16:775–8, 2004.
13. Nash SV, Bourgeault R, Sands M. Colonic disease associated with a positive assay for *Clostridium difficile* toxin: a retrospective study. J Clin Gastro 25:476–9, 1997.
14. Rodemann JF, Dubberke ER, Reske KA, et al. Incidence of *Clostridium difficile* infection in inflammatory bowel disease. Clin Gastroenterol Hepatol 5:339–44, 2007.
15. Schroeder MS. *Clostridium difficile*-associated diarrhea. Am Fam Physician 71:921–8, 2005.
16. Shen BO, Jiang ZD, Fazio VW, et al. *Clostridium difficile* infection in patients with ileal pouch-anal anastomosis. Clin Gastroenterol Hepatol 6:782–8, 2008.
17. Surawicz CM, McFarland LV. Pseudomembranous colitis: causes and cures. Digestion 60:91–100, 1999.

C. perfringens (welchii)

18. Arseculeratne SN, Panabokke RG, Navaratnam C. Pathogenesis of necrotizing enteritis with special reference to intestinal hypersensitivity reactions. Gut 21:265–78, 1980.

19. Gomez L, Martino R, Rolston KV. Necrotizing enterocolitis: spectrum of the disease and comparison of definite and possible cases. Clin Infect Dis 27:695–9, 1998.

20. Gui L, Subramony C, Fratkin J, Hughson MD. Fatal enteritis necroticans (pigbel) in a diabetic adult. Mod Pathol 15:66–70, 2002.

21. Lawrence G, Walker PD. Pathogenesis of enteritis necroticans in Papua New Guinea. Lancet 1(7951):125–6, 1976.

22. Lawrence G, Cooke R. Experimental pigbel: the production and pathology of necrotizing enteritis due to *Clostridium welchii* type C in the guinea-pig. Brit J Exp Pathol 61:261–71, 1980.

23. Matsuda T, Okada Y, Inagi E, et al. Enteritis necroticans "pigbel" in a Japanese diabetic adult. Pathol Int 57:622–6, 2007.

24. Murrell TGC, Roth L, Adelaide MB, et al. Pig-bel: enteritis necroticans. Lancet 1(7431):217–22, 1966.

25. Petrillo TM, Beck-Sague CM, Songer JG, et al. Enteritis necroticans (pig-bel) in a diabetic child. N Engl J Med 342(17):1250–3, 2000.

C. septicum

26. Al Otaibi A, Barker C, Anderson R, Sigalet DL. Neutropenic enterocolitis (typhlitis) after pediatric bone marrow transplant. J Pediatr Surg 37:770–2, 2002.

27. Anonymous. *Clostridium septicum* and neutropenic enterocolitis. Lancet 2(8559):608, 1987.

28. Kirchner JT. *Clostridium septicum* infection: beware of associated cancer. Postgrad Med 90:157–60, 1991.

29. Lev R, Sweeney KG. Neutropenic enterocolitis: two unusual cases with review of the literature. Arch Path Lab Med 117:524–7, 1993.

30. Rifkin GD. Neutropenic enterocolitis and *Clostridium septicum* infection in patients with agranulocytosis. Arch Intern Med 140(6):834–5, 1980.

Chapter 11

Spirochetes

Keywords Spirochete • Spirochetosis • Syphilis • *Treponema pallidum* • Proctitis • Gastritis

Gastrointestinal syphilis (Treponema pallidum). Gastrointestinal syphilis commonly involves the anorectum, although the stomach is perhaps the most frequently reported site of involvement in the GI tract. Homosexual males are at particularly high risk of infection, and many authorities believe that syphilis, particularly anorectal syphilis, is markedly underdiagnosed due to the variability of the clinical findings (syphilis is, after all, known as "the great mimicker") and a low index of suspicion.

Common presenting symptoms in syphilitic proctitis include pain, (often with defecation), tenesmus, constipation, bleeding, and anal discharge, which may be mucoid or bloody. Luetic gastritis commonly presents with upper gastrointestinal bleeding, which can occur early or late in the course of disease. Melena and coffee-ground emesis may be present, along with nausea, fever, malaise, anorexia, early satiety, and epigastric pain.

Pathologic features. Gross findings in primary anorectal syphilis include anal chancres (indurated, circular lesions up to 2 cm in diameter, single or multiple, with variable tenderness) and/or a mild proctitis. Signs of secondary syphilis typically present 6–8 weeks later and include masses, mucocutaneous rash, or condyloma lata (raised, moist, smooth warts that secrete mucus and are associated with itching and a foul odor). Inguinal adenopathy is typical. The gross features of primary and secondary infection sometimes coexist. The mass lesions of secondary syphilis may mimic malignancy, and surgical removal without a prior biopsy should be avoided.

Histologically, syphilitic proctitis features a dense plasmacytic cell infiltrate (Fig. 11.1). Cryptitis and crypt abscesses are often present as well, along with gland destruction and reactive epithelial changes (Fig. 11.2). Granulomas have been reported rarely, and occasionally prominent, proliferative capillary endothelial cells may be noted (proliferative endarterteriolitis) (Fig. 11.3). Syphilitic proctitis can be very

non-specific, showing only features of acute infectious-type colitis without a significant increase in plasma cells.

Macroscopic findings in gastric syphilis include antral erosions, ulcers, or features of gastritis including mucosal erythema and friability. The antrum is most commonly involved. The ulcers may have irregular, heaped up margins that mimic malignancy; sometimes the edges have an erythematous or violaceous color. Late in the course of disease, there may be marked fibrosis and rigidity of the gastric wall, with associated rugal hypertrophy and adenopathy that

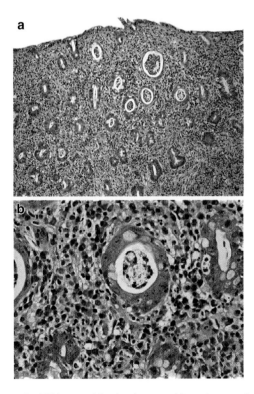

Fig. 11.1 Syphilitic proctitis showing cryptitis and crypt abscesses with a dense plasma cell infiltrate in the lamina propria, visible even at low power (**a**). Higher power view showing dense plasma cell infiltrate and damage to glandular epithelium (**b**). (Courtesy Dr. Amy Hudson)

L.W. Lamps, *Surgical Pathology of the Gastrointestinal System: Bacterial, Fungal, Viral, and Parasitic Infections*, DOI 10.1007/978-1-4419-0861-2_11, © Springer Science+Business Media, LLC 2009

Fig. 11.2 Diffuse cryptitis and numerous crypt abscesses, along with glandular epithelial damage, apoptotic epithelial cells, and reactive epithelial changes (**a**, courtesy Dr. Amy Hudson; **b**, courtesy Dr. Rodger C. Haggitt)

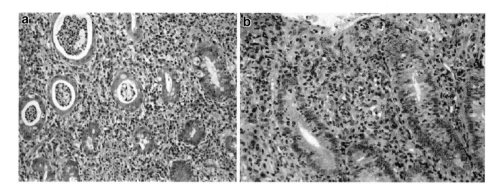

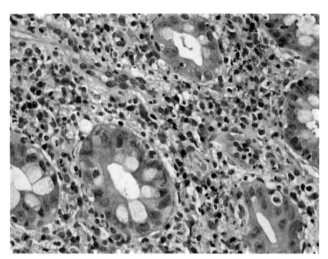

Fig. 11.3 Small vessel in the lamina propria infiltrated by plasma cells and neutrophils with markedly reactive endothelial cells. (Courtesy Dr. Amy Hudson)

Fig. 11.4 Warthin-Starry silver impregnation stain shows numerous tightly coiled spirochetes characteristic of *T. pallidum*. (Courtesy Dr. Rodger Haggitt)

mimic linitis plastica adenocarcinoma or lymphoma both clinically and radiographically.

Syphilitic gastritis also features a dense plasmacytic infiltrate, which may extend into the submucosa. The glands may be infiltrated by neutrophils with crypt abscesses, or may be relatively spared. Granulomas have been reported, and proliferative endarterteriolitis is variably present. Fibrosis may be very prominent as the disease progresses.

Differential diagnosis. The gross differential diagnosis of chancre includes anal fissures, fistulas, or traumatic lesions. Syphilitic proctitis also can mimic many other sexually transmitted proctocolitides on physical examination. In general, condyloma acuminata are more dry and keratinized than condyloma lata. As mentioned above, both anorectal and gastric syphilis can mimic malignancy.

The histologic differential diagnosis primarily includes other infectious processes, including *Helicobacter pylori* infection in the stomach. If the plasma cell infiltrate is very prominent and monomorphic, and effaces the normal architecture, a hematopoietic neoplasm with plasmacytic differen-

tiation should also be considered. *T. pallidum* stains with silver impregnation stains such as Warthin–Starry (Fig. 11.4), Steiner, and Dieterle stains, and immunohistochemistry is also available. Darkfield examination of anorectal discharge may show organisms, although care must be taken in interpretation since spirochetes are also present in the normal gut flora as well as in intestinal spirochetosis. Serologic studies (RPR, VDRL, and FTA-ABS) are extremely helpful in confirming the diagnosis.

Intestinal spirochetosis . This condition is characterized by the presence of spirochetal microorganisms on the luminal surface of the large bowel mucosa. The prevalence of spirochetosis ranges from 2 to 16% in Western nations, but is significantly higher in developing countries and homosexual and HIV-infected patients, where prevalence is reportedly as high as 50% based on both biopsy findings and stool culture. Spirochetosis has been described in association with a wide variety of conditions including diverticular disease, chronic idiopathic inflammatory bowel disease, hyperplastic polyps, and adenomatous polyps, and it also has been found in children. Spirochetosis represents infection by a heterogeneous group of related organisms, most importantly *Brachyspira aalborgi* and *Brachyspira pilosicoli*, which are genetically unrelated to *T. pallidum*. Patients with spirochetosis may harbor one or both of these species.

The clinical significance of spirochetosis in humans remains controversial. Patients with spirochetosis are often asymptomatic, but may have symptoms such as diarrhea, which can be chronic and watery, abdominal pain, lower GI bleeding, signs and symptoms of appendicitis, and anorectal pain and discharge. It is not clear, however, that spirochetosis actually causes these symptoms, and many immunocompromised patients have other concomitant infections (especially gonorrhea) that complicate the clinical picture. Many symptomatic patients do appear to respond to antimicrobial therapy, however, and ultrastructural studies have suggested that the spirochetes cause epithelial damage at the ultrastructural level despite the usual lack of concomitant inflammation. Some authorities believe that *B. pilosicoli* is a true opportunistic pathogen, as it has been isolated from the blood of seriously ill patients, whereas *B. aalborgi* (the more commonly detected species) is a commensal. This remains controversial, however.

Pathologic findings. Any level of the colon may be involved, including the appendix. Typically, endoscopic abnormalities are either mild (such as mucosal edema or erythema) or completely absent. Histologically, spirochetosis produces a fuzzy, "fringed" 2–3-μm thick blue line at the luminal border of the colonic mucosa on routine H&E sections (Fig. 11.5). The presence of organisms can be patchy and very focal, and multiple sites may be involved. Most cases show no associated inflammatory infiltrate, although occasionally an associated cryptitis is present (Fig. 11.6). In general, it is believed that the organisms do not invade, although there are rare reports of minimal invasion when many organisms are present.

The spirochetes stain intensely with Warthin–Starry or similar silver impregnation stains (Fig. 11.7), which also highlight their spirillar morphology (Fig. 11.8). They also stain with Alcian blue (pH 2.5) and PAS stains, but do not stain distinctly with tissue Gram stain (Fig. 11.9). Electron microscopy has been used in the past to identify the organisms as well (Fig. 11.10). Currently there is an excellent immunohistochemical stain available, and many authorities argue that the immunostain is superior as the quality of silver impregnation stains vary widely depending on the freshness

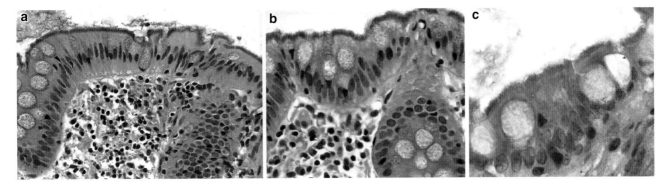

Fig. 11.5 The fuzzy, fringed-like 2–3-μm thick blue line at the luminal border of the colonic mucosa characteristic of intestinal spirochetosis (**a–c**)

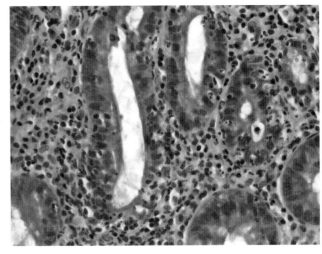

Fig. 11.6 Cryptitis underlying spirochetosis in the rectum

Fig. 11.7 Spirochetes stain intensely with silver impregnation stains. The organisms involve the surface epithelium and may involve the superficial crypt epithelium (**a** and **b**). The surface openings of goblet cells are spared

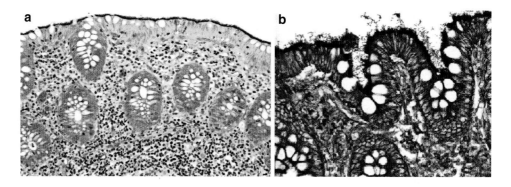

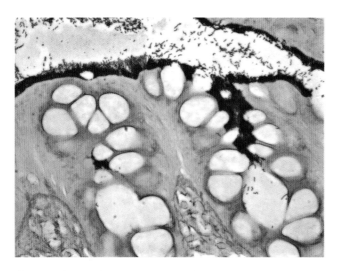

Fig. 11.8 A Warthin–Starry stain highlights the spirillar morphology of the spirochetes

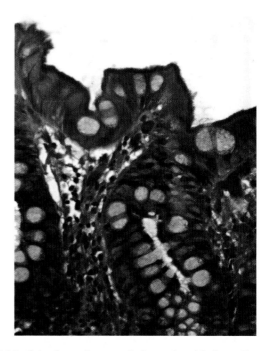

Fig. 11.9 Spirochetes do not stain intensely with tissue Gram stain (Twort tissue Gram stain)

Fig. 11.10 Scanning (**a**) and transmission (**b**) electron micrographs showing the spirillar organisms at the surface of the large bowel mucosa. (Courtesy Drs. George F. Gray, Jr., and Dr. Margie Scott)

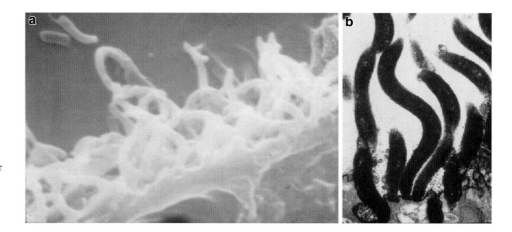

of the reagents and the ability of the technician. PCR and in situ hybridization assays also exist for identification of the organisms.

Differential diagnosis. The differential diagnosis primarily consists of a prominent glycocalyx, which does not stain with silver impregnation stains or immunohistochemistry directed against the bacteria. Some type of special stain or immunostain is recommended in the evaluation of cases where spirochetosis is suspected, both to avoid underdiagnosis and to avoid mistaking a prominent glycocalyx for organisms. Occasionally, enteroadherent *Escherichia coli* can induce a similar histologic appearance, but *E. coli* are Gram negative and lack spirillar morphology.

Selected References

Gastrointestinal Syphilis

1. Akdamar K, Martin RJ, Ichinose H. Syphilitic proctitis. Dig Dis 22:701–4, 1977.
2. Baker RW, Peppercorn MA. Gastrointestinal ailments of homosexual men. Medicine 61:390–405, 1982.
3. Butz WC, Watts JC, Rosales-Quintana S, Hicklin MD. Erosive gastritis as a manifestation of secondary syphilis. Am J Clin Pathol 63:895–900, 1975.
4. Fyfe B, Poppiti RJ, Lubin J, Robinson M. Gastric syphilis: primary diagnosis by gastric biopsy. Arch Pathol Lab Med 117:820–23, 1993.
5. Kasmin F, Reddy S, Mathur-Wagh U, et al. Syphilitic gastritis in an HIV-infected individual. Am J Gastroenterol 87:1820–2, 1992.
6. Lichtenstein JE. Case: syphilitic gastritis. Gastrointest Radiol 6:371–4, 1981.
7. Long BW, Johnston JH, Wetzel JH, et al. Gastric syphilis: endoscopic and histological features mimicking lymphoma. Am J Gastroenterol 90:1504–7, 1995.
8. Reisman TN, Leverett FL, Hudson JR, Kaiser MH. Syphilitic gastropathy. Am J Dig Dis 20:588–93, 1975.
9. Wexner SD. Sexually transmitted diseases of the colon, rectum, and anus. Dis Col Rect 33:1048–59, 1990.

Intestinal Spirochetosis

10. Esteve M, Salas A, Fernandez-Banares F, et al. Intestinal spirochetosis and chronic watery diarrhea: clinical and histological response to treatment and long term follow up. J Gastroenterol Hepatol 21:1326–33, 2006.
11. Henrik-Nielsen R, Lundbeck FA, Teglbjaerg PS, et al. Intestinal spirochesosis of the vermiform appendix. Gastroenterol 88:971–7, 1985.
12. Korner M, Gebbers J-O. Clinical significance of human intestinal spirochetosis-a morphological approach. Infection 31:341–9, 2003.
13. Koteish A, Kannangai R, Abraham S, Torbenson M. Colonic spirochetosis in children and adults. Am J Clin Pathol 120:828–32, 2003.
14. Rotterdam H. Intestinal spirochetosis. In Connor DH, Chandler FW et al. (eds): Pathology of Infectious Diseases, Stamford, CT: Appleton and Lange, 1997, pp. 583–9.
15. Surawicz CM. Intestinal spirochetosis in homosexual men. Am J Med 82:587–92, 1988.
16. Tanahashi J, Daa T, Gamachi A, et al. Human intestinal spirochetosis in Japan; its incidence, clinicopathologic features, and genotypic identification. Mod Pathol 21:76–84, 2008.
17. Uhlemann ER, Fenoglio-Preiser C. Intestinal spirochetosis (letter). Am J Surg Pathol 29:982, 2005.
18. Weisheit B, Bethke B, Stolte M. Human intestinal spirochetosis: analysis of the symptoms of 209 patients. Scand J Gastroenterol 42:1422–7, 2007.

Chapter 12

Whipple's Disease

Keywords Whipple's disease • Macrophage • PAS • *Tropheryma whipplelii* • Diarrhea • Malabsorption

Whipple's disease is named after Dr. George H. Whipple, who first described it in 1907. Eighty-four years after Whipple initially reported the disease, the actinobacterium named *Tropheryma whippelii,* and also known as the Whipple's bacillus, was identified. Whipple's disease is now considered to be a chronic, insidious multisystem infection.

The clinical presentation is extremely variable, because the disease can affect virtually any organ system. Whipple's disease typically presents in middle-aged Caucasian patients, with a striking male to female predominance of 8:1. Typical signs and symptoms include low-grade fever, chronic weight loss, arthritis, malabsorption, and lymphadenopathy. Many patients also have significant neuropsychiatric manifestations. The polyarthritis of Whipple's disease is often the first manifestation and may precede gastrointestinal symptoms by years. Immunosuppressive therapy may significantly exacerbate both the intestinal and systemic manifestations of the disease.

Pathologic features. The small bowel is most often affected, although esophageal, gastric, colonic, and appendiceal involvement have been described rarely. Endoscopically, mucosal folds are thickened and coated with yellow–white plaques, often with surrounding erythema, friability, and mucosal erosion. Endoscopy may be normal, however.

Histologically, the characteristic lesion is massive infiltration of the lamina propria and submucosa by foamy macrophages that are packed with bacilli (Fig. 12.1), which are strongly PAS-positive (Fig. 12.2). The infiltrate often blunts and distends villi (Figs. 12.2 and 12.3). Involvement may be diffuse or patchy. There is usually no associated mononuclear inflammatory infiltrate, but varying numbers of neutrophils may be present (Fig. 12.4). The lamina propria often contains small foci of fat (Figs. 12.2 and 12.5), and overlying vacuolization of enterocytes may occur as well (Fig. 12.6). Epithelioid granulomas are present in a minority of cases, with or without multinucleated giant cells.

PAS-positive macrophages may persist in biopsies for years, even in patients who have been treated with long-term antibiotic therapy.

Mesenteric adenopathy is common in Whipple's disease, and lymph node biopsy may be useful in diagnosis. Involved lymph nodes commonly show aggregates of foamy macrophages containing PAS-positive bacilli (Fig. 12.7), as well as small foci of fat, similar to the morphologic findings in the bowel. In addition, non-caseating granulomas may be seen that are similar to sarcoidosis (Fig. 12.8);

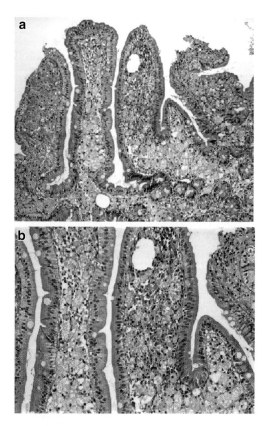

Fig. 12.1 The lamina propria is packed with an infiltrate of foamy macrophages. Rare fat vacuoles are also present (**a**). Higher power view shows the lamina propria distended by foamy macrophages, along with fat vacuoles and a patchy neutrophilic infiltrate (**b**)

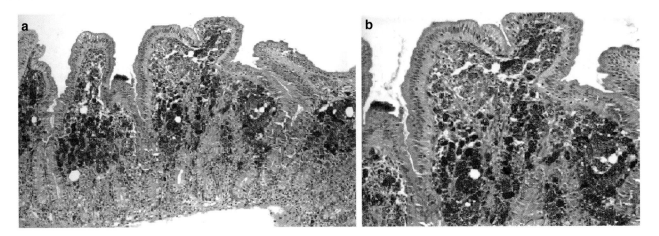

Fig. 12.2 The macrophages are intensely PAS positive (**a** and **b**)

PAS-positive bacilli may or may not be present within the granulomas.

Differential diagnosis. The differential diagnosis predominantly includes other infectious processes, most importantly MAI. However, other intracellular organisms such as *Histoplasma* and *Rhodococcus* may simulate Whipple's disease rarely. MAI are acid-fast, whereas the Whipple's bacillus is not. *Histoplasma* may produce a similar histiocytic infiltrate, and are GMS as well as PAS positive, but the morphology (small yeast with budding at the more pointed pole) easily distinguishes histoplasmosis from Whipple's disease. *Rhodococcus*, which is exceedingly rare, stains with PAS and Gram stains, and may be partially acid-fast as well. In cases of Whipple's disease with granulomatous features, granulomatous infections and sarcoidosis also enter the differential diagnosis. The most valuable tool for confirming the diagnosis of Whipple's disease is the PCR assay, which can be performed from the paraffin block. The bacillus also can be identified by electron microscopy (Fig. 12.9).

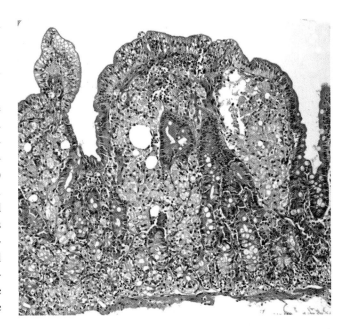

Fig. 12.3 The foamy macrophage infiltrate causes distension and blunting of small bowel villi

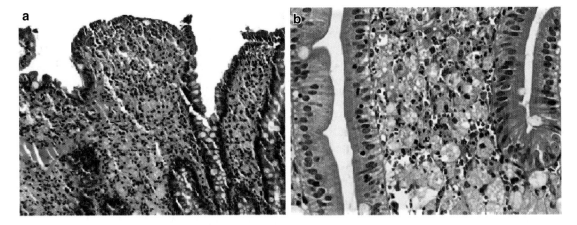

Fig. 12.4 Although there is no significant associated mononuclear cell infiltrate, a patchy neutrophilic infiltrate is common in Whipple's disease

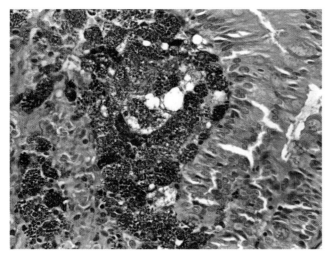

Fig. 12.5 Fat vacuoles in the lamina propria are a common feature of Whipple's disease

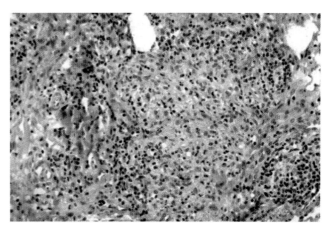

Fig. 12.8 Granulomas may be present in Whipple's disease, in both lymph nodes and bowel. (Courtesy Dr. George F. Gray, Jr)

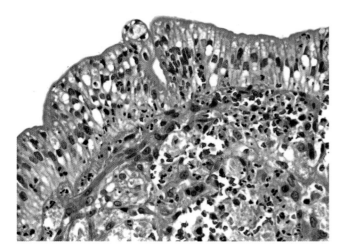

Fig. 12.6 The surface epithelium is often vacuolated. Note associated neutrophilic infiltrate

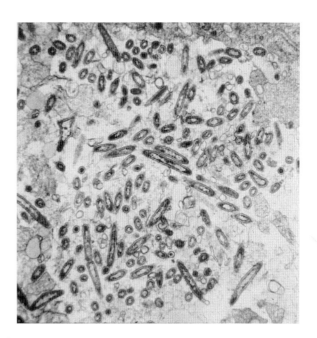

Fig. 12.9 Transmission electron micrograph of the Whipple's bacillus. (Courtesy Dr. George F. Gray, Jr)

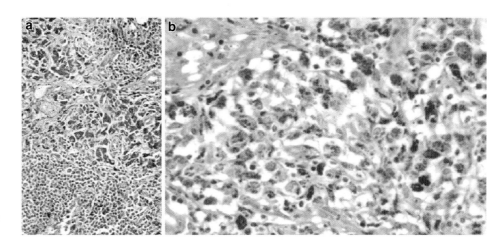

Fig. 12.7 Mesenteric lymph node in Whipple's disease, containing an infiltrate of strongly PAS-positive macrophages (**a** and **b**). (Courtesy Dr. George F. Gray, Jr)

Selected References

1. Babaryka I, Thorn L, Langer E, Epithelioid cell granulomata in the mucosa of the small intestine in Whipple's disease. Virch Arch A 382:227–35, 1979.
2. Bai JC, Mazure RM, Vazquez H, et al. Whipple's disease. Clin Gastroenterol Hepatol 2:849–60, 2004.
3. Cho C, Linscheer WG, Hirschkorn MA, Ashutosh K. Sarcoidlike granulomas as an early manifestation of Whipple's disease. Gastroenterol 87:941–7, 1984.
4. Dobbins WO. Whipple's Disease. Springfield, IL: Charles C. Thomas, 1987.
5. Dutly F, Altwegg M. Whipple's disease and "Tropheryma whippelii." Clin Microbiol Rev 14:561–83, 2001.
6. Ectors NL, Geboes KJ, De Vos RM, et al. Whipple's disease: a histological, immunocytochemical, and electron microscopic study of the small intestinal epithelium. J Pathol 172:73–9, 1994.
7. Geboes K, Ectors N, Heidbuchel H, et al. Whipple's disease: endoscopic aspects before and after therapy. Gastrointest Endosc 36:247–52, 1990.
8. Gras E, Matias-Guiu X, Garcia A, et al. PCR analysis in the pathological diagnosis of Whipple's disease: emphasis on extraintestinal involvement or atypical morphologic features. J Pathol 188:318–21, 1999.
9. Hamrock D, Azmi F, O'Donnell E, et al. Infection by *Rhodococcus equi* in a patient with AIDS: histological appearance mimicking Whipple's disease and *MAI* infection. J Clin Pathol 52: 68–71, 1999.
10. Mahnel R, Kalt A, Ring S, et al. Immunosuppressive therapy in Whipple's disease patients is associated with the appearance of gastrointestinal manifestations. Am J Gastroenterol 100:1167–73, 2005.
11. Weizsackher Fv, Blum HE. Impact of molecular biology in gastroenterology. Digestion 54:125–9, 1993.
12. Wilcox GM, Tronic BS, Schecter DJ, et al. Periodic acid-Schiff-negative granulomatous lymphadenopathy in patient with Whipple's disease. Am J Med 83:165–70, 1987.

Chapter 13

Miscellaneous Bacterial Infections

Keywords Esophagitis • Actinomyces • Actinomycosis • *Brucella* sp. • Brucellosis • Granuloma • *Rhodococcus equi* • Macrophage • Gram stain • *Rickettsia* sp. • Rocky mountain spotted fever • Arthropod • *Erlichia* sp. • Erlichiosis • Malakoplakia • Michaelis–Gutmann body • Vasculitis • *Bartonella* sp. • Lymphogranuloma venereum • *Neisseria gonorrhea* • Proctitis

Bacterial esophagitis. Bacterial esophagitis is rare and usually found in immunocompromised or debilitated patients, including those with AIDS, neutropenia, hematologic malignancies, and bone marrow or solid organ transplants. Implicated bacteria include *Staphylococcus aureus, Lactobacillus acidophilus*, and *Klebsiella pneumoniae*. By definition, the bacteria should invade the mucosa or deeper layers of the esophageal wall, and there should be no evidence of fungal or viral infection, neoplasia, or history of previous esophageal surgery.

Endoscopic findings include ulceration, pseudomembrane formation, and hemorrhage. Histologic findings include acute inflammation, ulceration, and necrosis of the mucosa, and clusters of bacteria are often visible on routine H&E staining (Fig. 13.1). Gram stain demonstrates bacteria within the wall of the esophagus (Fig. 13.2). The differential diagnosis includes more common causes of infectious esophagitis, particularly *Candida* and viral infections. Once these have been excluded, it is important to remember that bacterial esophagitis is a rare but important cause of infectious esophagitis in debilitated or immunocompromised patients.

Actinomycosis (Actinomyces israelii). This filamentous anaerobic Gram-positive bacterium is a normal inhabitant of the oral cavity and upper GI tract. It occasionally produces a chronic, non-opportunistic gastrointestinal infection, often after trauma or other disruption of normal mucosa barriers, and thus risk factors include previous abdominal surgery, neoplasia, and diverticular disease. A specific portal of entry for the organism is seldom identified, however. Symptoms include fever, weight loss, abdominal pain, and, occasionally, a palpable mass. Perianal fistulas and chronic (often granulomatous) appendicitis have been described in association with

actinomycosis. Complications include bowel obstruction and perforation, which may further mimic a malignancy.

Pathologic features. Most commonly, only a single intra-abdominal organ is affected; the appendix, terminal ileum, right colon, and stomach are preferentially involved, although infection may occur at any level of the GI tract. Grossly, inflammation may produce a large, solitary mass (Fig. 13.3), either with or without mucosal ulceration. The inflammatory process often infiltrates surrounding structures, mimicking malignancy, and may produce abscesses or sinus tracts.

Transmural inflammation, lymphoid hyperplasia, and marked fibrosis are common histologic features (Fig. 13.4), along with mucosal ulceration and architectural distortion (Fig. 13.5). The inflammatory reaction is often neutrophilic, with occasional abscess formation. Palisading histiocytes and giant cells, as well as frank granulomas, are often present as well (Fig. 13.6). The organism typically produces actinomycotic ("sulfur") granules, consisting of irregular round clusters of bacteria rimmed by eosinophilic, club-like projections of proteinaceous material (Splendore-Hoeppli material) (Fig. 13.7). Gram stain reveals the filamentous, Gram-positive organisms (Fig. 13.8). Actinomyces may stain with GMS and Warthin-Starry as well.

Commensal actinomyces may be present at the lumenal surface, and these do not necessarily imply invasive infection, particularly if there is no inflammatory response.

Invasive actinomycosis requires several weeks of intravenous antibiotic therapy; therefore, a definite diagnosis of invasive actinomycosis (rather than the presence of commensals) is important, and requires demonstration of the organisms within the wall of the bowel with an associated inflammatory response. This may require multiple levels of lesional tissue sections.

Differential diagnosis. The macroscopic differential diagnosis includes peptic ulcer (in the stomach), lymphoma, and carcinoma. The histologic differential primarily includes other infectious processes, particularly *Nocardia*. *Nocardia* are partially acid-fast and do not form the typical sulfur granules of actinomycosis; however, cultures may be required to

L.W. Lamps, *Surgical Pathology of the Gastrointestinal System: Bacterial, Fungal, Viral, and Parasitic Infections*,
DOI 10.1007/978-1-4419-0861-2_13, © Springer Science+Business Media, LLC 2009

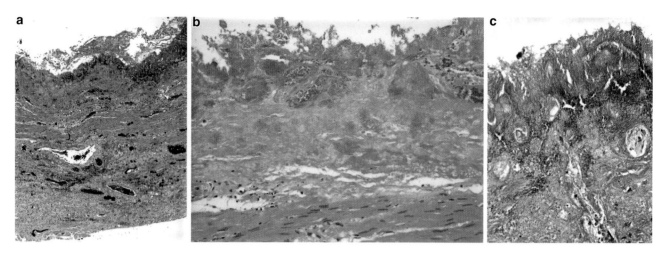

Fig. 13.1 Deep ulceration and mucosal necrosis characterize bacterial esophagitis; clusters of bacteria are visible at the surface and within the wall of the esophagus (**a–c**)

Fig. 13.2 Twort Gram stain highlights clusters of bacteria within the esophageal wall

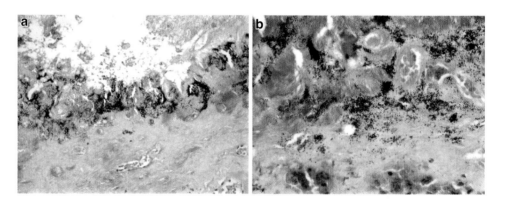

distinguish these two filamentous organisms. Even though actinomyces are GMS positive, they have a more slender morphology than fungi, and do not bud or produce hyphae. Care should be taken not to confuse actinomycosis with other bacteria that form clusters and chains but are not truly fila-

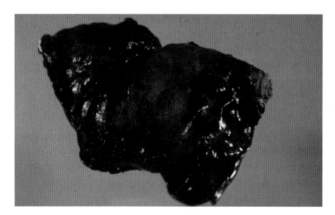

Fig. 13.3 Appendiceal actinomycosis. The proximal appendiceal margin is on the right; the remainder of the organ is encased in a thick fibrotic mass that mimicked malignancy (Courtesy Dr. George F. Gray)

mentous, such as *Pseudomonas* and *Escherichia coli*. Occasionally, the transmural inflammation, fibrosis, and granulomatous inflammation produced by actinomycotic infection may mimic Crohn's disease.

Brucellosis. Worldwide, brucellosis is a widespread and economically important zoonotic bacterial disease, particularly in developing countries. Human infections are linked to methods of animal husbandry, hygiene, and food preparation, particularly lack of pasteurization of dairy products. Although human *Brucella* infections are common, and the GI tract is believed to be an important portal of entry for these bacteria, reports of gastrointestinal manifestations are quite rare. Many patients recover spontaneously, but these small, Gram-negative bacteria are capable of surviving and multiplying for extended periods of time within macrophages, leading to chronic or relapsing infections in some patients.

Brucellosis is a systemic infection with a wide range of presentations. Symptomatic patients usually have fever, chills, arthralgias, myalgais, malaise, and night sweats. Approximately 30–80% of patients have gastrointestinal complaints, including anorexia, abdominal pain, diarrhea, vomiting, and GI bleeding.

Fig. 13.4 Actinomycosis of the right colon, with transmural inflammation and dense mural fibrosis (**a** and **b**, courtesy Dr. Dianne Johnson)

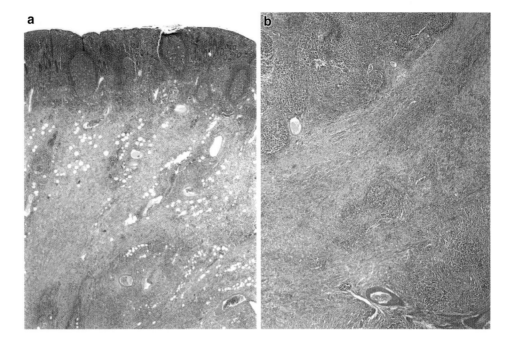

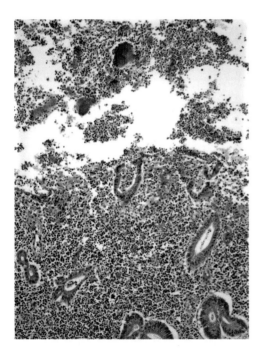

Fig. 13.5 Mucosal ulceration and underlying architectural distortion in a case of appendiceal actinomycosis

Pathologic features. The ileum and right colon are preferentially involved, most likely due to the abundant lymphoid tissue, but any level of the alimentary tract may be affected. Endoscopic findings include mild mucosal hyperemia and focal ulcerations, often overlying Peyer's patches and similar to typhoid fever. Endoscopy may be unremarkable, however. Histologic findings have not been well described, and appear to consist of non-specific mucosal inflammatory changes (acute infectious-type colitis) without granulomas. Serologic studies are valuable aids to diagnosis; as the organism is difficult to recover, microbiological culture is often not helpful.

Rhodacoccus equi. These Gram-positive coccobacilli, formerly known as *Corynebacterium equi*, are well known to infect animals. Human infection is rare, and usually affects immunocompromised persons. Patients often have exposure to horses. The lung is the most common site of infection, but extrapulmonary foci of infection have been well documented, either with or without concomitant pulmonary disease. Gastrointestinal infection presents as chronic (often bloody) diarrhea and is generally a manifestation of systemic involvement.

Pathologic features. R. equi produces inflammatory polyps, sometimes with associated mesenteric adenitis. Histologically, polyps consist of organism-laden macrophages (Fig. 13.9) that pack the mucosa and submucosa, often with an associated granulomatous response. The histiocytes have eosinophilic, granular cytoplasm. A spindled histiocytic response is rarely seen, and scattered microabscesses are common. Organisms stain with PAS, GMS, and Gram stains (Fig. 13.10), and may be partially acid-fast. The histologic features may mimic infection with MAI or Whipple disease. *Rhodococcus* is more granular on PAS than the bacilli of MAI, however, and is negative with routine Ziehl–Neelsen stain. In addition, *R. equi* is Gram positive, whereas the Whipple bacillus is Gram negative. Microbiological culture may be a helpful aid to diagnosis.

Rickettsial disease. Authorities on rickettsial illnesses have frequently noted that both gastrointestinal symptoms

Fig. 13.6 Scattered giant cells (**a**) and epithelioid granulomas (**b**) are often present within the inflammatory infiltrate in actinomycosis

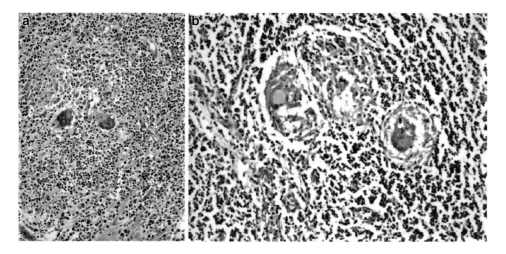

Fig. 13.7 Actinomycotic ("sulfur") granules, consisting of clusters of bacteria (**a**), sometimes associated with proteinaceous Splendore-Hoeppli material (**b**) and neutrophilic inflammation (**c**)

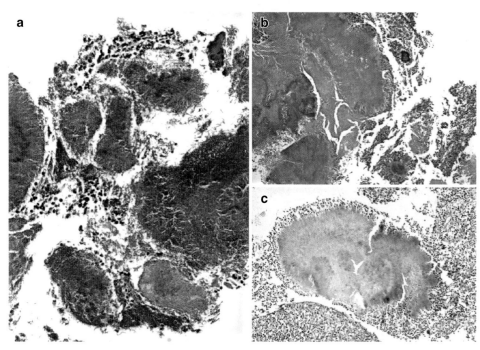

Fig. 13.8 Gram stain reveals the Gram-positive, filamentous organisms (**a** and **b**)

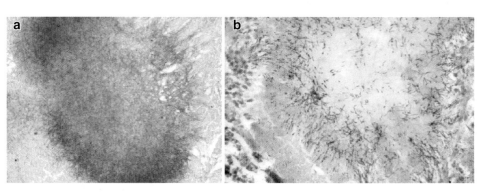

and lesions are common in the rickettsial diseases, yet receive surprisingly little attention. *Rickettsiae* are obligate intracellular bacteria that are associated with an arthropod host. This group of diseases includes Rocky Mountain spot- ted fever (*R. rickettsii*) scrub typhus (*R. tsutsugamushi*), and murine typhus (*R. typhi*). All diseases caused by these organisms have similar tissue targets (blood vessels), par- ticularly those of the skin, lung, brain, and gastrointestinal tract. Rickettsial disease begins when bacteria, or feces left by lice or fleas, are inoculated into the skin by an arthropod bite or by scratching. During the incubation period, the organisms spread via the blood stream and infect endothelial cells.

Patients generally initially present with non-specific generalized symptoms including fever, headache, rash, myalgias, and arthralgias. Gastrointestinal symptoms are very common, and include abdominal pain, nausea, vomiting, diarrhea, and GI bleeding. Gastrointestinal symptoms may precede the development of a rash in many patients. More severe illness is associated with older age and delayed diagnosis and therapy.

Pathologic features. Any level of the GI tract may be involved. Endoscopic findings include mucosal hyperemia, petechiae, purpura, hemorrhage, and erosions, along with active bleeding in some cases. The pathologic lesions are a result of vascular infection and injury to the endothelium and to the vascular smooth muscle in cases of RMSF. The vascular lesions may be present in the mucosa, submucosa, or muscularis propria. Early changes include perivascular edema and prominent endothelial cells. Later alterations include a perivascular mononuclear cell infiltrate (Fig. 13.11) and occasional non-occlusive thrombi (Fig. 13.12), with associated hemorrhage. Scattered neutrophils are variably present. If the course of infection is fulminant and rapidly fatal, there may be little if any inflammatory response. These small organisms are difficult to detect with Giemsa or tissue Gram stains, and thus immunohistochemical (Fig. 13.13) or immunofluorescence stains (Fig. 13.14) may be required. Serologic and molecular studies also may aid in diagnosis.

Differential diagnosis. The differential diagnosis is virtually limitless, as patients present with non-specific sys-

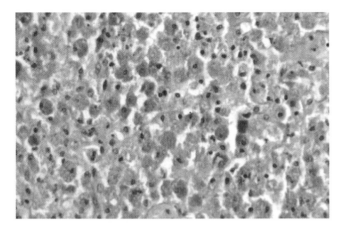

Fig. 13.9 *Rhodococcus equi* infection, featuring a dense histiocytic infiltrate (courtesy Dr. Margie Scott)

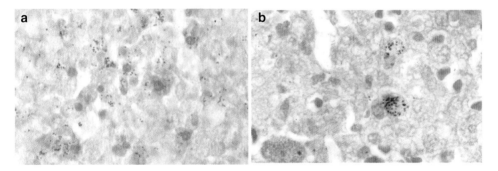

Fig. 13.10 Gram stains highlight the Gram-positive, intracellular coccobacilli (**a** and **b**, courtesy of Dr. Margie Scott)

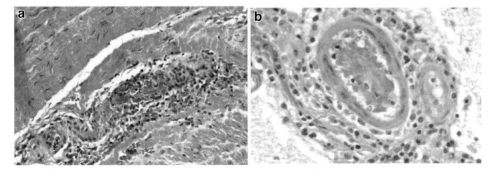

Fig. 13.11 Mononuclear cell infiltrate surrounding a vessel in the lamina propria of the stomach (**a**, courtesy Dr. David Walker). An early fibrin thrombus is present within a small vessel surrounded by a mononuclear cell infiltrate (**b**, courtesy Dr. Margie Scott)

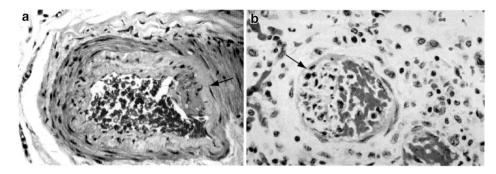

Fig. 13.12 Eccentric, non-occlusive thrombi are present within small vessels, with a surrounding mononuclear cell infiltrate and hemorrhage (**a**, courtesy Dr. David Walker; **b**, courtesy Dr. Margie Scott)

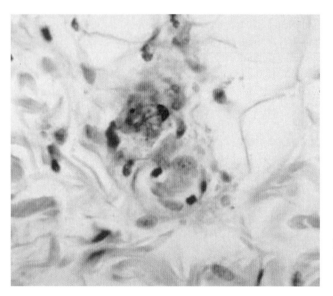

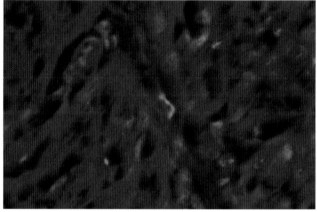

Fig. 13.14 Immunofluorescence staining of the organism in RMSF (courtesy Dr. Margie Scott)

Fig. 13.13 An immunohistochemical stain highlights the organisms in RMSF (courtesy Dr. Margie Scott)

temic symptoms. The histologic differential diagnosis is also extremely large, since many infectious and non-infectious entities cause vasculitis. It is important to include the rickettsial illnesses in the differential diagnosis of severe systemic febrile illnesses with prominent GI symptoms, however, because a delay in therapy may be fatal.

Ehrlichiosis. Ehrlichia are small, Gram-negative, pleomorphic intracellular bacteria that are transmitted by arthropod bites. Ehrlichiosis is most common in the southeastern, south central, and mid-Atlantic United States. They infect leukocytes, and the type of leukocyte infected is an important criterion in the differentiation of species and the classification of disease. *Ehrlichia sennetsu, E. chaffeensis, E. equi,* and *E. phagocytophila* are believed to be the species that cause human disease. Ehrlichiosis typically presents with the abrupt onset of fever, headache, myalgia, and shaking chills; GI symptoms are common and include nausea, vomiting, diarrhea, abdominal pain, and anorexia. The labo-

ratory hallmarks of erlichiosis include leukopenia, thrombocytopenia, and elevated transaminases. The pathologic features of gastrointestinal ehrlichiosis in humans have not been well studied or described. Unlike many of the rickettsial illnesses, there is no vasculitis. Helpful diagnostic tests include serologic studies, examination of blood smears or buffy coat preparations for morulae (the characteristic inclusions within leukocytes), and molecular assays.

Malakoplakia. Malakoplakia is an unusual inflammatory disorder originally believed to be restricted to the urinary tract, but subsequently described in almost all organs of the body. Although the exact pathogenesis remains unknown, it is believed to be secondary to a defect in the ability of the macrophage to process intracellular bacteria. It can affect any portion of the gastrointestinal tract, and the majority of cases are associated with colorectal adenocarcinoma or an immunocompromising condition. Mesenteric lymph nodes may also be involved. Numerous bacteria have been associated with gastrointestinal malakoplakia, including *E. coli, Klebsiella, Yersinia, R. equi,* and mycobacterial organisms.

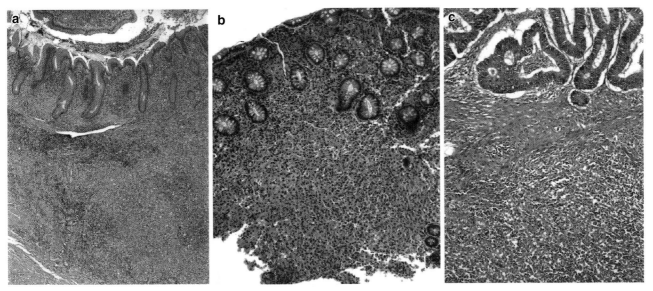

Fig. 13.15 Gastrointestinal malakoplakia. A dense histiocytic infiltrate within the wall of the appendix (**a**, courtesy Dr. Elizabeth Montgomery), a colon biopsy with the infiltrate in the lamina propria (**b**, courtesy Dr. Elizabeth Montgomery), and a colon resection specimen also containing adenocarcinoma of the colon (**c**)

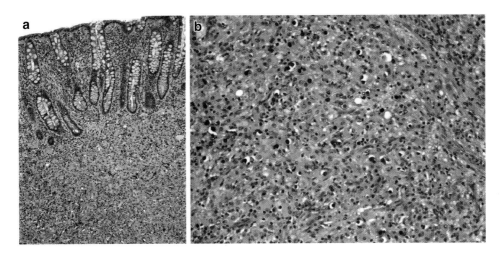

Fig. 13.16 The histiocytic infiltrate contains numerous histiocytes with eosinophilic cytoplasm, and admixed plasma cells, lymphocytes, and granulocytes (**a** and **b**, courtesy Dr. Joel Greenson)

Pathologic features. Grossly, the lesions consist of soft, yellow plaques (hence the name from Greek: malakos, meaning soft and plakos, meaning plaque). Histologically, there is a dense histiocytic infiltrate (Fig. 13.15) featuring histiocytes with eosinophilic cytoplasm, admixed with numerous plasma cells, lymphocytes, and scattered granulocytes (Fig. 13.16). The macrophages contain characteristic Michaelis–Gutmann bodies (Fig. 13.17), which are calcospherites that may be small with clear centers, or large and prominently laminated. The calcospherites stain with von Kossa, iron, and PAS stains. Special stains for organisms are virtually always negative. The differential diagnosis includes Whipple's disease, *Rhodococcus* infection, MAI infection, but the characteristic Michaelis–Gutmann bodies and the inability to identify organisms help to distinguish malakoplakia from other infectious diseases.

Bartonella species. Bartonella (formerly *Rochalimaea*) species (either *quintana* or *henselae*) are small, fastidious, Gram-negative bacteria. They occasionally cause disease in the GI tract, most commonly manifested as bacillary angiomatosis, a vascular proliferation that usually occurs in the skin. These pyogenic granuloma-like lesions occur in immunocompromised patients and mimic Kaposi's sarcoma. Patients characteristically present with bloody diarrhea or hematemesis.

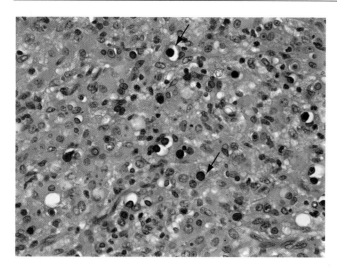

Fig. 13.17 The macrophages contain characteristic Michaelis–Gutmann bodies, which are calcospherities that may be prominently laminated

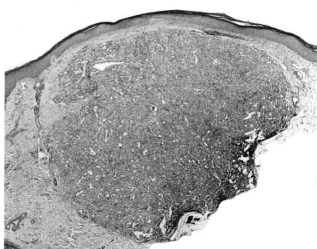

Fig. 13.18 A nodular, dome-shaped mucocutaneous lesion in bacillary angiomatosis (courtesy Dr. Bruce Smoller)

Pathologic features. Macroscopic findings include erythematous mucosal nodules with associated ulceration. Bacillary angiomatosis can be found anywhere in the GI tract, and may or may not be associated with cutaneous lesions. Lesions are often dome-shaped (Fig. 13.18) and may be polypoid, and range in size from pinpoint to several centimeters in largest diameter. The proliferating small vessels may have a lobular configuration (Fig. 13.19), and usually have associated acute and chronic inflammation with an appearance similar to granulation tissue (Fig. 13.20). Endothelial cells may be plump, with vacuolated cytoplasm and focal nuclear atypia (Fig. 13.21). Silver impregnation stains (such as Warthin-Starry) sometimes reveal organisms (Fig. 13.22). Molecular assays and immunohistochemical stains are also available for diagnosis. The inflammatory infiltrate and presence of bacteria help to distinguish bacillary angiomatosis from Kaposi sarcoma. However, the two lesions may be very difficult to distinguish morphologically and may coexist in the same patient.

Bacillary angiomatosis is usually associated with *Bartonella quintana*. Although the stellate granulomatous lesions of cat scratch disease (most often associated with *Bartonella henselae*) rarely affect the gastrointestinal tract itself, affected mesenteric nodes may impinge on the gut and cause ulceration (Figs. 13.23 and 13.24.).

Sexually transmitted bacterial proctocolitis. Herpes simplex virus is the most common etiologic agent of infectious proctocolitis among homosexual men (see Chapter 21), but there are many bacterial causes.

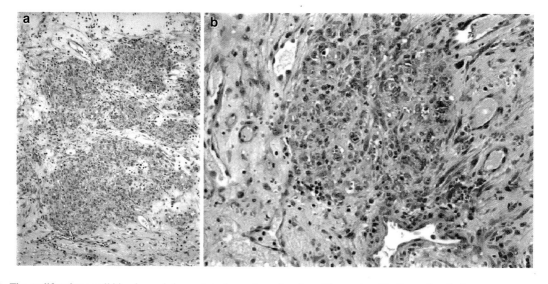

Fig. 13.19 The proliferating small blood vessels have a lobular configuration (**a** and **b**, courtesy Dr. Bruce Smoller)

Fig. 13.20 The vascular and inflammatory lesions of bacillary angiomatosis may resemble granulation tissue (**a**), with numerous admixed neutrophils (**b** and **c**)

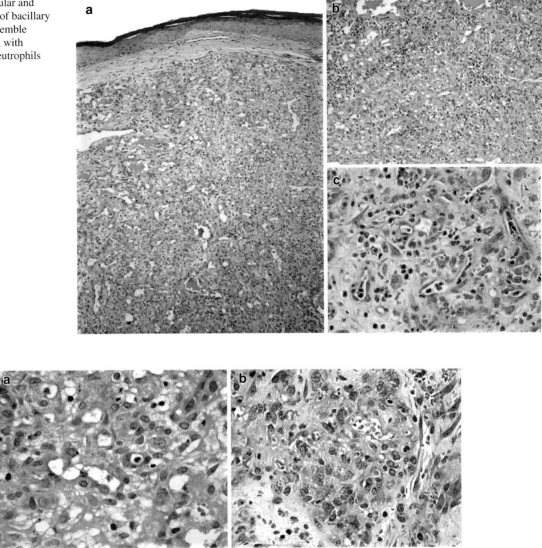

Fig. 13.21 Endothelial cells are often plump, with enlarged nuclei and vacuolated cytoplasm (**a** and **b**). Endothelial cells may have some degree of cytologic atypia, with irregular nuclear outlines (**b**)

Chlamydia trachomatis. Serotypes L1, L2, and L3 cause lymphogranuloma venereum (LGV). The anorectum is the most common gastrointestinal site, but LGV has been described in the ileum and colon as well. Anal pain is usually severe and accompanied by bloody discharge and tenesmus. Inguinal lymphadenopathy is usually present, and patients may have malaise, fever, and headache. Some patients with gastrointestinal LGV lack the classic genital ulcerations. Complications of chronic, untreated disease include lymphedema from repeated episodes of inflammation and scarring, anorectal fistulas, and strictures.

Pathologic features. Macroscopic findings include mucosal granularity, erythema, friability, and ulceration. Strictures and inflammatory mass lesions have been described. The inflammatory infiltrate is variable; most patients have a lymphoplasmacytic infiltrate in the mucosa and submucosa (Fig. 13.25), but neutrophils may be prominent as well. Granulomatous inflammation is sometimes present, and histologic features (including transmural inflammation, fibrosis, and neural hyperplasia) may mimic Crohn's disease. In addition, LGV may produce a striking "follicular" proctitis, as well as significant architectural distortion, that can mimic ulcerative colitis. Culture, immunofluorescence studies, serologic studies, molecular assays, and immunohistochemistry may serve as valuable diagnostic aids.

Neisseria gonorrhea. Anorectal gonococcal infection is reportedly present in over 40% of both women and men with uncomplicated gonorrhea. Infection is frequently asymptomatic. When present, symptoms are non-specific

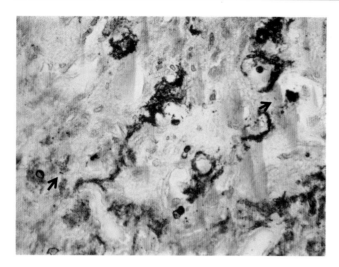

Fig. 13.22 Cocco-bacillary forms may be found on silver impregnation stains such as the Warthin-Starry

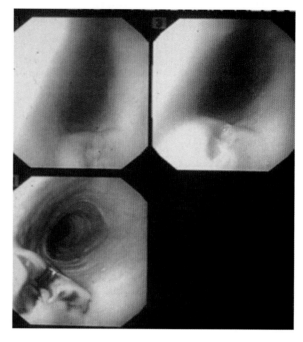

Fig. 13.23 An enlarged para-esophageal lymph node in a child with cat scratch disease, which eroded through the esophagus to produce an ulcer (courtesy Dr. William A. Webb)

and include mucoid stools, purulent discharge, anal bleeding, anal itching/irritation, rectal discomfort or fullness, and painful defecation. Classically, the rectum is involved while the squamous-lined anal canal proper is spared, although a classic finding is the ability to express mucoid pus from the anal crypt glands. Perirectal abscesses are a rare complication. *N. meningitidis* also has been isolated from the anorectum, but it remains unclear if this represents colonization or an actual pathogen in this location.

Pathologic features. Proctoscopic findings include mucosal erythema, friability, erosions, and fissures, along with a mucupurulent discharge in the anal canal. Proctoscopic examination may be entirely unremarkable, however, even in symptomatic patients. Most biopsies in rectal gonorrhea are normal; some contain a mild increase in neutrophils and mononuclear cells or focal cryptitis and crypt abscesses.

Gram-negative intracellular diplococci occasionally can be seen on a Gram stain of anal discharge, but culture is the "gold standard" for diagnosis.

The macroscopic differential diagnosis includes ulcerative proctitis, other infectious disorders (particularly other sexually transmitted proctocolitides), radiation proctitis, and early involvement by carcinoma. Ultimately, symptoms, physical findings, and histologic findings in cases of rectal gonorrhea are non-specific, and thus appropriate cultures should be done in symptomatic patients who practice anorectal intercourse.

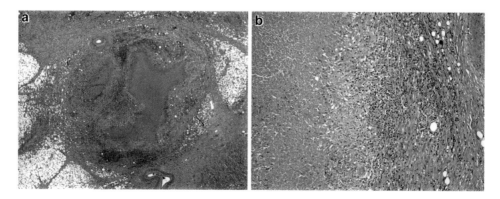

Fig. 13.24 A mesenteric lymph node with the characteristic lesion of cat scratch disease, consisting of a stellate, necrotizing granuloma with central necrosis (**a**), and well-delineated layers of palisading histiocytes and mononuclear cells (**b**)

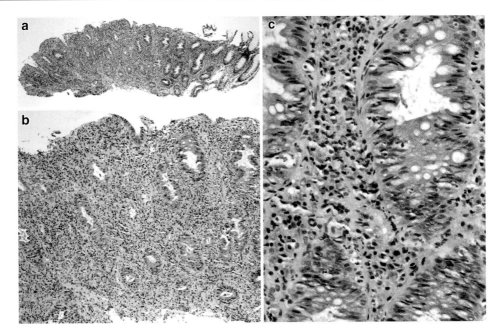

Fig. 13.25 Distal colon biopsies from a patient with LGV proctitis. Biopsies show a dense lymphoplasmacytic infiltrate with mild architectural distortion (**a** and **b**), along with cryptitis (**c**), mimicking chronic idiopathic inflammatory bowel disease. (Courtesy Dr. Greg Lauwers)

Selected References

Bacterial Esophagitis

1. Ezzell JH, Bremer J, Adamec TA. Bacterial esophagitis: an often forgotten cause of odynophagia. Am J Gastroenterol 85:296–8, 1990.
2. Walsh TJ, Belitsos NJ, Hamilton SR. Bacterial esophagitis in immunocompromised patients. Arch Intern Med 146:1345–8, 1986.

Actinomycosis

3. Ferrari TC, Couto CA, Murta-Oliveira C, et al. Actinomycosis of the colon: a rare form of presentation. Scand J Gastroenterol 35:108–9, 2000.
4. Mueller MC, Ihrler S, Degenhart C, Bogner JR. Abdominal actinomycosis. Infection 36:191, 2008.
5. Schmidt P, Koltai JL, Weltzien A. Actinomycosis of the appendix in childhood. Pediatr Surg Int 15:63–5, 1999.
6. Skoutelis A, Panagopoulos C, Kalfarentzos F, Bassaris H. Intramural gastric actinomycosis. South Med J 88:647–50, 1995.
7. Valko P, Busolini E, Donati N, et al. Severe large bowel obstruction secondary to infection with *Actinomyces israelii*. Scand J Infect Dis 38:231–4, 2006.

Brucellosis

8. Ablin J, Mevorach D, Eliakim R. Brucellosis and the gastrointestinal tract: the odd couple. J Clin Gastroenterol 24:25–9, 1997.
9. Colmenero JD, Reguera JM, Martos F, et al. Complications associated with *Brucella melitensis* infection: a study of 530 cases. Medicine 75:195–211, 1996.
10. Jorens PG, Michielsen PP, Van den Enden EJ, et al. A rare cause of colitis-*Brucella melitensis*. Dis Colon Rectum 34:194–6, 1991.
11. Mousa AR, Elhag KM, Khogali M, Marafie AA. The nature of human brucellosis in Kuwait: a study of 379 cases. Rev Infect Dis 10:211–7, 1988.
12. Petrella R, Young EJ. Acute brucella ileitis. Am J Gastroenterol 83:80–2, 1988.
13. Young EJ. Human brucellosis. Rev Infect Dis 5:821–42, 1983.

Rhodococcus equi

14. Hamrock D, Azmi F, O'Donnell E, et al. Infection by *Rhodococcus equi* in a patient with AIDS: histological appearance mimicking Whipple's disease and *MAI* infection. J Clin Pathol 52:68–71, 1999.
15. Scott MA, Graham BS, Verrall R, et al. *Rhodococcus equi* – an increasingly recognized opportunistic pathogen. Report of 10 cases and review of the literature. Am J Clin Pathol 103:649–55, 1995.
16. Verville TD, Huycke MM, Greenfield RA, et al. *Rhodococcus equi* infections of humans: 12 cases and review of the literature. Medicine 73:119–32, 1994.

Rickettsial Disease

17. Dumler JS, Taylor JP, Walker DH. Clinical and laboratory features of murine typhus in South Texas, 1980–1987. JAMA 266: 1365–70, 1991.

18. Kim SJ, Chung IK, Chung IS, et al. The clinical significance of upper gastrointestinal endoscopy in gastrointestinal vasculitis related to scrub typhus. Endoscopy 32:950–5, 2000.
19. Randall MB and Walker DH. Rocky mountain spotted fever: gastrointestinal and pancreatic lesions and rickettsial infection. Arch Pathol Lab Med 108:963–7, 1984.
20. Walker DH, Dumler JS. Rickettsial infections. In Connor DH, Chandler FW et al. (eds): Pathology of Infectious Diseases, Stamford, CT: Appleton and Lange, 1997, pp. 789–99.

Ehrlichiosis

21. Dumler SJ, Walker DH. Ehrlichial infections. In Connor DH, Chandler FW et al. (eds): Pathology of Infectious Diseases, Stamford, CT: Appleton and Lange, 1997, pp. 543–8.
22. Fritz CL, Glaser CA. Ehrlichiosis. Infect Dis Clin North Am 12(1):123–36, 1998.
23. Harkess JR. Ehrlichosis. Infect Dis Clin North Am 5(1):37–51, 1991.
24. Nutt AK, Raufman JP. Gastrointestinal and hepatic manifestations of human erlichiosis: 8 cases and a review of the literature. Dig Dis 17:37–43, 1998.

Malakoplakia

25. Birkenstock W, Louw JH. Malakoplakia of the colon. Brit J Surg 59:662–4, 1972.
26. Finlay-Jones LR, Blackwell JB, Papadimitriou JM. Malakoplakia of the colon. Am J Clin Pathol 50:320–9, 1968.
27. Joyeuse R, Lott JV, Michaelis M, Gumucio CC. Malakoplakia of the colon and rectum: report of a case and review of the literature. Surgery 81:189–92, 1977.
28. Mcclure J. Malakoplakia of the gastrointestinal tract. Post Med J 57:95–103, 1981.
29. Nakabayashi H, Ito T, Izutsu K, et al. Malakoplakia of the stomach. Report of a case and review of the literature. Arch Pathol Lab Med 102:136–9, 1978.

Bartonella species

30. Chang AD, Drachenberg CI, James SP. Bacillary angiomatosis associated with extensive esophageal polyposis: a new mucocutaneous manifestation of acquired immunodeficiency disease (AIDS). Am J Gastroenterol 91:2220–3, 1996.
31. Chetty R, Sabaratnam RM. Upper gastrointestinal bacillary angiomatosis causing hematemesis: a case report. Int J Surg Pathol 11:241–4, 2003.
32. Huh YB, Rose S, Schoen RE, et al. Colonic bacillary angiomatosis. Ann Intern Med 124:735–7, 1996.
33. Lamps LW, Scott MA. Cat scratch disease: historical, clinical, and pathological perspectives. Am J Clin Pathol Suppl 121:S71–80, 2004.
34. Spach DH, Koehler JE. *Bartonella*-associated infections. Infect Dis Clin North Am 12(1):137–55, 1998.

Sexually Transmitted Bacterial Proctocolitis

35. Baker RW, Peppercorn MA. Gastrointestinal ailments of homosexual men. Medicine 61:390–405, 1982.
36. Davis BT, Thiim M, Zukerberg LR, et al. Case records of the Massachusetts General Hospital (Case 2-2006). A 31-year-old, HIV-positive man with rectal pain. N Engl J Med 354(3): 284–9, 2006.
37. de la Monte SM, Hutchins GM. Follicular proctocolitis and neuromatous hyperplasia with lymphogranuloma venereum. Hum Pathol 16:1025–32, 1985.
38. Geller SA, Zimmerman MJ, Cohen A. Rectal biopsy in early lymphogranuloma venereum proctitis. Am J Gastro 74:433–5, 1980.
39. Jaffe LR, Stavis JAS. Isolation of *Neisseria meningitides* from anogenital sites in adolescents: clinical implications. J Adolesc Health Care 4:171–3, 1983.
40. Klein EJ, Fisher LS, Chow AW, Guze LB. Anorectal gonococcal infection. Ann Intern Med 86:340–6, 1977.
41. Lebedeff DA, Hochman EB. Rectal gonorrhea in men: diagnosis and treatment. Ann Intern Med 92:463–6, 1980.
42. McMillan A, McNeillage G, Gilmour HM, Lee FD. Histology of rectal gonorrhea in men, with a note on anorectal infection with *Neisseria meningitidis*. J Clin Pathol 36:511–14, 1983.
43. Quinn TC, Corey L, Chaffee RG, et al. The etiology of anorectal infections in homosexual men. Am J Med 71:395–406, 1981.
44. Rompalo AM. Diagnosis and treatment of sexually acquired proctitis and proctocolitis. Clin Infect Dis 28(Suppl 1):S84–90, 1999.
45. Surawicz CM, Goodell SE, Quinn TC, et al. Spectrum of rectal biopsy abnormalities in homosexual men with intestinal symptoms. Gastroenterol 91:651–9, 1986.
46. Tinmouth J, Rachlis A, Wesson T, Hseih E. Lymphogranuloma venereum in North America: case reports and an update for gastroenterologists. Clin Gastroenterol Hepatol 4:469–73, 2006.
47. Wexner SD. Sexually transmitted diseases of the colon, rectum, and anus. Dis Colon Rectum 33:1048–59, 1990.
48. Zellner SR, Trudeau WL. Anorectal gonorrhea presenting as ulcerative proctitis. South Med J 66:706–8, 1973.

Part II
Fungal Infections of the Gastrointestinal Tract

Abstract The incidence of fungal infections of the gastrointestinal tract has increased significantly as the number of patients with organ transplants, AIDS and other immunodeficiency states, and on long-term chemotherapy has risen. Tissue biopsy remains one of the most important tools available in the diagnosis of fungal infections, particularly as fungal cultures may require days to weeks for adequate growth and analysis. This section addresses common and uncommon fungal infections affecting the gastrointestinal tract, including clinical setting, macroscopic and histologic features, differential diagnoses, and useful laboratory tests that can aid in diagnosis.

Chapter 14

General Approach to Diagnosis of Fungal Infections of the Gastrointestinal Tract

Keywords Fungus • Mycosis • Invasive • Immunocompromised • GMS • PAS

The incidence of invasive fungal infections, including fungal infections of the gastrointestinal tract, has increased significantly over the past 20 years as the number of patients with organ transplants, AIDS and other immunodeficiency states, and on long-term chemotherapy has risen. Gastrointestinal fungal infections occur most commonly in immunocompromised patients, but virtually all fungi have been reported to cause infection in immunocompetent persons as well. Fungal infections of the gastrointestinal tract can be roughly divided into two categories: those caused by transmucosal invasion and those that disseminate following primary infection of another site (usually pulmonary). In addition, invasive fungal infections are associated with repetitive abdominal surgeries, widespread use of antimicrobial agents, intrusive vascular lines, diabetes, total parenteral nutrition, neonatal prematurity, and advancing age.

Signs and symptoms of gastrointestinal fungal infections are in general similar, regardless of the type of fungus, and include diarrhea, vomiting, melena, frank GI bleeding, abdominal pain, and fever. Esophageal fungal infections usually present with odynophagia and dysphagia. It is important to note that fungal infections of the GI tract are often a part of a disseminated disease process, but gastrointestinal symptoms and signs may be the presenting manifestations.

Tissue biopsy remains one of the most important tools available in the diagnosis of fungal infections, particularly as fungal cultures may require days to weeks for adequate growth and analysis. In addition, cultures are often not obtained as often as pathologists might wish or expect. Although organisms may be identifiable on H&E sections in heavy infections, GMS and PAS stains remain invaluable diagnostic aids. Fungi usually can be correctly classified in tissue sections based on morphologic criteria (Table 14.1). It is important to note, however, that fungi exposed to antifungal therapy or ambient air may produce bizarre and unusual forms. Microbiological culture remains the gold standard for speciation, especially as antifungal therapy may vary according to the specific type of fungus isolated.

Helpful diagnostic aids, in addition to culture, include serologic assays, antigen tests, immunohistochemistry, and molecular assays, although the latter two methodologies are less widely available. The development of diagnostic assays is currently focused on detecting fungal cell wall elements and their antibodies in host tissue and body fluids. Molecular tests may be over-sensitive in some settings due to fungal colonization, and some immunohistochemical and serologic tests suffer from cross-reactivity between fungal species. However, these are promising areas of active clinical research. Knowledge of the patient's geographic and/or travel history also may be very helpful in diagnosing fungal infections.

A detailed discussion of the major mycoses affecting the gastrointestinal tract is presented in the following sections. Other fungal infections that occasionally involve the gastrointestinal tract, but are not discussed in detail here, include *Fusarium* (an emerging pathogen in neutropenic patients, similar to *Aspergillus*), *Blastomyces dermatididis*, and *Paracoccidiodes brasiliensis* (South American blastomycosis), which can mimic chronic idiopathic inflammatory bowel disease both clinically and radiographically.

L.W. Lamps, *Surgical Pathology of the Gastrointestinal System: Bacterial, Fungal, Viral, and Parasitic Infections*,
DOI 10.1007/978-1-4419-0861-2_14, © Springer Science+Business Media, LLC 2009

Table 14.1 Morphologic features of fungi involving the gastrointestinal tract

Organism	Primary geographic distribution	Morphologic features	Host reaction	Major differential diagnoses
Aspergillus species	Worldwide	Hyphae – septate Uniform width Branching – regular Acute angles Conidial head formation in cavitary lesions	Ischemic necrosis with angioinvasion Acute inflammation Occasionally granulomatous	Zygomycetes *Fusarium* *Pseudallescheria boydii*
Blastomyces dermatitidis (North American blastomycosis)	Similar to histoplasmosis; rare cases from Africa and Central America	Large pleomorphic (8–15 μm) spherical to ovoid yeast Intra- or extracellular Broad-based buds Multinucleate	Mixed suppurative and granulomatous reaction	*Histoplasma* sp. *Cryptococcus neoformans* (especially capsule-deficient) *Coccidioides immitis*
Candida albicans *Candida tropicalis*	Worldwide	Mixture of budding yeast and pseudohyphae; occasional septate hyphae	Usually suppurative, with variable necrosis and ulceration Occasionally granulomatous Occasional angioinvasion	*Trichosporon*
Candida (Torulopsis) glabrata	Worldwide	Budding yeast No hyphae No "halo" effect	Similar to other *Candida* species	*Histoplasma* *Cryptococcus*
Cryptococcus neoformans	Worldwide	Highly pleomorphic (4–7 μm) Uninucleate Narrow-based buds Usually mucicarmine positive	Usually suppurative; may have extensive necrosis Sometimes granulomatous	Histoplasmosis Blastomycosis *C. glabrata*
Histoplasma capsulatum var. capsulatum	Worldwide, but endemic in Ohio, Mississippi river basins; parts of Central and South America; St. Lawrence river basin in Canada	Uniform small (2–5 μm), uninucleate ovoid yeast Narrow-based buds Intracellular "Halo" effect around organism on H&E	Lymphohistiocytic infiltrate with parasitized histiocytes Occasional granulomas	*Cryptococcus* *P. marneffei* *C. glabrata* *P. carinii* Intracellular parasites
Pneumocystis carinii	Worldwide	Ovoid Cup or crescent shaped if collapsed No buds Internal enhancing detail	Characteristic foamy casts May have suppurative or granulomatous inflammation as well	Histoplasmosis Small parasites
Zygomycetes	Worldwide, associated with diabetics more than any other mycosis	Hyphae-Pauciseptate Ribbon-like Thin walls Branching– haphazard	Similar to *Aspergillus*	Similar to *Aspergillus*

Selected References

1. Anand AR, Madhavan HN, Neelam V, Lily TK. Use of polymerase chain reaction in the diagnosis of fungal endopthalmitis. Opthalmol 108:326–30, 2001.
2. Chandler FW, Watts JC. Pathologic Diagnosis of Fungal Infections. Chicago, IL: ASCP Press, 1987.
3. Cherniss EI, Waisbren BA. North American blastomycosis: a clinical study of 40 cases. Ann Intern Med 44:105–23, 1956.
4. Dictar MO, Maiolo E, Alexander B, et al. Mycoses in the transplanted patient. Med Mycol 38(Suppl 1):251–8, 2000.
5. Ellis M. Invasive fungal infections: evolving challenges for diagnosis and therapeutics. Mol Immunol 38:947–57, 2001.
6. Fleming RV, Walsh TJ, Anaissie EJ. Emerging and less common fungal pathogens. Infect Dis Clin North Am 16:915–33, 2002.
7. Kaufman L. Immunohistologic diagnosis of systemic mycoses: an update. Eur J Epidemiol 8:377–92, 1992.
8. Khandekar A, Moser D, Fidler WJ. Blastomycosis of the esophagus. Ann Thorac Surg 30:76–9, 1980.
9. Martino P, Gastaldi R, Raccah R, Girmenia C. Clinical patterns of *Fusarium* infections in immunocompromised patients. J Infection 28(Suppl 1):7–15, 1994.
10. Penna FJ. Blastomycosis of the colon resembling clinically ulcerative colitis. Gut 20: 896–9, 1979.
11. Prescott RJ, Harris M, Banerjee SS. Fungal infections of the small and large intestine. J Clin Pathol 45:806–11, 1992.
12. Reed JA, Hemann BA, Alexander JL, Brigati DJ. Immunomycology: rapid and specific immunocytochemical identification of fungi in formain-fixed, paraffin-embedded material. J Histochem Cytochem 41:1217–21, 1993.
13. Schwarz J. The diagnosis of deep mycoses by morphologic methods. Hum Pathol 13:519–33, 1982.
14. Shin JH, Nolte FS, Holloway BP, Morrison CJ. Rapid identification of up to three *Candida* species in a single reaction tube by a 5' exonuclease assay using fluorescent DNA probes. J Clin Microbiol 37:165–70, 1999.
15. Smith JMB. Mycoses of the alimentary tract. Gut 10:1035–40, 1969.
16. Turenne CY, Sanche SE, Hoban DJ, et al. Rapid identification of fungi by using the ITS2 genetic region and an automated fluorescent capillary electrophoresis system. J Clin Microbiol 37:1846–51, 1999.
17. Washburn RG, Bennett JE. Deep Mycoses. In: Blaser MJ, Smith PD, Ravdin JI, et al. (eds): Infections of the Gastrointestinal Tract. New York: Raven Press, 1995, pp. 957–66.

Chapter 15

Candida Species

Keywords *Candida* sp. • Esophagitis • Immunocompromise • Pseudohyphae • Budding yeast

Candida is the most common infection of the esophagus, but may infect any level of the GI tract; in fact, some authors believe, based on autopsy studies, that *Candida* infection of the gastrointestinal tract is increasing in frequency. Common risk factors for invasive *Candida* infection include immunosuppression, chemotherapy, corticosteroids, and major abdominal surgery. The gastrointestinal tract is a major portal for disseminated candidiasis, since *Candida* often superinfects ulcers that develop from other causes. It is important to morphologically differentiate between invasive candidiasis and superficial colonization, as *Candida* is capable of colonizing benign ulcers and mucosal surfaces without invasion. *C. albicans* is most commonly isolated, but *C. tropicalis* and *C. (Torulopsis) glabrata* may produce similar clinical and pathologic manifestations. In addition, other non-*albicans* species (such as *C. krusei* and *C. parapsilosis*) are emerging as important causes of invasive fungal infection.

Pathologic features. Grossly, the esophagus typically contains white plaques that easily scrape away to reveal ulcerated mucosa underneath (Figs. 15.1, 15.2, and 15.3). The gross features of candidiasis in the remainder of the GI tract are variable and include ulceration, pseudomembrane formation, and inflammatory masses (Figs. 15.4, 15.5, and 15.6). Ulcers are often multiple, irregular, and hemorrhagic, and may be confluent in advanced cases (Figs. 15.5 and 15.6). Deep linear ulcers also have been described. If vascular invasion is prominent, the bowel may appear infarcted. Involvement may be diffuse or segmental.

The associated inflammatory response ranges from minimal (especially in immunocompromised patients) to marked with prominent neutrophilic infiltrates, abscess formation, erosion/ulceration, and necrosis (Figs. 15.7 and 15.8). When pseudomembranes are present, they are composed of a mixture of yeast, necrotic debris, and fibrin. Granulomas are occasionally present as well. The presence of numerous intraepithelial neutrophils in the squamous mucosa of the

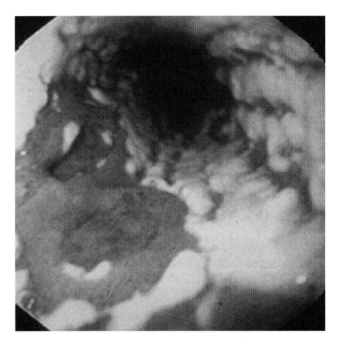

Fig. 15.1 Endoscopic photograph of esophageal candidiasis showing white plaques that are easily scraped away to reveal ulcerated mucosa. (Courtesy Dr. William A. Webb)

esophagus is a common finding in esophageal candidiasis, and should provoke the use of fungal stains (Figs. 15.9, 15.10, and 15.11). Fungi may invade any level of the gut wall, and invasion of mucosal and submucosal blood vessels is sometimes a prominent feature.

Morphologic features of the organism. *C. albicans* and *C. tropicalis* produce a mixture of budding yeast forms intermingled with pseudohyphae and occasional true hyphae (Figs. 15.12, 15.13, 15.14, 15.15, and 15.16). *Candida* stains with GMS, and is bright fuchsia on PAS stain (Fig. 15.15). *C. (Torulopsis) glabrata* features tiny budding yeast forms similar to *Histoplasma*, but does not produce hyphae or pseudohyphae (Fig. 15.17).

Differential diagnosis. The differential diagnosis primarily includes other infectious processes (see

L.W. Lamps, *Surgical Pathology of the Gastrointestinal System: Bacterial, Fungal, Viral, and Parasitic Infections*,
DOI 10.1007/978-1-4419-0861-2_15, © Springer Science+Business Media, LLC 2009

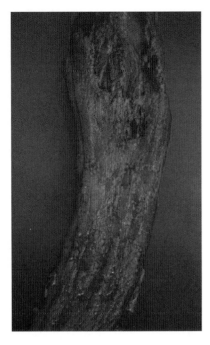

Fig. 15.2 An esophagus removed at autopsy showing *Candida* infection, with extensive yellow–white membranes and adjacent areas of ulceration

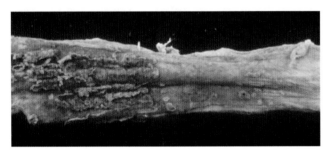

Fig. 15.3 Severely ulcerated esophagus removed at autopsy showing virtually denuded mucosa with hemorrhagic exudates. (Courtesy Dr. Margie Scott)

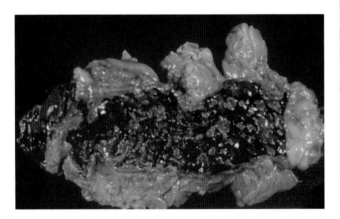

Fig. 15.4 A segment of colon removed at autopsy in a patient with invasive candidiasis, showing ulcerated mucosa with patchy overlying pseudomembranes. (Courtesy Dr. Cole Elliott)

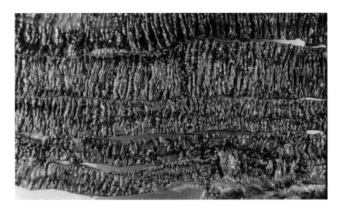

Fig. 15.5 Bowel removed at autopsy with *C. tropicalis* infection, showing confluent areas of ulceration with adjacent extensively hemorrhagic mucosa. (Courtesy Dr. Margie Scott)

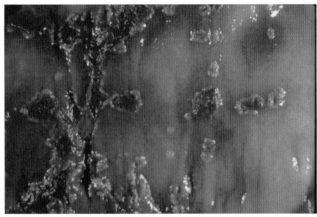

Fig. 15.6 High-power gross photograph of *C. tropicalis* colitis, with confluent and linear ulcers with associated areas of white-tan exudates. (Courtesy Dr. Margie Scott)

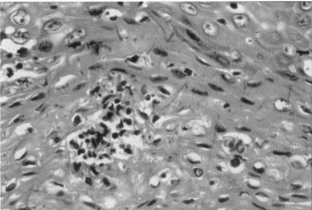

Fig. 15.7 High-power photomicrograph of lightly basophilic intraepithelial budding yeast and pseudohyphae within esophageal squamous mucosa, with little associated inflammatory infiltrate

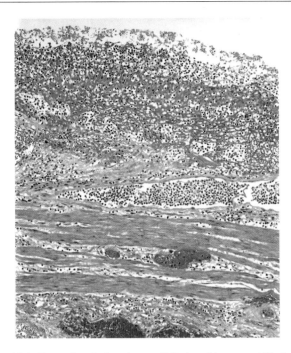

Fig. 15.8 Deep ulcer in invasive candidiasis, with neutrophilic infiltrate extending into the muscular wall of the esophagus, and an overlying pseudomembrane composed of necrotic debris and fibrin

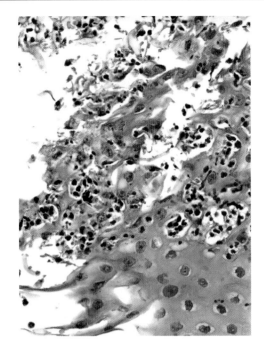

Fig. 15.10 High-power view of acantholytic squamous mucosa with intraepithelial neutrophils, neutrophilic microabscesses, and rare budding yeast forms

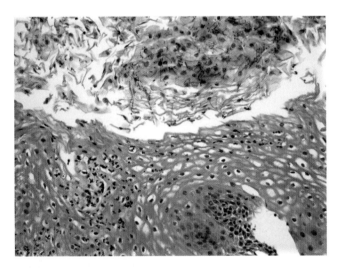

Fig. 15.9 Esophageal biopsy showing squamous mucosa with intraepithelial neutrophils, along with sloughing squamous cells and characteristic basophilic buds and pseudohyphae within the sloughing mucosa

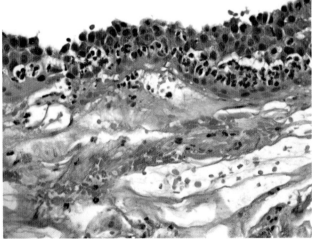

Fig. 15.11 High-power view of neutrophilic infiltrate undermining reactive squamous mucosa

Table 14.1). Grossly, intestinal candidiasis may mimic other inflammatory process including chronic idiopathic inflammatory bowel disease, pseudomembranous colitis, and ischemic colitis. Furthermore, fungal stains should be strongly considered in any immunocompromised patient with ischemic lesions of the gastrointestinal tract .

In the esophagus, care should be taken to avoid confusing oral contamination by *Candida* for true invasive *Candida* esophagitis. In invasive candidiasis, fungi should be present within the squamous epithelium, with associated acute inflammation. In oral contamination, fungi are seen at the surface of the epithelium or adjacent to detached squamous cells, with no associated acute inflammation.

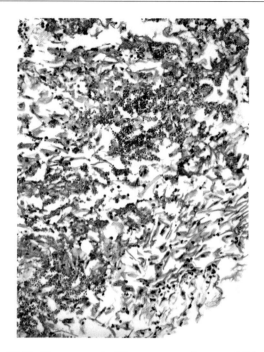

Fig. 15.12 Numerous budding yeast forms visible on hematoxylin/eosin within sloughed squamous cells and associated neutrophils

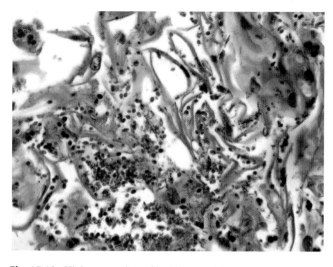

Fig. 15.13 High-power view of budding yeast forms within squamous cells in an esophageal biopsy

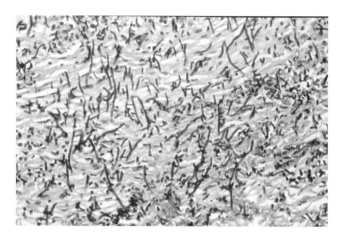

Fig. 15.15 PAS stain shows numerous bright pink *Candida* within the esophageal mucosa

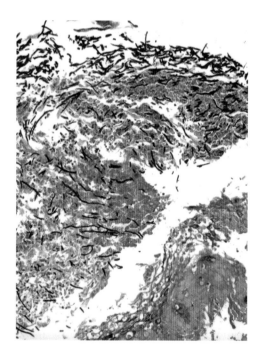

Fig. 15.14 Low-power GMS stain shows characteristic budding yeast and pseudohyphae typical of *Candida albicans*

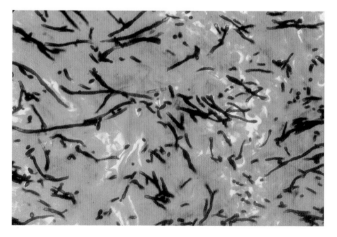

Fig. 15.16 High-power view of *C. albicans* showing characteristic buds and pseudohyphae (GMS stain)

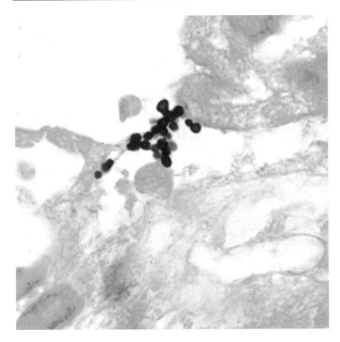

Fig. 15.17 *C.* (*Torulopsis*) *glabrata*. Small extracellular yeast forms have buds but no hyphae or pseudohyphae (GMS stain)

Selected References

1. Chandler FW, Watts JC. Pathologic Diagnosis of Fungal Infections. Chicago, IL: ASCP Press, 1987.

2. Chandler FW, Ajello L. *Torulopsis.* In: Conner DH, Chandler FW (eds): Pathology of Infectious Diseases. Stamford, CT: Appleton and Lange, 1997, pp. 1105–8.

3. Dictar MO, Maiolo E, Alexander B, et al. Mycoses in the transplanted patient. Med Mycol 38(Suppl 1):251–8, 2000.

4. Ellis M. Invasive fungal infections: evolving challenges for diagnosis and therapeutics. Mol Immunol 38:947–57, 2001.

5. Eras P, Goldstein MJ, Sherlock P. *Candida* infection of the gastrointestinal tract. Medicine 51:367–79, 1972.

6. Joshi SN, Garvin PJ, Sunwoo YC. Candidiasis of the duodenum and jejunum. Gastroenterol 80:829–33, 1981.

7. Kullberg BJ, Oude Lashof AM. Epidemiology of opportunistic invasive mycoses. Eur J Med Res 7:183–91, 2002.

8. Luna M. Candidiasis. In: Conner DH, Chandler FW (eds): Pathology of Infectious Diseases. Stamford, CT: Appleton and Lange, 1997, pp. 953–64.

9. Ostrosky-Zeichner L, Rex JH, Bennett J, Kullberg BJ. Deeply invasive candidiasis. Infect Dis Clin North Am 16:821–35, 2002.

10. Prescott RJ, Harris M, Banerjee SS. Fungal infections of the small and large intestine. J Clin Pathol 45:806–11, 1992.

11. Schwesinger G, Junghans D, Schroder G, et al. Candidosis and aspergillosis as autopsy findings from 1994 to 2003. Mycoses 48:176–80, 2005.

12. Shin JH, Nolte FS, Holloway BP, Morrison CJ. Rapid identification of up to three *Candida* species in a single reaction tube by a 5' exonuclease assay using fluorescent DNA probes. J Clin Microbiol 37:165–70, 1999.

13. Walsh TJ, Merz WG. Pathologic features in the human alimentary tract associated with invasiveness of *Candida tropicalis*. Am J Clin Pathol 85:498–502, 1986.

14. Washburn RG, Bennett JE. Deep Mycoses. In: Blaser MJ, Smith PD, Ravdin JI, et al. (eds): Infections of the Gastrointestinal Tract. New York: Raven Press, 1995, pp. 957–66.

Chapter 16

Aspergillus Species and Zygomycetes

Keywords *Aspergillus* sp. • Zygomycetes • Mucor • Immunocompromise • Hyphae

Aspergillus infection of the gastrointestinal tract occurs almost exclusively in immunocompromised patients, particularly those with prolonged neutropenia, and thus bone marrow transplant recipients are at particular risk for invasive aspergillosis. The majority of patients with aspergillosis also have coexistent lung lesions. *Aspergillus* species have replaced *Candida* species as the most common fungal pathogen at some institutions.

Pathologic features. The bowel (particularly colon) is the most frequent site of gastrointestinal involvement, followed by the esophagus and stomach. Multiple sites of concomitant involvement are common. Aspergillosis is much less frequently seen in the esophagus compared to candidiasis, however. The characteristic histologic lesion of aspergillosis is a nodular infarction consisting of a zone of ischemic necrosis centered on blood vessels containing fungi (Figs. 16.1 and 16.2). These nodular infarctions may produce mucosal

"target lesions" with a central necrotic zone surrounded by a ring of hemorrhage (Fig. 16.3). Fungal hyphae often extend outward from the infarct in parallel or radial arrays (Figs. 16.4, 16.5, and 16.6). The inflammatory response is variable and ranges from minimal to marked, with a prominent neutrophilic infiltrate (Fig. 16.7). Granulomatous inflammation may develop as well. Transmural infarction of the bowel wall is common. The typical hyphae of *Aspergillus* are septate, have parallel walls, and branch at acute angles (Figs. 16.8 and 16.9).

Zygomycetes. Gastrointestinal zygomycosis is relatively uncommon, and the lesions caused by *Mucor* and related zygomycetes are extremely similar to those seen in aspergillosis (Figs. 16.10 and 16.11). Zygomycosis is associated with diabetes and other causes of metabolic acidosis, deferoxamine therapy, skin and soft tissue breakdown from other causes, intravenous drug use, neonatal prematurity, and malnourishment. Although any portion of the alimentary tract can be affected, gastric and colonic involvement are the most frequent. Ulcers are the most common

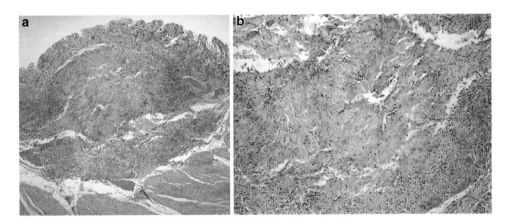

Fig. 16.1 Nodular infarction consisting of a zone of ischemic necrosis centered on a blood vessel (**a**). Higher power view showing central necrosis with surrounding neutrophilic infiltrate and admixed necrotic debris (**b**)

L.W. Lamps, *Surgical Pathology of the Gastrointestinal System: Bacterial, Fungal, Viral, and Parasitic Infections*, DOI 10.1007/978-1-4419-0861-2_16, © Springer Science+Business Media, LLC 2009

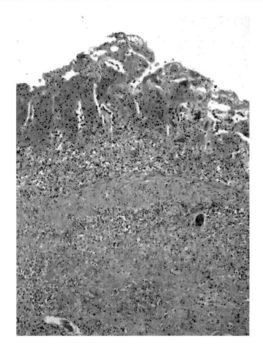

Fig. 16.2 Nodular submucosal gastric infarction centered on submucosal vessel occluded by *Aspergillus*, with overlying mucosal ischemia

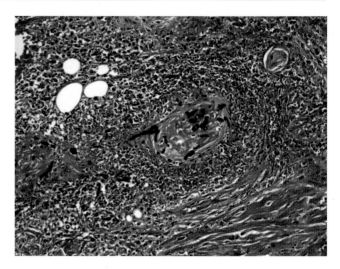

Fig. 16.4 *Aspergillus* fill a vessel, with associated blood and fibrinous debris (hematoxylin and eosin/methenamine silver stain)

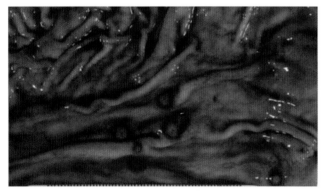

Fig. 16.3 Characteristic target lesion in the stomach of a bone marrow transplant patient with disseminated aspergillosis. Note central necrotic area and surrounding hemorrhage. (Courtesy Dr. George F. Gray, Jr)

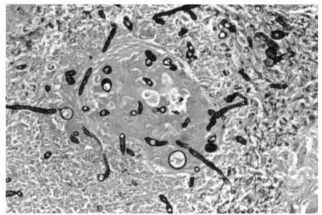

Fig. 16.5 *Aspergillus* fill a submucosal vessel and extend outward in a radial pattern (hematoxylin and eosin/methenamine silver stain)

gross manifestation, often large, with rolled, irregular edges that may mimic malignancy. These fungi may also superinfect previously ulcerated tissues.

Differential diagnosis. The differential diagnosis primarily includes other infectious processes (see Table 14.1), and *Aspergillus* and the zygomycetes can certainly mimic each other morphologically. In contrast to *Aspergillus*, zygomycetes have broad, ribbon-like, pauciseptate hyphae with irregular walls, which branch randomly at various angles (Fig. 16.12). *Fusarium*, an emerging filamentous fungal pathogen that is also associated with neutropenia, also closely mimics aspergillosis both clinically and radiographically, and is indistinguishable from *Aspergillus* on morphologic grounds alone.

As mentioned previously, fungal stains should be strongly considered in any immunocompromised patient with ischemic lesions of the gastrointestinal tract, particularly ischemic lesions of the stomach; because of its rich blood supply, the stomach is not usually affected by ischemia due to atherosclerosis.

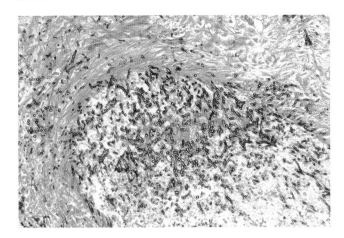

Fig. 16.6 *Aspergillus* occlude a large vessel and extend outward from it. Note parallel walls and branching at acute angles (GMS stain)

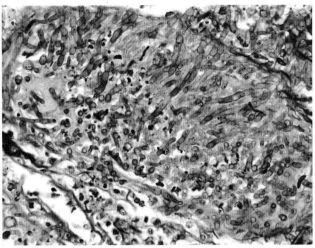

Fig. 16.8 High-power view of *Aspergillus* occluding a mucosal vessel. Note septate hyphae and branching at acute angles (GMS stain)

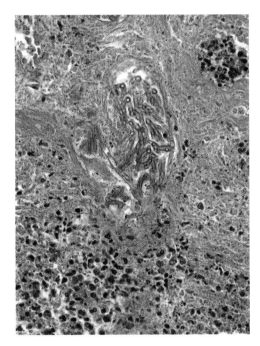

Fig. 16.7 Small gastric vessel filled with *Aspergillus*, with surrounding neutrophilic infiltrate and necrotic debris

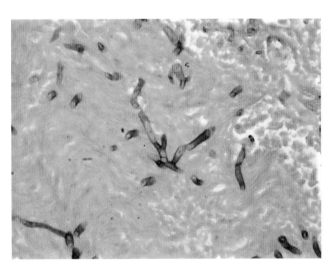

Fig. 16.9 High-power photomicrograph of *Aspergillus* illustrating filamentous fungi with parallel walls, septate hyphae, and branching at acute angles (GMS stain)

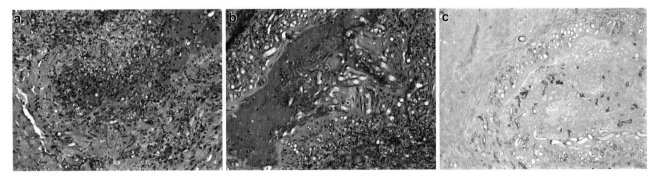

Fig. 16.10 *Mucor* within a large submucosal vessel (**a**). Higher power view showing the typical ribbon-like hyphae of *Mucor* invading the vessel wall (**b**). GMS stain demonstrates characteristic organisms in and around a large submucosal vessel. (Courtesy Dr. Neriman Gokden)

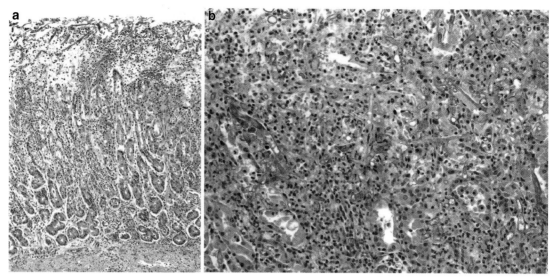

Fig. 16.11 Numerous zygomycetes are present within the gastric mucosa of a patient with an indwelling feeding tube, surrounded by a neutrophilic infiltrate (**a**). Higher power view showing the zygomycetes invading the mucosa and small vessels (**b**). (Courtesy Dr. Owen Middleton)

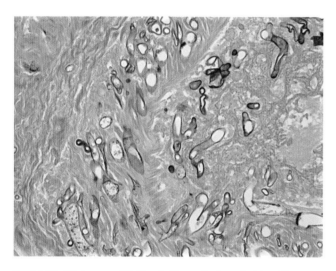

Fig. 16.12 High-power GMS stain illustrating broad, ribbon-like, pauciseptate hyphae with irregular walls branching randomly at various angles that are characteristic of the zygomycetes

Selected References

1. Chandler FW, Watts JC: Pathologic Diagnosis of Fungal Infections. Chicago, IL: ASCP Press, 1987.
2. Cohen R, Heffner JE. Bowel infarction as the initial manifestation of disseminated aspergillosis. Chest 101:877–9, 1992.
3. Dictar MO, Maiolo E, Alexander B, et al. Mycoses in the transplanted patient. Med Mycol 38(Suppl 1):251–8, 2000.
4. Ellis M. Invasive fungal infections: evolving challenges for diagnosis and therapeutics. Mol Immunol 38:947–57, 2001.
5. Fleming RV, Walsh TJ, Anaissie EJ. Emerging and less common fungal pathogens. Infect Dis Clin North Am 16:915–33, 2002.
6. Gonzalez CE, Rinaldi MG, Sugar AM. Zygomycosis. Infect Dis Clin North Am 16:895–914, 2002.
7. Hosseini M, Lee J. Gastrointestinal mucormycosis mimicking ischemic colitis in a patient with systemic lupus erythematosus. Am J Gastroenterol 93:1360–2, 1998.
8. Kaufman L. Immunohistologic diagnosis of systemic mycoses: an update. Eur J Epidemiol 8:377–92, 1992.
9. Kahn LB. Gastric mucormycosis: report of a case with a review of the literature. S Afr Med J 37(December 14):1265–9, 1963.
10. Kullberg BJ, Oude Lashof AM. Epidemiology of opportunistic invasive mycoses. Eur J Med Res 7:183–91, 2002.
11. Lyon DT, Schubert TT, Mantia AG. Phycomycosis of the gastrointestinal tract. Am J Gastroenterol 72:379–94, 1979.
12. Martino P, Gastaldi R, Raccah R, Girmenia C. Clinical patterns of *Fusarium* infections in immunocompromised patients. J Infection 28(Suppl 1):7–15, 1994.
13. Phillips P, Weiner MH. Invasive aspergillosis diagnosed by immunohistochemistry with monoclonal and polyclonal reagents. Hum Pathol 18:1015–24, 1987.
14. Prescott RJ, Harris M, Banerjee SS. Fungal infections of the small and large intestine. J Clin Pathol 45:806–11, 1992.
15. Schwesinger G, Junghans D, Schroder G, et al. Candidosis and aspergillosis as autopsy findings from 1994 to 2003. Mycoses 48:176–80, 2005.
16. Smith JMB. Mycoses of the alimentary tract. Gut 10:1035–40, 1969.
17. Thomson SR, Bade PG, Taams M, Chrystal V. Gastrointestinal mucormycosis. Brit J Surg 78:952–4, 1991.
18. Walsh TJ, Merz WG. Pathologic features in the human alimentary tract associated with invasiveness of *Candida tropicalis*. Am J Clin Pathol 85:498–502, 1986.
19. Washburn RG, Bennett JE. Deep Mycoses. In: Blaser MJ, Smith PD, Ravdin JI, et al. (eds): Infections of the Gastrointestinal Tract. New York: Raven Press, 1995, pp. 957–66.
20. Young RC, Bennett JE, Vogel CL, et al. Aspergillosis: the spectrum of the disease in 98 patients. Medicine 49:147–73, 1970.

Chapter 17

Histoplasmosis

Keywords *Histoplasma capsulatum* • Histoplasmosis • Budding yeast • Intracellular • Disseminated fungal infection

Histoplasma capsulatum var. capsulatum is endemic to the central United States, especially within the Ohio, Missouri, and Mississippi river valleys; other endemic areas in the Western hemisphere include Mexico, Guatemala, Peru, and Venezuela. Histoplasmosis has been reported in many non-endemic areas as well. It is most plentiful in soil enriched by avian or bat droppings. It has a marked affinity for dissemination through the mononuclear phagocyte system, and gastrointestinal involvement occurs in more than 80% of patients with disseminated infection. Isolated gastrointestinal histoplasmosis has been reported rarely. Although most patients with disseminated histoplasmosis are immunocompromised, dissemination can occur in apparently immunocompetent hosts. Of note, it is the most common endemic mycosis in patients with AIDS. Histoplasmosis has also been described in association with infliximab therapy, an anti-tumor necrosis factor alpha drug used in the treatment of Crohn's disease and rheumatoid arthritis.

Patients may initially present with signs and symptoms of gastrointestinal illness and do not always have concomitant pulmonary involvement. Notable presenting gastrointestinal symptoms include diarrhea, gastrointestinal bleeding, abdominal pain, dysphagia, nausea, vomiting, weight loss, and signs of small bowel obstruction. The majority of patients are febrile, and many have had symptoms for weeks to months. Gastrointestinal bleeding and anorectal disease are more common in patients with AIDS and other immunocompromising conditions.

Pathologic features. The ileum is the most common site of involvement, followed by colon, stomach, and esophagus; any portion of the gastrointestinal tract may be involved. Associated lymphadenopathy is common. The esophagus may also be impinged upon by mediastinal lymphadenopathy secondary to histoplasmosis or by *Histoplasma*-associated mediastinal fibrosis. Ulcers are the most common gross lesion; they are often multiple, with annular raised borders, associated hemorrhage, and necrosis at the base

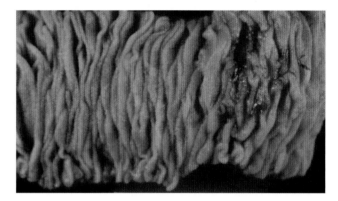

Fig. 17.1 Cecal ulcer secondary to histoplasmosis, with rolled edges and hemorrhagic, necrotic base

(Fig. 17.1). Nodules (often centered on lymphoid aggregates) and obstructive masses or strictures are also common (Figs. 17.2 and 17.3). Often, a combination of lesions is present.

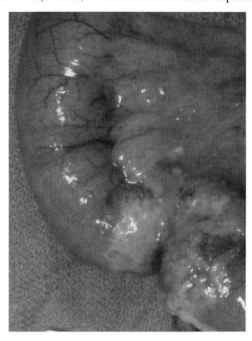

Fig. 17.2 Ileal stricture in an AIDS patient due to histoplasmosis; note extension of the lesion into the mesentery

L.W. Lamps, *Surgical Pathology of the Gastrointestinal System: Bacterial, Fungal, Viral, and Parasitic Infections*, DOI 10.1007/978-1-4419-0861-2_17, © Springer Science+Business Media, LLC 2009

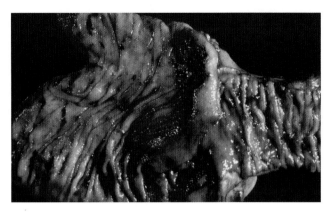

Fig. 17.3 Obstructive "histoplasmoma" at the ileocecal valve. (Courtesy Dr. David Walker)

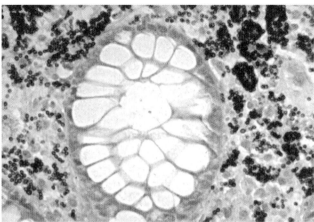

Fig. 17.5 GMS stain shows innumerable intracellular *Histoplasma* within the histiocytes of the lamina propria in a colon biopsy. (Courtesy Dr. Patrick Dean)

Histologic findings include diffuse lymphohistiocytic infiltrates (Figs. 17.4 and 17.5) and nodules (Figs. 17.6, 17.7, 17.8, and 17.9), usually involving the mucosa and submucosa, with associated overlying ulceration. In addition to histiocytes and lymphocytes, there may be numerous associated eosinophils, neutrophils, and plasma cells. These lesions are usually associated with Peyer's patches (Fig. 17.9). Nonspecific ulceration and inflammation with numerous organisms present in the bowel wall also may be seen (Figs. 17.10 and 17.11). Discrete granulomas and giant cells are

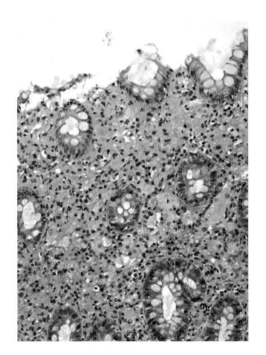

Fig. 17.4 The lamina propria of the colon is expanded by a diffuse histiocytic infiltrate with accompanying plasma cells and lymphocytes. The histiocytes contain numerous *Histoplasma*. (Courtesy Dr. Maria Porter)

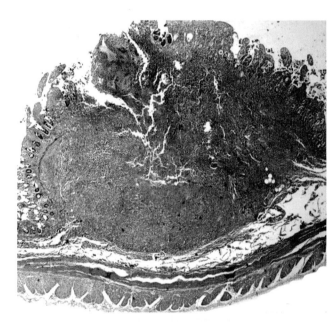

Fig. 17.6 A lymphohistiocytic nodule centered on a Peyer's patch in the small bowel, with overlying ulceration (H&E/methenamine silver stain)

present in only a minority of cases (Figs. 17.12 and 17.13). In contrast to gastrointestinal lesions, abdominal lymph nodes often show necrotizing granulomas (Figs. 17.14 and 17.15). In immunocompromised patients or very young children, macroscopic findings may be normal, and large numbers of organisms may be seen with virtually no tissue reaction histologically (Fig. 17.16). Occasionally, the histiocytic infiltrate associated with small bowel histoplasmosis may mimic Whipple's disease (Fig. 17.17).

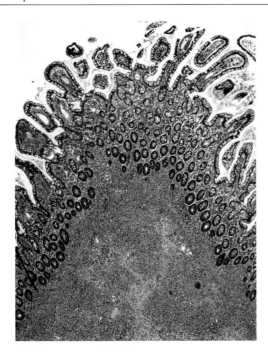

Fig. 17.7 Submucosal lymphohistiocytic nodule in the ileum of an AIDS patient

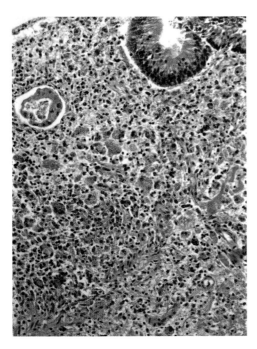

Fig. 17.8 High-power view of an ulcerated lymphohistiocytic nodule in the small bowel, with numerous *Histoplasma* visible within macrophages

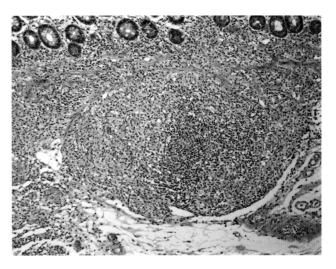

Fig. 17.9 Lymphohistiocytic infiltration of a Peyer's patch in the ileum in an AIDS patient with histoplasmosis

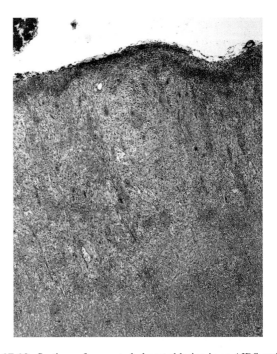

Fig. 17.10 Sections of a resected ulcerated lesion in an AIDS patient with a small bowel stricture secondary to histoplasmosis

Morphologic features of the organism. Histoplasma organisms are small (2–5 μm), ovoid, usually intracellular yeast forms with single small buds at the more pointed pole (Figs. 17.18 and 17.19). Multiple organisms are often clustered within a macrophage (Fig. 17.20). On H&E staining, organisms have a surrounding "halo," reflecting the thin, poorly stained cell wall in contrast to the basophilic cytoplasm (Fig. 17.21). Organisms stain with GMS and PAS stains.

Several other laboratory methods are available for diagnosing histoplasmosis. Fungal cultures are definitive, but are not useful for rapid diagnosis. Histoplasmin skin testing and serologic tests may be useful in immunocompetent adults, but are unreliable in immunocompromised patients, young

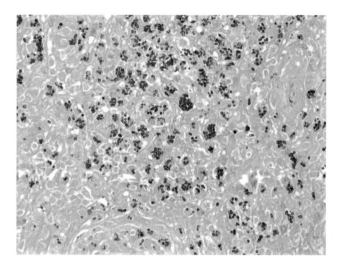

Fig. 17.11 GMS stain revealed numerous *Histoplasma*, even though the features of the ulcer were very non-specific

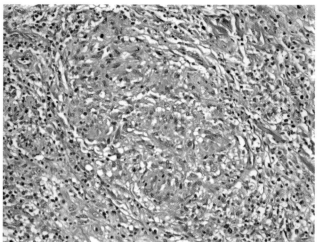

Fig. 17.13 Well-formed granulomas are seen in a minority of cases of gastrointestinal histoplasmosis

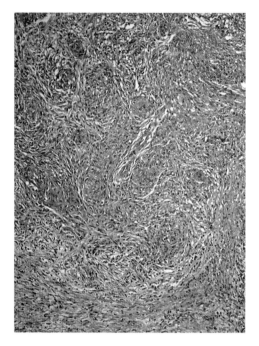

Fig. 17.12 Loosely formed epithelioid granulomas are present in the wall of a stricture secondary to histoplasmosis

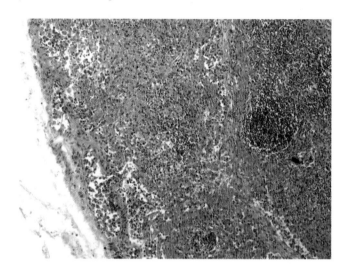

Fig. 17.14 Necrotizing granulomatous inflammation within a mesenteric lymph node

children, elderly patients, and those with disseminated disease. Urine antigen detection may be helpful.

Differential diagnosis. The differential diagnosis for the inflammatory lesions of histoplasmosis includes idiopathic inflammatory bowel disease, sarcoidosis, and other infections. Obstructive masses may clinically mimic neoplasia as well. Special stains should easily identify organisms.

Other organisms that should be distinguished from *H. capsulatum* (see Table 14.1) include *Pneumocystis carinii*, which lacks buds, is extracellular, and has a characteris-

tic internal structure and a different inflammatory reaction (see Chapter 18); *Cryptococcus neoformans*, which is more variable in size than the uniformly small *H. capsulatum*, and has a mucicarmine and Fontana-Masson positive capsule (see Chapter 18); Blastomyces, which are much larger and have broad-based buds; and *Leishmania*, which have a characteristic kinetoplast and are GMS negative. *Candida* (or *Torulopsis) glabrata* may be the most difficult to distinguish from *H. capsulatum*, as they are similarly sized; however, *C. glabrata* are slightly larger, have more frequent buds, and are often extracellular (Fig. 17.22). In addition, they lack the "halo" effect that *H. capsulatum* has in tissue sections. *Penicillium marneffei*, an emerging pathogen primarily affecting HIV-infected patients living or traveling in Southeast Asia, also mimics histoplasmosis both clinically and morphologically. However, *P. marneffei* has a single, centrally located transverse septum (Fig. 17.23), and extracellular organisms become elongated and sausage-shaped. Erythrocytes and naked cell nuclei may mimic *Histoplasma* in sections over-stained with GMS; comparison with H&E slides often helps to resolve this.

Selected References

1. Assi M, McKinsey DS, Driks MR, et al. Gastrointestinal histo-plasmosis in the acquired immunodeficiency syndrome: report of 18 cases and literature review. Diag Microbiol Infect Dis 55:195–201, 2006.
2. Cappell MS, Mandell W, Grimes MM, et al. Gastrointestinal histo-plasmosis. Dig Dis Sci 33:353–60, 1988.
3. Chandler FW, Watts JC. Histoplasmosis capsulati. In: Pathologic Diagnosis of Fungal Infections. Chicago, IL: ASCP Press, 1987, pp 123–39.
4. Cooper CR, McGinnis MR. Pathology of *Penicillium marneffei*: an emerging acquired immunodeficiency syndrome-related pathogen. Arch Pathol Lab Med 121:798–804, 1997.
5. Fleming RV, Walsh TJ, Anaissie EJ. Emerging and less common fungal pathogens. Infect Dis Clin North Am 16:915–33, 2002.
6. Goodwin RA, Des Prez RM. Histoplasmosis. Am Rev Respir Dis 117:929–55, 1978.
7. Goodwin RA, Shapiro JL, Thurman GH, et al. Disseminated histo-plasmosis: clinical and pathological correlations. Medicine 59:1–33, 1980.
8. Goodwin RA, Loyd JE, Des Prez RM. Histoplasmosis in normal hosts. Medicine 60:231–66, 1981.
9. Jain S, Koirala J, Castro-Pavia F. Isolated gastrointestinal histo-plasmosis: case report and review of the literature. South Med J 97:172–4, 2004.
10. Kahi CJ, Wheat LJ, Allen SD, Sarosi GA. Gastrointestinal histo-plasmosis. Am J Gastroenterol 100:220–31, 2005.
11. Lamps LW, Molina CP, West AB, et al. The pathologic spectrum of gastrointestinal and hepatic histoplasmosis. Am J Clin Pathol 113:64–72, 2000.
12. Lee JT, Dixon MR, Murrell Z, et al. Colonic histoplasmosis pre-senting as colon cancer in the nonimmunocompromised patient:

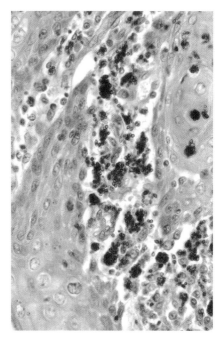

Fig. 17.16 Numerous *Histoplasma* are seen within histiocytes in the esophagus of a patient with disseminated histoplasmosis, with virtually no attendant inflammatory infiltrate (H&E/methenamine silver stain)

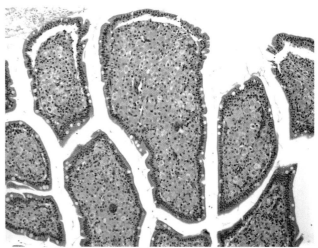

Fig. 17.17 Occasionally, the histiocytic infiltrate associated with histo-plamsosis can mimic Whipple's disease in the small bowel

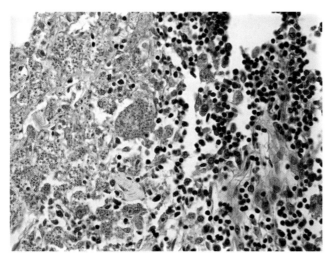

Fig. 17.15 High-power view showing collections of macrophages con-taining *Histoplasma* in a mesenteric node

report of a case and review of the literature. Am Surg 70:959–63, 2004.
13. Shull HJ. Human histoplasmosis: a disease with protean mani-festations, often with digestive system involvement. Gastroenterol 25:582–95, 1953.
14. Soper RT, Silber DL, Holcomb GW. Gastrointestinal histoplasmo-sis in children. J Pediatr Surg 5:32–9, 1970.
15. Suh KN, Anekthananon T, Mariuz PR. Gastrointestinal histoplas-mosis in patients with AIDS: case report and review. Clin Infect Dis 32:483–91, 2001.

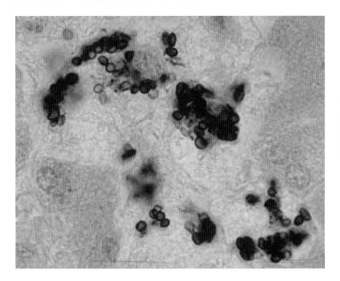

Fig. 17.18 *Histoplasma* form narrow-based buds at the more pointed pole (GMS stain; courtesy Dr. Brian West)

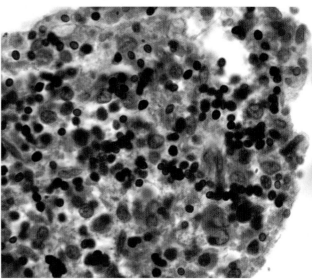

Fig. 17.20 Many *Histoplasma* are often present within individual macrophages

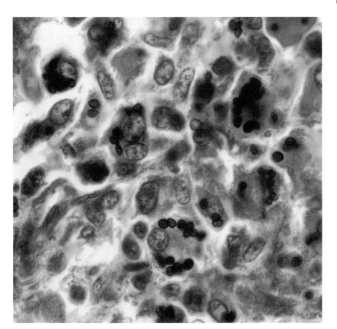

Fig. 17.19 *Histoplasma* are intracellular and uniformly small at 2–5 μm (H&E/methenamine silver)

16. Sunanda K, Brasitus T. *Histoplasmosis capsulatum* as a cause of lower gastrointestinal bleeding in common variable immunodeficiency. Dig Dis Sci 45:2133–5, 2000.
17. Wheat J, French MLV, Kohler RB, et al. The diagnostic laboratory tests for histoplasmosis. Ann Intern Med 97:680–5, 1982.

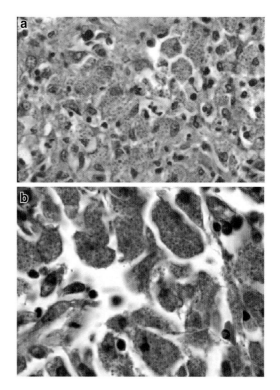

Fig. 17.21 a and **b:** On H&E staining, organisms have a surrounding "halo," reflecting the thin, poorly stained cell wall in contrast to the basophilic cytoplasm. (Courtesy Dr. Rodger C. Haggitt)

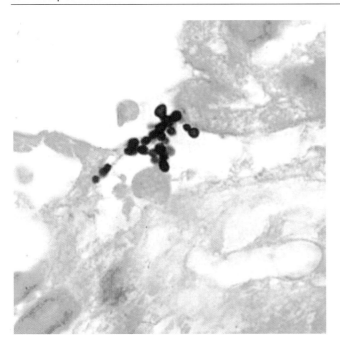

Fig. 17.22 *Candida (Torulopsis) glabrata* may be difficult to distinguish from *H. capsulatum*, as they are similarly sized; however, *C. glabrata* are slightly larger, have more frequent buds, and are often extracellular

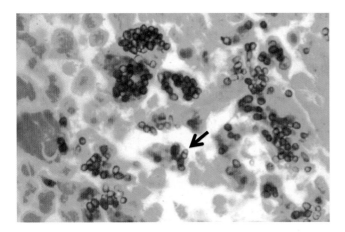

Fig. 17.23 *P. marneffei* mimics histoplasmosis both clinically and histologically, but has a central transverse septum. (Courtesy Dr. David Walker)

Chapter 18

Cryptococcus neoformans

Keywords *Cryptococcus neoformans* • AIDS • Mucicarmine • Pleomorphic yeast

This fungus is a rare but important cause of gastrointestinal infection. Virtually all patients with gastrointestinal cryptococcosis have hematogenously disseminated disease with multisystem organ involvement, and most have associated pulmonary and meningeal disease. Cryptococcosis is associated with AIDS as well as other immunosuppressive states.

Pathologic features. Grossly, cryptococcal infection may be located anywhere in the gastrointestinal tract; the colon is the most frequently involved site, followed by the esophagus. Endoscopic lesions include nodules and ulcers, sometimes associated with thick white exudates. However, the mucosa is normal in many cases, even when deeply invasive organisms are present, as the organisms are often located within lymphatics. Inflammatory polypoid masses have been described rarely.

Histologically, the inflammatory reaction is variable and depends on the immune status of the host, ranging from a suppurative, necrotizing inflammatory reaction, often with granulomatous features (Fig. 18.1), to virtually no reaction in anergic hosts (Fig. 18.2). Both superficial and deep involvement may occur, and lymphatic involvement is common. Fungal cells are surrounded by optimally clear, smooth "halos" that represent the unstained or weakly stained capsules, and impart a "soap bubble" appearance (Fig. 18.3).

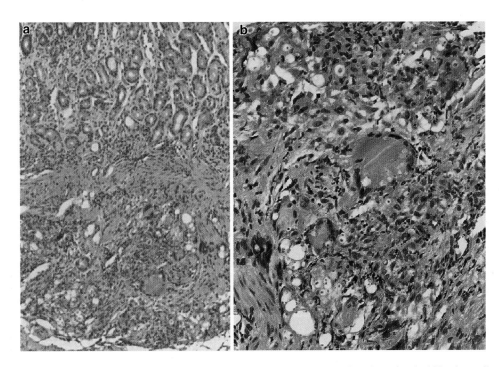

Fig. 18.1 Submucosal granulomas due to *Cryptococcus* in a gastric biopsy (**a**). Higher power view shows fungi within giant cells, with surrounding clear "halos" (**b**). (Courtesy Dr. Kay Washington)

L.W. Lamps, *Surgical Pathology of the Gastrointestinal System: Bacterial, Fungal, Viral, and Parasitic Infections*,
DOI 10.1007/978-1-4419-0861-2_18, © Springer Science+Business Media, LLC 2009

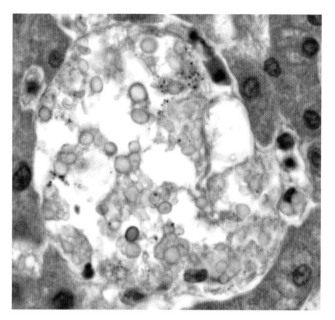

Fig. 18.2 Capsule-deficient *Cryptococci* distend a lymphatic, with virtually no attendant inflammatory reaction. Note rare mucin-positive organisms (mucicarmine stain)

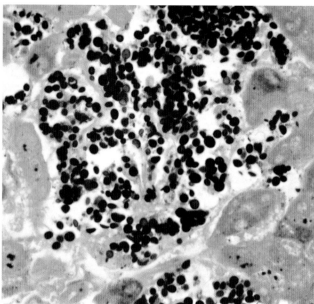

Fig. 18.4 High-power GMS stain illustrates the narrow-based budding and marked pleomorphism in size characteristic of cryptococcosis

Morphologic features of the organism. Yeast forms measure on average 4–7 μm and are highly pleomorphic in size. The yeast forms are round-to-oval with narrow-based buds. Occasionally, they produce hyphae and pseudohyphae. The mucopolysaccharide capsule stains with GMS, Alcian blue, mucicarmine, Fontana-Masson, and colloidal iron (Figs. 18.4 and 18.5). Unfortunately, capsule-deficient cryptococci may

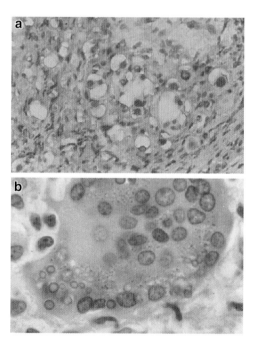

Fig. 18.5 *Cryptococci* routinely stain strongly with mucicarmine staining. Note "soap-bubble" appearance around organisms (**a**, courtesy Dr. Kay Washington). High-power mucicarmine stain showing *Cryptococci* within a giant cell (**b**, courtesy Dr. George F. Gray, Jr)

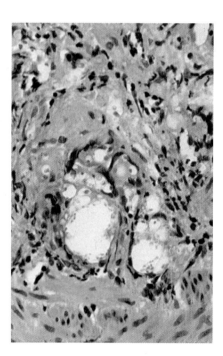

Fig. 18.3 *Cryptococci* are surrounded by optimally clear, smooth "halos" that represent the unstained or weakly stained capsules, and impart a "soap bubble" appearance. (Courtesy Dr. Kay Washington)

pose a diagnostic challenge, but most have sufficient capsular material to be at least focally appreciated on mucin stains (Fig. 18.6).

Differential diagnosis. The differential diagnosis primarily includes other dimorphic fungi (see Table 14.1). Blastomycosis, which rarely infects the gastrointestinal tract, may

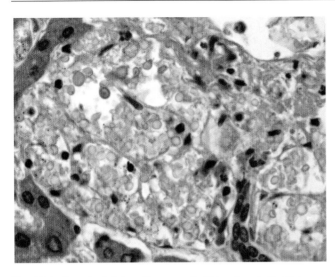

Fig. 18.6 Capsule-deficient *Cryptococci* within a lymphatic. Note rare mucin-positive organisms (mucicarmine stain)

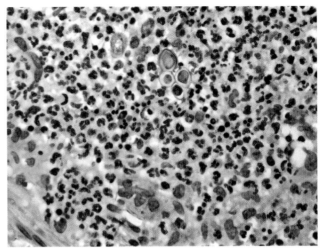

Fig. 18.8 Multiple nuclei, broad-based budding, and double-contoured walls are features of *B. dermatididis* (PAS stain). (Courtesy Dr. Bruce Smoller)

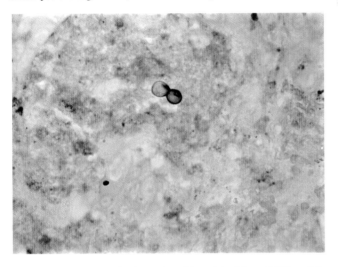

Fig. 18.7 Blastomycosis. Note broad-based budding (GMS stain). (Courtesy Dr. Bruce Smoller)

show some variation in size, and occasionally stains with mucicarmine. However, it has broad-based buds (Figs. 18.7 and 18.8) and is multinucleate (Fig. 18.8). Cryptococci are on average smaller, more pleomorphic in size, and have narrow-based buds. *Histoplasma* are uniformly small and do not stain with mucicarmine.

Selected References

1. Bonacini M, Nussbaum J, Ahluwalia C. Gastrointestinal, hepatic, and pancreatic involvement with *Cryptococcus neoformans* in AIDS. J Clin Gastroenterol 12:295–7, 1990.
2. Chalasani N, Wilcox CM, Hunter HT, et al. Endoscopic features of gastroduodenal cryptococcosis in AIDS. Gastrointest Endosc 45:315–7, 1995.
3. Chandler FW, Watts JC: Pathologic Diagnosis of Fungal Infections. Chicago, IL: ASCP Press, 1987.
4. Chandler FW, Watts JC. Cryptococcosis. In: Conner DH, Chandler FW: Pathology of Infectious Diseases. Stamford, CT: Appleton and Lange, 1997, pp. 989–97.
5. Daly JS, Porter KA, Chong FK, Robillard RJ. Disseminated, nonmeningeal gastrointestinal cryptococcal infection in an HIV-negative patient. Am J Gastroenterol 85:1421–4, 1990.
6. Hutto JO, Bryan CS, Greene FL, et al. Cryptococcosis of the colon resembling Crohn's disease in a patient with the hyperimmunoglobulinemia E-recurrent infection (Job's) syndrome. Gastroenterol 94:808–12, 1988.
7. Jacobs DH, Macher AM, Handler R, et al. Esophageal cryptococcosis in a patient with the hyperimmunoglobulin E-recurrent infection (Job's) syndrome. Gastroenterol 87:201–3, 1984.
8. Kovacs JA, Dovacs AA, Polis M, et al. Cryptococcosis in the acquired immunodeficiency syndrome. Ann Intern Med 103:533–8, 1985.
9. Lazcano O, Speights VO Jr., Strickler JG, et al. Combined histochemical stains in the differential diagnosis of *Cryptococcus neoformans*. Mod Pathol 6:80–4, 1993.
10. Melato M, Gorji N. Primary intestinal cryptococcosis mimicking adenomatous polyp in an HIV-negative patient. Am J Gastroenterol 93:1592–3, 1998.
11. Schwarz J. The diagnosis of deep mycoses by morphologic methods. Hum Pathol 13:519–33, 1982.
12. Unat EK, Pars B, Kosyak JP. A case of cryptococcosis of the colon. Br Med J Nov 19:1501–2, 1960.
13. Washington K, Gottfried MR, Wilson ML. Gastrointestinal cryptococcosis. Mod Pathol 4: 707–11, 1991.
14. Washburn RG, Bennett JE. Deep Mycoses. In: Blaser MJ, Smith PD, Ravdin JI, et al. Infections of the Gastrointestinal Tract. New York: Raven Press, 1995, pp. 957–66.

Chapter 19

Pneumocystis carinii

Keywords *Pneumocystis carinii* • AIDS • Foamy exudate

Pneumocystis carinii pneumonia is a major cause of morbidity in the AIDS population, and extrapulmonary (including gastrointestinal) involvement is not uncommon. In addition to patients with AIDS, *Pneumocystis* infection rarely has been reported in the context of organ transplant, hematologic malignancy, other immunodeficiency states, and steroid therapy. *Pneumocystis* infection has also been reported in association with infliximab therapy, an immunosuppressive treatment for Crohn's disease and rheumatoid arthritis. Risk factors for extrapulmonary infection include severe underlying immunodeficiency, overwhelming pulmonary infection, and aerosolized pentamindine prophylaxis for *Pneumocystis* pneumonia. Although the life cycle of this organism more closely resembles that of a protozoan, there is convincing molecular evidence that *P. carinii* has greater homology with fungi.

Pathologic features. Macroscopically, *P. carinii* infection produces a non-specific, often erosive, esophagogastritis or colitis, occasionally with small polypoid nodules. Any portion of the gastrointestinal tract may be involved. Microscopically, granular, foamy eosinophilic casts identical to those seen in pulmonary disease, and often referred to as "honeycomb exudates," may be seen within mucosal vessels or within the lamina propria (Figs. 19.1, 19.2, 19.3, 19.4, 19.5, and 19.6). Mesenteric lymph nodes may also be involved (Fig. 19.7). As in the lung, a wide variety of inflammatory responses may occur, including granulomatous inflammation, prominent macrophage infiltrates, and necrosis. However, because granulomatous reactions are rare with *Pneumocystis*, concurrent pathogens should be excluded when granulomas are seen. The organisms are 5–7 μm spherules

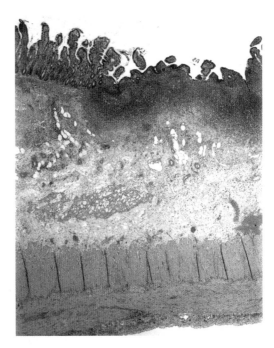

Fig. 19.1 The submucosa is expanded by the characteristic foamy "honeycomb" exudates of *Pneumocystis* in this resection from an AIDS patient. (Courtesy Dr. Henry Appelman)

that have cup or crescent shapes when collapsed (Figs. 19.8 and 19.9). Many contain characteristic single or paired comma-shaped internal structures. Organisms stain with GMS and toluidine blue.

Pneumocystis can usually be correctly classified in tissue sections based on morphologic criteria and the characteristic foamy casts. The differential diagnosis primarily includes other infectious processes (see Table 14.1).

L.W. Lamps, *Surgical Pathology of the Gastrointestinal System: Bacterial, Fungal, Viral, and Parasitic Infections*,
DOI 10.1007/978-1-4419-0861-2_19, © Springer Science+Business Media, LLC 2009

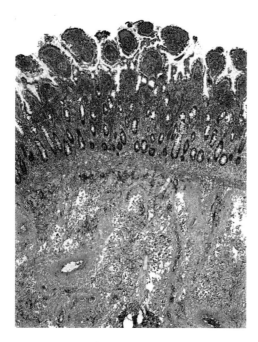

Fig. 19.2 Foamy exudate fills the submucosa in this case of gastrointestinal *Pneumocystis*. (Courtesy Dr. Henry Appelman)

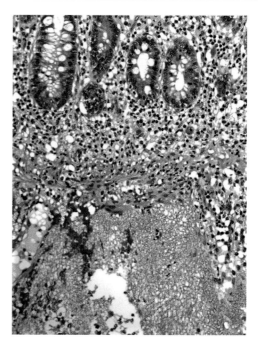

Fig. 19.4 High-power view of submucosal "honeycomb" exudates, with overlying neutrophilic infiltrate in the mucosa. (Courtesy Dr. Henry Appelman)

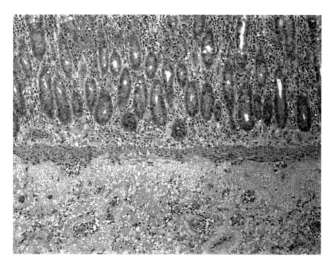

Fig. 19.3 Higher power view of foamy exudates of *Pneumocystis* within the submucosa. The overlying mucosa shows a neutrophilic inflammatory exudates. (Courtesy Dr. Henry Appelman)

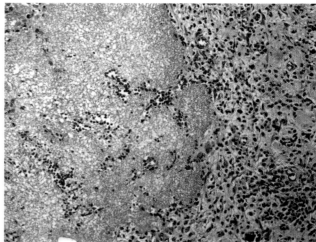

Fig. 19.5 The foamy exudates extend into the lamina propria, where they are surrounded by neutrophils and macrophages. (Courtesy Dr. Henry Appelman)

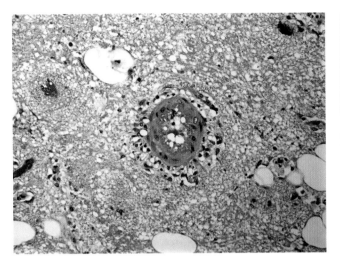

Fig. 19.6 Submucosal vessel completely surrounded by "honeycomb" exudates, with no other significant inflammatory infiltrate. (Courtesy Dr. Henry Appelman)

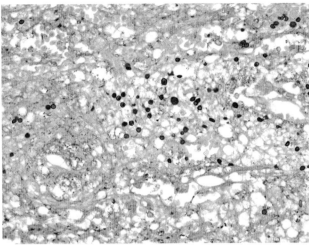

Fig. 19.8 GMS stain shows numerous organisms characteristic of *Pneumocystis carinii* within the exudates. (Courtesy Dr. Henry Appelman)

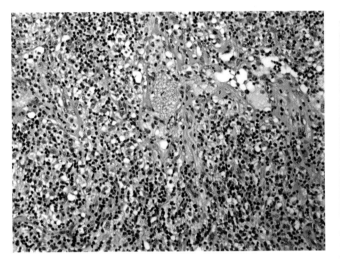

Fig. 19.7 A mesenteric lymph node is focally involved by the characteristic exudates of *Pneumocystis* infection. (Courtesy Dr. Henry Appelman)

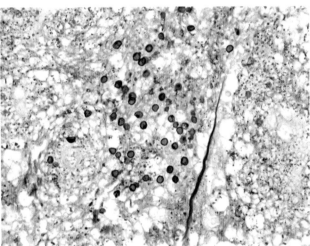

Fig. 19.9 High-power GMS stain shows 5–7 μm spherules that have cup or crescent shapes when collapsed, as well as characteristic single or paired comma-shaped internal structures. (Courtesy Dr. Henry Appelman)

Selected References

1. Chandler FW, Watts JC: Pathologic Diagnosis of Fungal Infections. Chicago, IL: ASCP Press, 1987.
2. DeRoux SJ, Adsay V, Ioachim HL. Disseminated pneumocystosis without pulmonary involvement during prophylactic aerosolized pentamidine therapy in a patient with the acquired immunodeficiency syndrome. Arc Pathol Lab Med 115:1137–40, 1991.
3. Dieterich DT, Lew EA, Bacon DJ, Pearlman KI, Scholes JV. Gastrointestinal pneumocystosis in HIV-infected patients on aerosolized pentamidine: report of five cases and review of the literature. Am J Gastroenterol 87:1763–70, 1992.
4. Gal AA, Koss MN, Strigle S, Angritt P. *Pneumocystis carinii* infection in the acquired immunodeficiency syndrome. Sem Diagn Pathol 6:287–99, 1989.
5. Hardy WD, Northfelt DW, Drake TA. Fatal, disseminated pneumocystosis in a patient with acquired immunodeficiency syndrome receiving prophylactic aerosolized pentamidine. Am J Med 87:329–31, 1989.
6. Kaur N, Mahl TC. *Pneumocystis jiroveci (carinii)* pneumonia after infliximab therapy: a review of 84 cases. Dig Dis Sci 52:1481–4, 2007.
7. Looney WJ, Windsor JJ. *Pneumocystis carinii* infection in human immunodeficiency virus-positive patients. Brit J Biomed Sci 56:39–48, 1999.
8. Telzak EE, Cote RJ, Gold JWM, et al. Extrapulmonary *Pneumocystis carinii* infections. Rev Infect Dis 12:380–6, 1990.
9. Watts JC, Chandler FW. Pneumocystosis. In: Conner DH, Chandler FW (eds): Pathology of Infectious Diseases. Stamford, CT: Appleton and Lange, 1997, pp. 1241–1251.
10. Watts JC, Chandler FW. Evolving concepts of infection by *Pneumocystis carinii*. Pathol Annu 26(part 1):93–138, 1991.

Part III
Viral Infections of the Gastrointestinal Tract

Abstract Viral infections of the gastrointestinal tract are an important cause of morbidity and mortality in immunocompromised patients and are also one of the most common causes of childhood illness worldwide. Tissue biopsy of the gastrointestinal tract is a valuable tool for the diagnosis of viral infection. This section addresses common and uncommon viral infections affecting the gastrointestinal tract, including clinical setting, macroscopic and histologic features, differential diagnoses, and useful laboratory tests that can aid in diagnosis.

Chapter 20

Cytomegalovirus

Keywords Cytomegalovirus • Inclusion • Immunocompromise • Transplant • Immunohistochemistry

Cytomegalovirus (CMV) is best known as an opportunistic pathogen in the context of a suppressed immune system; this includes patients with AIDS and other immunodeficiency disorders, solid organ and bone marrow transplant patients, those taking chronic immunosuppressive medications, and those with underlying malignancies. CMV is the most common gastrointestinal pathogen overall in patients with AIDS, and infection can develop anywhere in the gastrointestinal tract from mouth to anus. Symptoms vary with the immune status of the patient and the site of infection; the most common clinical symptoms of gastrointestinal infection are diarrhea (either bloody or watery), abdominal pain, fever, and weight loss. Patients with esophageal infection often have dysphagia and odynophagia.

Primary CMV infections in immunocompetent persons are generally asymptomatic. When symptomatic disease does occur, it is usually self-limited and may manifest as a mononucleosis-like syndrome of fever, myalgias, sore throat, rash, adenopathy, and hepatosplenomegaly. In most of these cases, gastrointestinal involvement is asymptomatic. Symptomatic gastrointestinal infection has been reported occasionally in immunocompetent patients, although many of these were elderly and/or were eventually found to have underlying malignancies or hematologic disorders, and thus may not have had entirely competent immune systems.

Pathologic features. CMV causes a remarkable variety of gross lesions. Ulceration is the most common; ulcers may be single or multiple and either superficial or deep. They may be very large (greater than 10.0 cm) and often have a well-circumscribed, "punched-out" appearance with intervening normal mucosa. Segmental ulcerative lesions and linear ulcers may mimic Crohn's disease grossly (Fig. 20.1). Other lesions include mucosal erosion, erythema, hemorrhage, pseudomembranes, and inflammatory polyps or masses (Fig. 20.2).

The histologic spectrum of CMV infection is also variable, ranging from minimal inflammation to deep ulcers

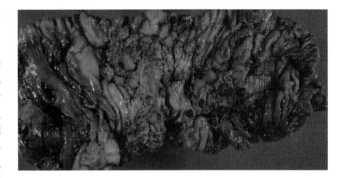

Fig. 20.1 Segmental ulceration mimicking Crohn's disease in a renal transplant patient with CMV colitis

with prominent granulation tissue and necrosis. Frequent histologic features include mucosal ulceration (Fig. 20.3), a mixed inflammatory infiltrate usually including numerous neutrophils, and cryptitis of glandular epithelium (Fig. 20.4). Crypt abscesses, crypt atrophy and loss, and numerous apoptotic enterocytes may be seen as well (Fig. 20.5). Prominent aggregates of macrophages may be seen surrounding viral inclusions, sometimes in a perivascular distribution within granulation tissue, or within the inflammatory exudate. Characteristic inclusions with virtually no associated inflammatory reaction may occur in severely immunocompromised patients.

Infected cells show both nuclear and cytoplasmic enlargement (Fig. 20.6), hence the name "cytomegalovirus." Characteristic "owl's eye" intranuclear viral inclusions (Fig. 20.7) and basophilic granular intracytoplasmic inclusions (Fig. 20.8) may be seen on routine H&E preparations. Inclusions are preferentially found in endothelial cells (Fig. 20.9), stromal cells (Figs. 20.2 and 20.4), and macrophages, and rarely in glandular epithelial cells (Fig. 20.10). Unlike adenovirus and herpes, CMV inclusions are often found deep within ulcer bases rather than at the edges of ulcers or in the superficial mucosa. Adjacent nuclei may be enlarged, appear smudged, or have a "ground-glass" appearance, but lack typical inclusions. In biopsy specimens, the diagnosis may be easily missed when only rare inclusions are present.

L.W. Lamps, *Surgical Pathology of the Gastrointestinal System: Bacterial, Fungal, Viral, and Parasitic Infections,*
DOI 10.1007/978-1-4419-0861-2_20, © Springer Science+Business Media, LLC 2009

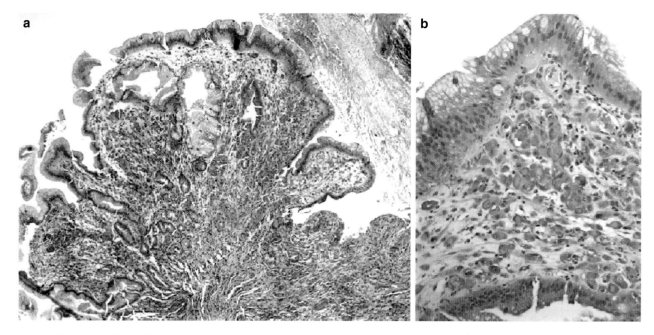

Fig. 20.2 Endoscopically visible inflammatory polyp removed from the gastric antrum of an immunocompromised patient (**a**). Higher power view shows innumerable CMV inclusions within the stroma and endothelial cells, along with a patchy mixed inflammatory exudate (**b**)

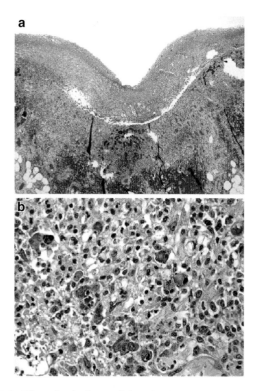

Fig. 20.3 Ulceration in the small bowel of a renal transplant patient (**a**). Numerous CMV inclusions are seen within granulation tissue at the base of the ulcer (**b**)

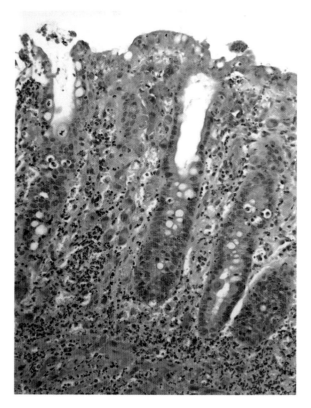

Fig. 20.4 Neutrophilic cryptitis and scattered apoptotic endothelial cells are seen in a case of CMV colitis. Note numerous inclusions within stromal and endothelial cells

CMV can cause several interesting clinicopathologic entities that bear special mention.

Hypertrophic gastropathy. A rare but important entity associated with CMV infection is transient protein-losing hypertrophic gastropathy resembling Menetrier's disease. Most of these cases have been described in pediatric patients and only rarely in adults. Patients have hypertrophic gastric

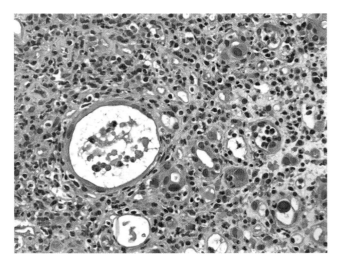

Fig. 20.5 A mixed inflammatory infiltrate and dilated, atrophic crypts containing apoptotic debris are present along with numerous CMV inclusions in a case of CMV colitis

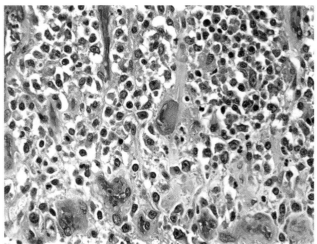

Fig. 20.6 CMV infection causes both nuclear enlargement and enlargement of the entire cell, as illustrated by this endothelial inclusion

rugae (Fig. 20.11), vomiting, and marked protein loss with peripheral edema, ascites, and pleural effusions. Inclusions have been identified within the gastric epithelium in these cases; in addition, CMV has been isolated by viral culture, and some patients have had serologic evidence of acute CMV infection.

Appendicitis. CMV has been described in the appendix with increasing frequency in immunocompromised patients. Patients typically have a longer pre-surgical course than immunocompetent patients with appendicitis, consisting of several weeks of fever, abdominal pain, and diarrhea; tenderness ultimately localizes to the right lower quadrant. Perforation is common. Histologic findings include mucosal ulceration with a transmural mixed inflammatory infiltrate and characteristic inclusions.

Vasculitis. The gastrointestinal tract is one of the most commonly affected organ systems in CMV vasculitis, along

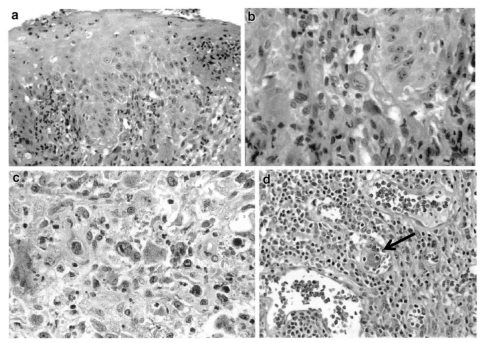

Fig. 20.7 Characteristic "owl's eye" nuclear CMV inclusions. Low-power view of a characteristic inclusion in an endothelial cell in a case of CMV esophagitis (**a**, courtesy Drs. Rodger C. Haggitt and Mary P. Bronner). Higher power view shows cytomegaly and characteristic "owl's eye" morphology (**b**, courtesy Drs. Rodger C. Haggitt and Mary P. Bronner). Characteristic nuclear inclusion in the granulation tissue in the base of an ulcer (**c**). Typical nuclear inclusion within an endothelial cell (**d**)

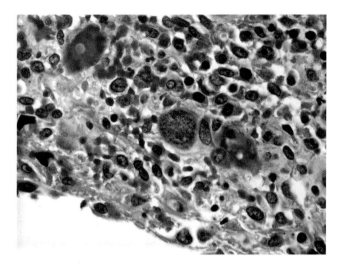

Fig. 20.8 Granular, basophilic cytoplasmic inclusions in the base of an ulcer

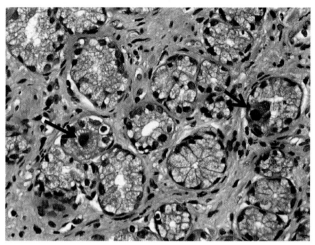

Fig. 20.10 Glandular epithelial inclusions are occasionally seen, as in this case of CMV gastritis in an AIDS patient

with the central nervous system and skin. Histologic findings include endothelial viral inclusions with associated inflammation, necrosis, and thrombosis of the affected vessel (Fig. 20.12). Surrounding tissue shows associated mucosal ulceration, hemorrhage, and ischemic necrosis (Fig. 20.13). CMV inclusions alone within vascular endothelial cells do not necessarily imply vasculitis; associated inflammation of the vessel wall and thrombosis should be present as well.

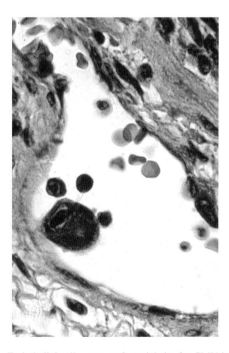

Fig. 20.9 Endothelial cells are a preferential site for CMV inclusions. (Courtesy Dr. Margie Scott)

Secondary CMV infection superimposed on chronic inflammatory bowel disease. Secondary CMV infection may be superimposed on chronic gastrointestinal diseases, particularly ulcerative colitis and Crohn's disease. In such cases, CMV superinfection is associated with exacerbations of the underlying disease, steroid-refractory disease, toxic megacolon, and a higher mortality rate. In fact, some authorities recommend immunohistochemical evaluation for CMV as part of the routine evaluation of biopsies in steroid-refractory chronic idiopathic inflammatory bowel disease patients. In addition, as mentioned above, CMV infection can mimic chronic idiopathic inflammatory bowel disease both grossly and microscopically (Figs. 20.1 and 20.14). The presence of CMV inclusions and acute inflammatory changes superimposed on well-developed features of chronicity, such as architectural distortion or neural hyperplasia (Fig. 20.15), helps to establish a background of chronic idiopathic inflammatory bowel disease with superimposed CMV infection, rather than CMV infection alone.

Bowel dysmotility. CMV infection (as well as several other viruses) has been implicated in some cases of intestinal pseudo-obstruction. Viral inclusions may be seen in ganglion cells, and there may be an inflammatory reaction surrounding ganglia and the myenteric plexus.

Differential Diagnosis. The differential diagnosis of CMV infection is primarily with other viral infections, particularly adenovirus (see Table 20.1). Adenovirus inclusions are usually crescent-shaped, located within surface epithelium, and exclusively intranuclear. CMV inclusions have an "owl's eye" morphology in the nucleus, are generally located within endothelial or stromal cells, and exist within either the nucleus or cytoplasm. As mentioned above, CMV infection can also mimic chronic idiopathic inflammatory bowel disease, ischemia, and other infectious processes.

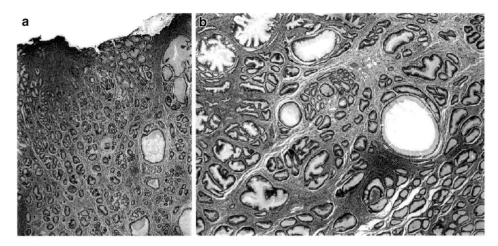

Fig. 20.11 Hypertrophic gastropathy secondary to CMV infection in a child, showing foveolar hyperplasia and cystic dilatation of glands (Courtesy Dr. David Parham)

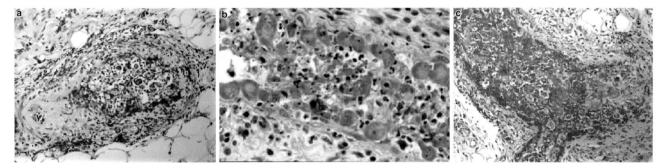

Fig. 20.12 CMV vasculitis causing small bowel ischemia in a renal transplant patient. CMV endothelial inclusions are accompanied by hemorrhage and acute inflammation of the vessel wall (**a**). Many inclusions within endothelial cells, along with acute inflammation and fibrinous debris (**b**, courtesy Dr. Margie Scott). CMV vasculitis with thrombosis (**c**)

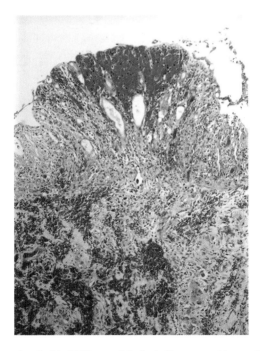

Fig. 20.13 Associated ischemic changes associated with CMV vasculitis, including mucosal hemorrhage, necrosis, and crypt withering

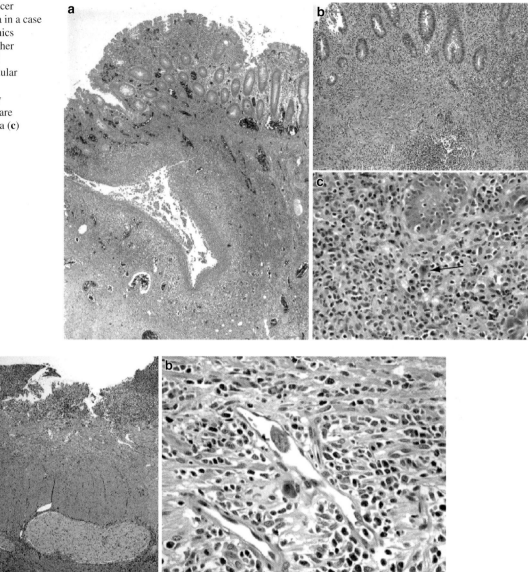

Fig. 20.14 Fissuring ulcer undermining the mucosa in a case of CMV colitis that mimics Crohn's disease (**a**). Higher power view shows basal plasmacytosis and glandular disarray (**b**). Basophilic inclusions, confirmed by immunohistochemistry, are present within the stroma (**c**)

Fig. 20.15 A patient with longstanding Crohn's disease and superimposed CMV infection. Note marked neural hyperplasia in the wall of the bowel (**a**). Characteristic inclusions are seen within the vessels at the base of the ulcers (**b**). (Courtesy Dr. Brian D. Quinn)

Table 20.1 Light microscopic comparison of CMV, adenovirus, and HSV infection

	CMV	Adenovirus	HSV
Cell involved	Stromal and endothelial cells; macrophages; rarely epithelial cells	Epithelial only - Predominantly surface - Predominantly goblet cells in colon	Epithelial cells, usually squamous
Location of inclusion	Nucleus and cytoplasm	Exclusively intranuclear	Intranuclear
Characteristics of inclusion	"Owl's eye" morphology in nucleus; basophilic and granular in cytoplasm	Basophilic "smudge cell" filling entire nucleus most common; rarely acidophilic inclusions with halos	Homogeneous with "ground glass" appearance or acidophilic with clear halo and peripheral chromatin margination
Associated changes	Cellular enlargement Apoptosis Mixed inflammatory infiltrate Vasculitis	Surface cell disorder, loss of orientation, degeneration; cells not enlarged	Sloughing of epithelial cells, neutrophilic infiltrate; multinucleated cells common

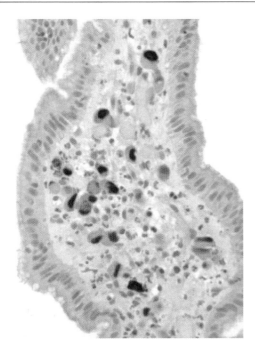

Fig. 20.16 Immunohistochemistry highlights many inclusions in the stroma of a small bowel villus

Distinction between CMV infection and graft-versus-host disease in bone marrow transplant patients may be particularly difficult, since the clinical and histologic features are similar. Immunohistochemistry or in situ hybridization studies should be employed to rule out CMV infection in this setting, since failure to identify CMV infection could result in delay of antiviral therapy. Furthermore, these conditions may coexist. Graft-versus-host disease is favored when there is abundant apoptosis associated with crypt necrosis and drop out, in the setting of minimal inflammation. The presence of viable nests of endocrine cells has also been reported to favor graft-versus-host disease.

Examination of multiple levels, and use of immunohistochemistry (Fig. 20.16), may be invaluable in detecting the rare cells containing an inclusion. Other diagnostic aids include viral culture, PCR assays, in situ hybridization, and serologic studies/antigen tests. Isolation of CMV in culture, however, does not imply active infection, since virus may be excreted for months to years after a primary infection. In addition, serologic studies often have limited utility due to the persistence of latent CMV infection.

Selected References

1. Balthazar EJ, Megibow AJ, Hulnick DH. Cytomegalovirus esophagitis and gastritis in AIDS. Am J Radiol 144:1201–4, 1985.

2. Buckner FS, Pomery C. Cytomegalovirus disease of the gastrointestinal tract in patients without AIDS. Clin Infect Dis 17:644–56, 1993.

3. Chetty R, Roskell DE. Cytomegalovirus infection in the gastrointestinal tract. J Clin Pathol 47:968–72, 1994.

4. Cieslak TJ, Mullett CT, Puntel RA, et al. Menetrier's disease associated with cytomegalovirus infection in children: report of two cases and review of the literature. Pediatr Infect Dis J 12:340–3, 1993.

5. Crespo MG, Arnal FM, Gomez M, et al. Cytomegalovirus colitis mimicking a colonic neoplasm or ischemia colitis 4 years after heart transplantation. Transplantation 66:1562–5, 1998.

6. Daniels JA, Lederman HM, Maitra A, Montgomery EA. Gastrointestinal tract pathology in patients with common variable immunodeficiency (CVID): a clinicopathologic study and review. Am J Surg Pathol 31:1800–12, 2007.

7. Dimitroulia E, Spanakis N, Konstantinidou AE, et al. Frequent detection of cytomegalovirus in the intestine of patients with inflammatory bowel disease. Infl Bowel Dis 12:879–84, 2006.

8. Fica A, Cervera C, Perez N, et al. Immunohistochemically proven cytomegalovirus end-organ disease in solid organ transplant patients: clinical features and usefulness of conventional diagnostic tests. Transpl Infect Dis 9:203–10, 2007.

9. Francis ND, Boylston AW, Roberts AHG, et al. Cytomegalovirus infection in gastrointestinal tracts of patients infected with HIV-1 or AIDS. J Clin Pathol 42:1055–64, 1989.

10. Golden MP, Hammer SM, Wanke CA, Albrecht MA. Cytomegalovirus vasculitis: case reports and review of the literature. Medicine 73:246–255, 1994.

11. Greenson JK. Macrophage aggregates in cytomegalovirus esophagitis. Hum Pathol 28:375–8, 1997.

12. Kambham N, Vig R, Cartwright CA, Longacre T. Cytomegalovirus infection in steroid-refractory ulcerative colitis; a case-control study. Am J Surgical Pathol 28:365–73, 2004.

13. Keates J, Lagahee S, Crilley P, et al. CMV enteritis causing segmental ischemia and massive intestinal hemorrhage. Gastro End 53:355–9, 2001.

14. Kraus MD, Feran-Doza M, Garcia-Moliner ML, et al. Cytomegalovirus infection in the colon of bone marrow transplant patients. Mod Pathol 11:29–36, 1998.

15. Laguna F, Garcia-Samaniego J, Alonso MJ, et al. Pseudotumoral apperance of cytomegalovirus esophagitis and gastritis in AIDS patients. Am J Gastroenterol 88:1108–11, 1993.

16. Lamps LW. Appendicitis and infections of the appendix. Sem Diag Pathol 21:86–97, 2004.

17. Mathias JR, Baskin GS, Reeves-Darby VG, et al. Chronic intestinal pseudoobstruction in a patient with heart-lung transplant. Therapeutic effect of leuprolide acetate. Dig Dis Sci 37:1761–8, 1992.

18. Meiselman MS, Cello JP, Margaretten W. Cytomegalovirus colitis: report of the clinical, endoscopic, and pathologic findings in two patients with the acquired immunodeficiency syndrome. Gastroenterol 88:171–5, 1985.

19. Neumayer La, Makar R, Ampel N, et al. Cytomegalovirus appendicitis in a patient with human immunodeficiency virus infection: case report and review of the literature. Arch Surg 128:467–8, 1993.

20. Occena RO, Taylor SF, Robinson CC. Association of cytomegalovirus with Menetrier's disease in childhood: report of two new cases with a review of literature. J Pediatr Gastroenterol Nutr 17:217–24, 1993.

21. Rafailidis PI, Mourtzoukou EG, Varbobitis IC, Falagas ME. Severe cytomegalovirus infection in apparently immunocompetent patients: a systematic review. Virol J 5:47, 2008.

22. Rich JD, Crawford JM, Kazanjian SN, Kazanjian PH. Discrete gastrointestinal mass lesions caused by cytomegalovirus in

patients with AIDS: report of three cases and review. Clin Infect Dis 15:609–14, 1992.

23. Sonsino E, Mouy R, Foucaud P, et al. Intestinal pseudoobstruction related to cytomegalovirus infection of myenteric plexus. N Engl J Med 311:196–7, 1984.

24. Suter WR, Neuweiler J, Borovicka J, et al. Cytomegalovirus-induced transient protein-losing hypertrophic gastropathy in an immunocompetent adult. Digestion 62:276–9, 2000.

25. Valerdiz-Casasola S, Pardo-Mindan FJ. Cytomegalovirus infection of the appendix in a patient with the acquired immunodeficiency syndrome. Gastroenterol 101:247–9, 1991.

26. Wilcox CM, Diehl DL, Cello JP, et al. Cytomegalovirus esophagitis in patients with AIDS. A clinical, endoscopic, and pathologic correlation. Ann Intern Med 113:589–93, 1990.

27. Xiao SY, Hart J. Marked gastric foveolar hyperplasia associated with active cytomegalovirus infection. Am J Gastroenterol 96:223–6, 2001.

Chapter 21

Herpes Simplex Virus

Keywords Herpes simplex virus • Inclusion • Proctitis • Esophagitis • Immunohistochemistry

Herpes simplex virus (HSV) is a member of the herpesvirus group that also includes varicella zoster virus, cytomegalovirus, Epstein–Barr virus, and human herpesviruses types 6 and 8 (see also Chapters 20, 22, and 26). HSV infection may occur throughout the gastrointestinal tract, but is most common in the esophagus and anorectum. HSV infections are often seen in immunocompromised patients, but they are not limited to this group. In immunocompetent patients, infection is often self-limited; immunocompromised persons may be at risk for dissemination and life-threatening illness. Herpes simplex virus remains one of the most common infections in persons with HIV.

Patients with HSV esophagitis present with odynophagia, dysphagia, chest pain, nausea, vomiting, fever, and gastrointestinal bleeding. Ulcers are the most common gross finding in the esophagus, and these are usually associated with an exudate. The ulcers are often shallow and sharply demarcated, with surrounding relatively normal mucosa. Some patients have vesicles surrounding the ulcers. Many patients, however, have a non-specific erosive esophagitis (Fig. 21.1). A protein-losing gastropathy resembling Menetrier's disease has been reported very rarely in association with HSV infection, similar to that associated with CMV infection.

HSV proctitis is the most common cause of nongonococcal proctitis in homosexual males. Patients generally present with severe anorectal pain, tenesmus, constipation, mucopurulent discharge, hematochezia, and fever, although some patients are asymptomatic. Concomitant neurologic symptoms (difficulty in urination and parasthesias of the buttocks and upper thighs) are also well described, as is inguinal lymphadenopathy. The presence of perianal vesicles, pustules, or shallow ulcers is common (Fig. 21.2). Vesicles are occasionally seen in the rectum or more proximal anal canal. Proctoscopic findings include mucosal ulceration and friability. HSV-associated colitis proximal to the anorectum has been rarely described, most often in the

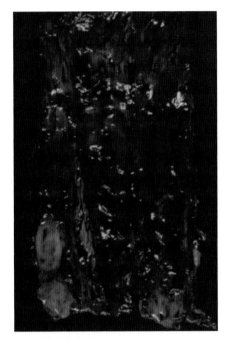

Fig. 21.1 Severe hemorrhagic erosive esophagitis in a case of herpes simplex esophagitis

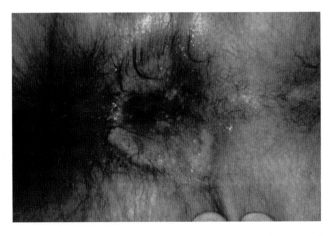

Fig. 21.2 Confluent perianal vesicles and shallow ulcers in a case of herpes simplex proctitis. (Courtesy Dr. Margie Scott)

L.W. Lamps, *Surgical Pathology of the Gastrointestinal System: Bacterial, Fungal, Viral, and Parasitic Infections*, DOI 10.1007/978-1-4419-0861-2_21, © Springer Science+Business Media, LLC 2009

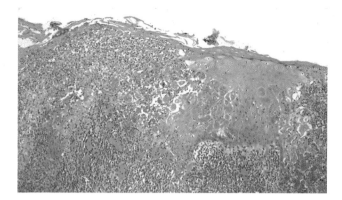

Fig. 21.3 Ulceration and discohesion of the squamous epithelium in a patient with herpetic proctitis. The patient had underlying chronic lymphocytic leukemia, represented by the dense lymphocytic infiltrate at the base of the lesion. (Courtesy Dr. Dianne Johnson)

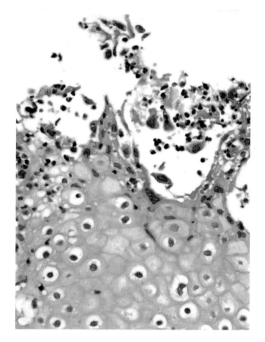

Fig. 21.5 Sloughing of epithelial cells and a neutrophilic infiltrate in a case of herpetic esophagitis. Inclusions are visible within the sloughed epithelial cells

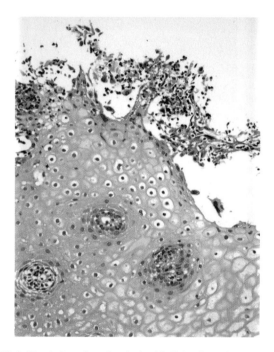

Fig. 21.4 Focal ulceration, sloughed epithelial cells, and a neutrophilic infiltrate in an esophageal biopsy from a patient with herpetic esophagitis

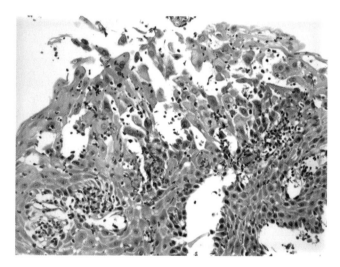

Fig. 21.6 Esophageal biopsy showing discohesion and sloughing of epithelial cells, intraepithelial neutrophils, and herpetic inclusions

context of underlying malignancy, immunodeficiency, or immunosuppression.

Histologic findings. Typical histologic findings, regardless of site, include ulceration (Figs. 21.3 and 21.4), an inflammatory exudate that often contains sloughed epithelial cells (Figs. 21.5 and 21.6), and a neutrophilic infiltrate in the lamina propria (Fig. 21.7). Prominent aggregates of macrophages may be seen within the inflammatory exudates as well. In the anorectum, perivascular lymphocytic cuffing (Fig. 21.8) and crypt abscesses in the lower rectal mucosa may be seen. The histologic features of HSV-1 and HSV-2 infection are indistinguishable (Fig. 21.9).

Characteristic viral inclusions and multinucleate giant cells are present in only a minority of biopsy specimens. The best place to search for viral inclusions is within the squamous epithelium at the edges of ulcers and in sloughed cells within the exudates (Fig. 21.10). Two types of nuclear inclusions may be found: the homogenous "ground glass" inclusion (Figs. 21.11 and 21.12) and the acidophilic inclusions with a surrounding clear halo and peripheral chromatin margination (Cowdry type-A inclusion, Fig. 21.13). Inclusions may be single or multinucleate (Fig. 21.14).

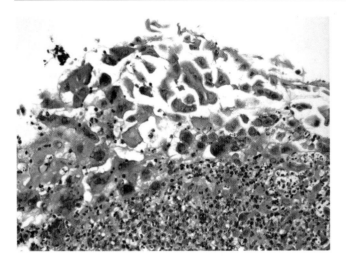

Fig. 21.7 Ulceration, sloughing of epithelial neutrophils, and a dense neutrophilic infiltrate in the lamina propria characterize herpetic esophagitis. Inclusions are visible within squamous cells

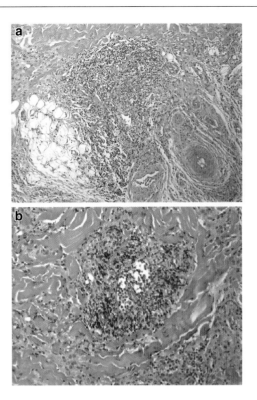

Fig. 21.8 Perivascular mononuclear cell infiltrate in the base of a biopsy from a case of herpetic proctitis (**a**). Higher power view shows lymphocytes and macrophages surrounding small submucosal vessels at the base of the ulcerative lesion (**b**)

Differential diagnosis. The differential diagnosis primarily includes other viral infections (see Table 20.1) including CMV, adenovirus, and herpes zoster/varicella, which also rarely infects the gastrointestinal tract. Herpes zoster/varicella produces histologic lesions identical to HSV, but patients often have a rash. Mixed infections are common in many clinical situations in which HSV infection is found.

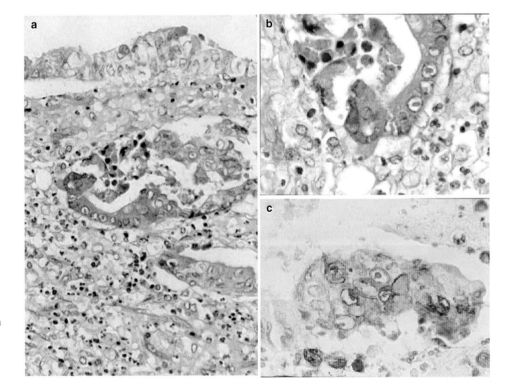

Fig. 21.9 Herpetic inclusions within rectal glandular epithelium in a patient with Crohn's disease (**a** and **b**); immunostain highlights infected cells (**c**). (Courtesy Dr. Brian West)

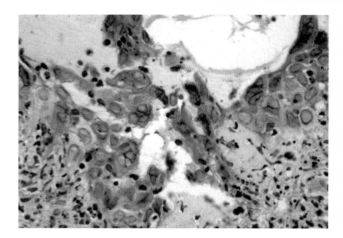

Fig. 21.10 Numerous "ground-glass" inclusions are seen at the edges of an ulcerative lesion in the esophagus

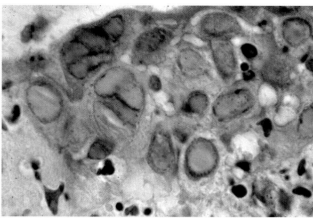

Fig. 21.12 The "ground glass" inclusion is intranuclear and homogeneous

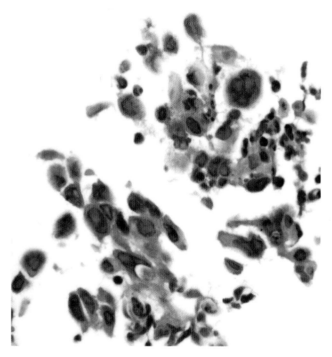

Fig. 21.11 "Ground glass" inclusions within squamous epithlelial cells in the ulcer exudate in an esophageal biopsy

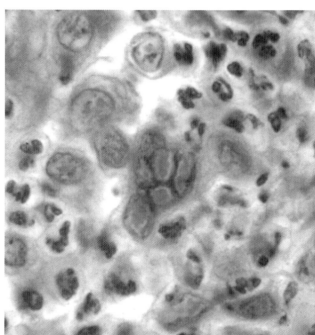

Fig. 21.13 The Cowdry type-A nuclear inclusion of herpes simplex is acidophilic with a surrounding clear halo and peripheral chromatin margination. (Photograph courtesy Dr. George F. Gray, Jr)

Viral culture is a valuable ancillary diagnostic aid. Immunohistochemistry and in situ hybridization assays may also be useful. Serologic studies may be useful if there is a very high or rising antibody titer. However, as latent infections can persist for years, serologic testing has limited use in routine clinical diagnosis.

Fig. 21.14 Multiple inclusions may be present within a single epithelial cell (polykaryon)

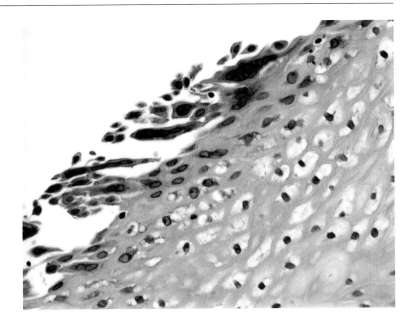

Selected References

1. Agha FP, Lee HL, Nostrant TT. Herpetic esophagitis: a diagnostic challenge in immunocompromised patients. Am J Gastroenterol 81:246–53, 1986.
2. Buss DH, Scharyj M. Herpes infection of the esophagus and other visceral organs in adults: incidence and clinical significance. Am J Med 66:457–62, 1979.
3. Colemont LJ, Pen JH, Pelckmans PA, et al. Herpes simplex virus type 1 colitis: an unusual cause of diarrhea. Am J Gastroenterol 85:1182–5, 1990.
4. Daley AJ, Craven P, Holland AJA, et al. Herpes simplex virus colitis in a neonate. Pediatr Infect Dis J 2:887–8, 2002.
5. El-Serag HB, Zwas FR, Cirillo NW, Eisen RN. Fulminant Herpes colitis in a patient with Crohn's disease. J Clin Gastroenterol 22:220–3, 1996.
6. Goodell SE, Quinn TC, Mkrtichian E, et al. Herpes simplex virus proctitis in homosexual men: clinical, sigmoidoscopic, and histopathological features. N Eng J Med 308:868–71, 1983.
7. Greenson JK, Beschorner WE, Boitnott JK, Yardley JH. Prominent mononuclear cell infiltrate is characteristic of herpes esophagitis. Hum Pathol 22:541–9, 1991.
8. Jun DW, Kim DH, Kim SH, et al. Menetrier's disease associated with herpes infection: response to treatment with acyclovir. Gastro Endosc 65:1092–5, 2007.
9. Kato S, Yamamoto R, Yoshimitsu S, et al. Herpes simplex esophagitis in the immunocompetent host. Dis Esoph 18:340–4, 2005.
10. Mallet E, Maitre M, Mouterde O. Complications of the digestive tract in varicella infection including two cases of erosive gastritis. Eur J Pediatr 165:64–5, 2006.
11. McBane RD, Gross JB. Herpes esophagitis: clinical syndrome, endoscopic appearance, and diagnosis in 23 patients. Gastrointest Endosc 37:600–3, 1991.
12. McDonald GB, Sharma P, Hackman RC, et al. Esophageal infections in immunosuppressed patients after marrow transplantation. Gastroenterol 88:1111–7, 1985.
13. Quinn TC, Corey L, Chaffee RG, et al. The etiology of anorectal infections in homosexual men. Am J Med 71:395–406, 1981.
14. Quinnan GV, Masur H, Rook AH, et al. Herpesvirus infections in the acquired immunodeficiency syndrome. JAMA 252:72–7, 1984.
15. Solammadevi SV, Patwardhan R. Herpes esophagitis. Am J Gastroenterol 77:48–50, 1982.

Chapter 22

Adenovirus

Keywords Adenovirus • Inclusion • Transplant • Immuno-histochemistry • Intussusception • Lymphoid hyperplasia • Appendicitis

Adenovirus infection is second only to rotavirus as a cause of childhood diarrhea and is associated with a broad spectrum of clinical disease in both children and adults. However, it has gained attention in recent years as a cause of diarrhea in immunocompromised patients, especially those with AIDS and patients who have undergone bone marrow or solid organ transplants. The incidence of adenovirus infection in bone marrow transplant patients has been reported at 5–20%; the incidence is lower in solid organ transplant patients. Pediatric transplant patients are affected more often than adults. Patients with severe combined immunodeficiency are also susceptible to gastrointestinal adenovirus infection. Virtually all patients present with diarrhea, sometimes accompanied by fever, weight loss, and abdominal pain. Risk factors for disseminated adenovirus infection include presence of concomitant graft-versus-host disease, use of immunosuppressive therapy, isolation of virus from multiple sites, and HLA-mismatched or unrelated transplants.

Adenovirus is also one of the more common viruses described in the appendix. It is associated with ileal and ileocecal intussusception, particularly in children. The virus is thought to cause intussusception by producing lymphoid hyperplasia, altering intestinal motility, or a combination of both. Most patients do not have symptoms of appendicitis, and adenovirus is found subsequent to resection for the intussusception.

Pathologic features. In the appendix, morphological changes are subtle, including lymphoid hyperplasia (Fig. 22.1) and overlying disorderly proliferation and degeneration of surface epithelium (Fig. 22.2). Histologic changes in adenovirus colitis include degenerative changes of the surface epithelium, such as epithelial cell disorder, loss of cell orientation (especially goblet cells), focal apoptosis, and sloughing of epithelial cells (Figs. 22.3 and 22.4). Adenovirus infection with similar histologic features has also been

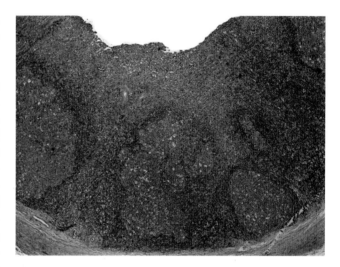

Fig. 22.1 Appendix with adenovirus infection shows marked lymphoid hyperplasia and overlying surface erosion with acute inflammatory exudates

described in the stomach and small bowel, in which mild villous blunting may be seen as well.

Characteristic inclusions (Figs. 22.3 and 22.4) are most often seen in areas with epithelial degenerative changes; inclusions may be widely scattered, with many apparently uninfected cells in between. Inclusions are usually present within surface epithelial cells, particularly goblet cells, in which the inclusions may be crescent-shaped (Figs. 22.3 and 22.4). Inclusions are rarely seen within the crypts (Fig. 22.5). The more common inclusions known as "smudge cells" have enlarged, basophilic nuclei without a clear nuclear membrane (Figs. 22.6 and 22.7). Homogenous, eosinophilic inclusions surrounded by halos with distinct nuclear membranes are much less common (Fig. 22.8). Adenovirus inclusions are exclusively intranuclear and fill the entire nucleus; however, the cell itself is not enlarged. In the appendix, inclusions are reportedly found in only one-third of patients with intussusception in which adenovirus is detected by other methods,

L.W. Lamps, *Surgical Pathology of the Gastrointestinal System: Bacterial, Fungal, Viral, and Parasitic Infections,* DOI 10.1007/978-1-4419-0861-2_22, © Springer Science+Business Media, LLC 2009

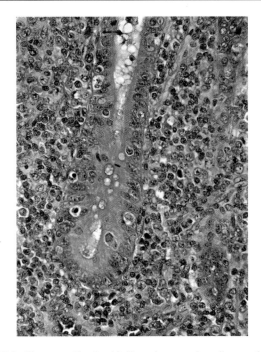

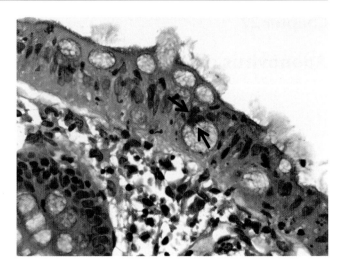

Fig. 22.4 Surface epithelial changes in adenovirus colitis include nuclear disarray and loss of polarity, goblet cell disorder, and a patchy mononuclear cell infiltrate. Note small crescent-shaped inclusion within goblet cell

Fig. 22.2 The appendiceal epithelium shows nuclear disarray, loss of nuclear polarity, and focal apoptosis

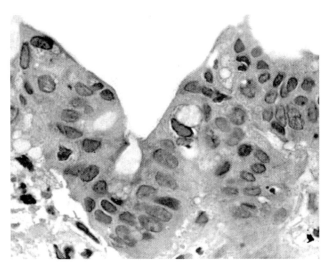

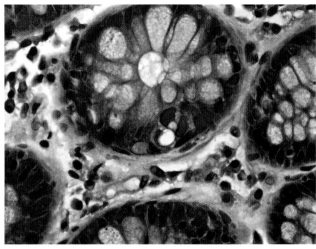

Fig. 22.5 Multiple characteristic adenovirus inclusions are seen within the colonic glandular epithelium in a case of adenovirus colitis in a patient with AIDS

Fig. 22.3 Adenovirus colitis showing surface nuclear disarray, loss of nuclear polarity, and characteristic inclusions within goblet cells and surface epithelial cells. (Courtesy Dr. Joel Greenson)

such as immunohistochemistry (Fig. 22.9), PCR, and in situ hybridization.

Differential diagnosis. The differential diagnosis of adenovirus infection is primarily with other viral infections, particularly CMV (see Table 20.1). Adenovirus inclusions are usually round to crescent shaped, generally located within surface epithelium, and exclusively intranuclear in location.

CMV inclusions have an "owl's eye" morphology in the nucleus, are generally located within endothelial or stromal cells, and exist within either the nucleus or cytoplasm.

Useful aids in the diagnosis of adenovirus infection include immunohistochemistry (Fig. 22.10), stool and/or tissue examination by electron microscopy, and viral culture. Positive serologies or fecal identification of the virus do not necessarily represent current infection, as viral shedding and elevated serological titers may persist for months.

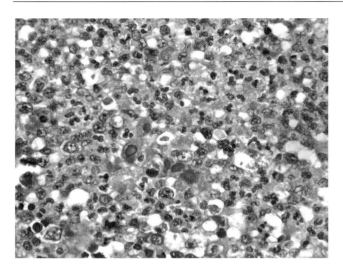

Fig. 22.6 Sloughed surface epithelial cells containing characteristic basophilic inclusions ("smudge cells") are seen within the inflammatory exudate in an appendix with adenovirus infection

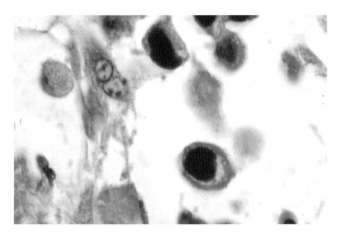

Fig. 22.7 The more common adenovirus inclusions known as "smudge cells" have enlarged, basophilic nuclei without a clear nuclear membrane. Adenovirus inclusions are intranuclear, and fill the entire nucleus, although the cell itself is not enlarged

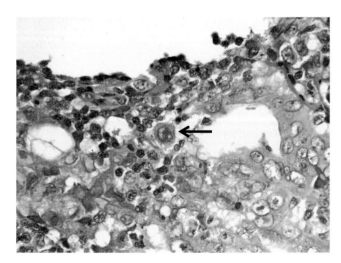

Fig. 22.8 Rare eosinophilic inclusions surrounded by halos with distinct nuclear membranes (Cowdry type A) are much less common

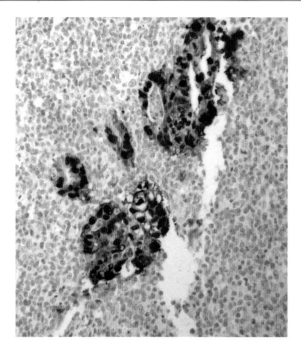

Fig. 22.9 Adenovirus immunostain shows strongly positive epithelial cells within the surface epithelium of the appendix

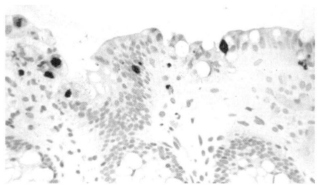

Fig. 22.10 Adenovirus immunostain highlights positive cells within the surface epithelium in a case of adenovirus colitis. (Courtesy Dr. Joel Greenson)

Selected References

1. de Mezerville MH, Tellier R, Richardson S, et al. Adenoviral infections in pediatric transplant recipients: a hospital-based study. Pediatr Infect Dis J 25:815–8, 2006.
2. Guarner J, de Leon-Bojorge B, Lopez-Corella E, et al. Intestinal intussusception associated with adenovirus infection in Mexican children. Am J Clin Pathol 120:845–50, 2003.
3. Ison MG. Adenovirus infections in transplant recipients. Clin Infect Dis 43:331–9, 2006.
4. Janoff EN, Orenstein JM, Manischewitz JF, Smith PD. Adenovirus colitis in the acquired immunodeficiency syndrome. Gastroenterol 100:976–9, 1991.
5. Lamps LW. Appendicitis and infection of the appendix. Semin Diagn Pathol 21:86–97, 2004.
6. Lamps LW. Beyond acute inflammation: a review of appendicitis and infections of the appendix. Diagn Histopathol 14:68–77, 2008.

7. Montgomery EA, Popek EJ. Intussusception, adenovirus, and children: a brief reaffirmation. Hum Pathol 25:169–74, 1994.

8. Porter HJ, Padfield CJH, Peres LC, et al. Adenovirus and intranuclear inclusions in appendices in intussusception. J Clin Pathol 46:154–8, 1993.

9. Reif RM. Viral appendicitis. Hum Pathol 12:193–6, 1981.

10. Shayan K, Saunders F, Roberts E, Cutz E. Adenovirus enterocolitis in pediatric patients following bone marrow transplantation: report of 2 cases and review of the literature. Arch Pathol Lab Med 127:1615–8, 2003.

11. Washington K. Immunodeficiency disorders of the GI tract. In: Odze RD, Goldblum JR, Crawford JM, (eds): Surgical Pathology of the GI Tract, Liver, Biliary Tract, and Pancreas. Philadelphia, PA: Elsevier, 2004, pp. 57–71.

12. Yan Z, Nguyen S, Poles M, Melamed J, Scholes JV. Adenovirus colitis in human immunodeficiency virus infection: an underdiagnosed entity. Am J Surg Pathol 22:1101–6, 1998.

13. Yunis EJ, Atchison RW, Michaels RH, et al. Adenovirus and ileocecal intussusception. Lab Invest 33:347–51, 1975.

Chapter 23

Miscellaneous Enteric Viruses

Keywords Viral enteritis • Acute viral gastroenteritis • Rotavirus • Coronavirus • Norwalk virus • Calicivirus • Echovirus • Enterovirus • Diarrhea

Acute viral gastroenteritis is second only to the common cold as a cause of illness in the United States. It often occurs in outbreaks, sometimes associated with food or water, and is a major recurrent problem in public health. Although most infections are self-limited, viral gastroenteritis can cause severe dehydration (particularly rotavirus), as well as chronic diarrhea in children with immunodeficiency syndromes such as severe combined immunodeficiency. Enteric viral infections are also a significant cause of diarrhea in patients with AIDS. Similar to adenovirus, rotavirus and enterovirus are associated with intussusception in children.

Many enteric viruses do not cause disease in humans; others seldom if ever cross the stage of the surgical pathologist, as they are detected in stool samples rather than biopsy specimens. Common enteric viruses known to cause diarrhea in humans include, but are not limited to, adenovirus, rotavirus, coronavirus, astrovirus, Norwalk virus and other enteric caliciviruses, and echovirus and other enteroviruses

(see Table 23.1). Interestingly, enteric involvement has been documented in the coronavirus-associated severe acute respiratory syndrome (SARS), and diarrhea was a common presenting symptom in that outbreak.

Pathologic findings. Many surgical pathologists are unfamiliar with the non-specific biopsy findings of viral enteritis, as we so rarely encounter these specimens. Pathologic studies are limited, and may not reflect the spectrum of changes in mild illness since most biopsy specimens are obtained from relatively sick patients.

Small bowel biopsy findings include villous fusion, broadening, and blunting (Figs. 23.1, 23.2, and 23.3); crypt hypertrophy (Fig. 23.4); and an increased mononuclear cell infiltrate within the lamina propria with variably present neutrophils (Fig. 23.5). There may be an increase in intraepithelial lymphocytes as well (Fig. 23.6). Reactive and degenerative epithelial changes are usually present, particularly at the surface, including epithelial cell disarray and loss of nuclear polarity (Figs. 23.7 and 23.8). Increased apoptosis may be seen in surface and glandular epithelium. In the limited number of human studies available, the severity of the histologic lesion does not appear to correlate with clinical

Table 23.1 Comparison of selected enteric viruses causing diarrheal illness in humans

	Average incubation period	Patient's age	Symptoms	Length of symptoms	Other features
Rotavirus	1–3 days	Peak age 6–24 months	Vomiting, fever, diarrhea	5–7 days	Most common cause of severe, dehydrating diarrhea in children Asymptomatic in neonates, older children, adults Peaks in winter in temperate zones
Norwalk virus	2 days	Any age	Mild vomiting, diarrhea, myalgias, headache	12–48 hour	Associated with shellfish, other food, water Associated with outbreaks in nursing homes, families, community settings
Astrovirus	3–4 days	Children	Mild vomiting, diarrhea, fever	2–4 days	Also affects elderly patients, immunocompromised patients
Enteric adenovirus	7 days	Infants and young children	Vomiting, fever, diarrhea	3–12 days	Also affects the immunocompromised

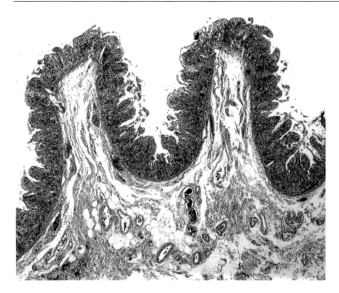

Fig. 23.1 A low-power view of severe viral enteritis shows villous blunting, broadening, and fusion in the small bowel mucosa

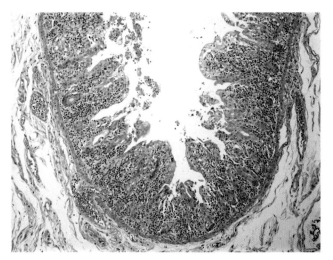

Fig. 23.2 Villous blunting, broadening, and fusion, along with an increased mononuclear cell infiltrate in the lamina propria and sloughing of surface epithelium

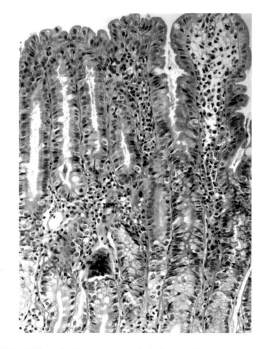

Fig. 23.3 Villous fusion in a case of viral enteritis

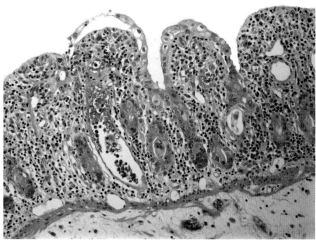

Fig. 23.4 Marked villous blunting and broadening, along with crypt hypertrophy and surface degenerative changes

severity of illness. Most human studies of the histopathology associated with enteric viral infection are limited to the duodenum. The rare reports that have evaluated the large bowel report histologic findings ranging from normal to focal cryptitis with increased apoptosis. With the exception of adenovirus infection in immunocompromised patients (see Chapter 22), inclusions are not seen on light microscopy.

Differential diagnosis. The differential diagnosis includes celiac disease, NSAID injury, and peptic ulcer disease. The histologic changes in viral enteritis rapidly return to normal as the patient's symptoms abate, and serologic assays for celiac disease should be negative. Peptic ulcer disease usually features more neutrophils and active inflammation than

viral enteritis, and lacks villous fusion and significant apoptosis. A history of NSAID usage (rare in pediatric patients) can help distinguish viral enteritis from NSAID injury, and again villous fusion is unusual in an adverse drug reaction. Viral culture and electron microscopic examination of tissue or feces may be valuable ancillary diagnostic tests.

Selected References

1. Agus SG, Dolin R, Wyatt RG, et al. Acute infectious nonbacterial gastroenteritis: intestinal histopathology. Ann Intern Med 79:18–25, 1973.

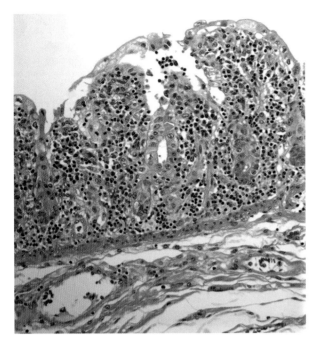

Fig. 23.5 Viral enteritis often shows an increase in mononuclear cells in the lamina propria, along with scattered granulocytes

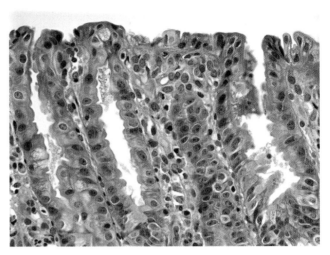

Fig. 23.7 Surface degenerative changes including pyknotic nuclei and loss of nuclear polarity

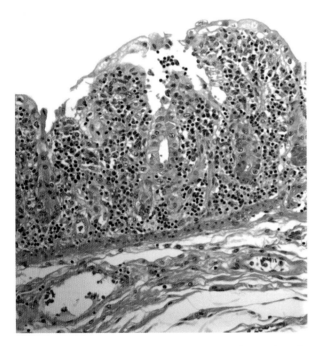

Fig. 23.6 Increased intraepithelial lymphocytes may be seen in surface and glandular epithelium

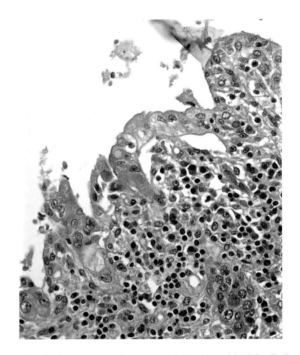

Fig. 23.8 Surface degenerative changes including epithelial cell disarray, loss of nuclear polarity, and sloughing of epithelial cells

2. Barnes GL, Townley RRW. Duodenal mucosal damage in 31 infants with gastroenteritis. Arch Dis Child 48:343, 1973.
3. Blacklow NR, Greenberg HB. Viral gastroenteritis. N Engl J Med 325:252–64, 1991.
4. Davidson GP, Barnes GL. Structural and functional abnormalities of the small intestine in infants and young children with rotavirus enteritis. Acta Paediatr Scand 68:181–6, 1979.
5. Estes MK, Hardy ME. Norwalk virus and other enteric caliciviruses. In: Blaser MJ, Smith PD, Ravdin JI, et al. (eds): Infections of the Gastrointestinal Tract. New York: Raven Press, 1995, pp. 1009–34.
6. Goldstein NS. Non-gluten sensitivity-related small bowel villous flattening with increased intraepithelial lymphocytes: not all that flattens is celiac disease. Am J Clin Pathol 121:546–50, 2004.
7. Guarner J, de Leon-Bojorge B, Lopez-Corella E, et al. Intestinal intussusception associated with adenovirus in Mexican children. Am J Clin Pathol 120:845–50, 2003.
8. Lack EE, Gang DL. In: Conner DH, Chandler FW: Pathology of Infectious Diseases. Stamford, CT: Appleton and Lange, 1997, pp. 101–106.

9. Leung WK, To KF, Chan PK, et al. Enteric involvement of severe acute respiratory syndrome-associated coronavirus infection. Gastroenterol 125:1011–7, 2003

10. Madely CR. The emerging role of adenoviruses as inducers of gastroenteritis. Pediatr Infect Dis 5:S63–74, 1986.

11. Matsui SM. Astroviruses. In: Blaser MJ, Smith PD, Ravdin JI, et al. Infections of the Gastrointestinal Tract. New York: Raven Press, 1995, pp. 1035–45.

12. Morotti RA, Kaufman SS, Fishbein TM, et al. Calicivirus infection in pediatric small intestine transplant recipients: pathological considerations. Hum Pathol 35:1236–40, 2004.

13. Rodriguez WJ, Kim HW, Brandt CD, et al. Fecal adenoviruses from a longitudinal study of families in metropolitan Washington, D.C.: laboratory, clinical, and epidemiologic observations. J Pediatr 107:514–20, 1985.

14. Saif LJ, Greenberg HG. Rotaviral gastroenteritis. In: Conner DH, Chandler FW. (eds): Pathology of Infectious Diseases. Stamford, CT: Appleton and Lange, 1997, pp. 297–302.

15. Schreiber DS, Blacklow NR, Trier JS. The mucosal lesion of the proximal small intestine in acute infectious nonbacterial gastroenteritis. N Engl J Med 288:1318–23, 1973.

16. Schreiber DS, Blacklow NR, Trier JS. The small intestinal lesion induced by Hawaii agent acute infectious nonbacterial gastroenteritis. J Infect Dis 129:705–8, 1974.

17. Thomas PD, Pollok RCG, Gazzard BG. Enteric viral infections as a cause of diarrhoea in the acquired immunodeficiency syndrome. HIV Med 1:19–24, 1999.

18. Vernacchio L, Vezina RM, Michell AA, et al. Diarrhea in American infants and young children in the community setting: incidence, clinical presentation and microbiology. Ped Infect Dis J 25:2–7, 2006.

19. Walter JE, Mitchell DK. Astrovirus infection in children. Cur Opin Infect Dis 16:247–53, 2003.

20. Washington K. Immunodeficiency disorders of the GI tract. In: Odze RD, Goldblum JR, Crawford JM. (eds): Surgical Pathology of the GI Tract, Liver, Biliary Tract, and Pancreas. Philadelphia, PA: Elsevier, 2004, pp. 57–71.

21. Winn WC. Adenoviruses. In: Conner DH, Chandler FW. (eds): Pathology of Infectious Diseases. Stamford, CT: Appleton and Lange, 1997, pp. 63–67.

Chapter 24

Human Papillomaviruses

Keywords Human papillomavirus • Papilloma • Squamous cell carcinoma • Condyloma • Dysplasia • Anal intraepithelial neoplasia

In the gastrointestinal tract, human papillomaviruses (HPV) have been implicated in the pathogenesis of esophageal papilloma, esophageal squamous cell carcinoma, anal condyloma and anal squamous intraepithelial lesions, and anal squamous cell carcinoma. Differences in reported rates of HPV positivity in these lesions may reflect differences in the investigative techniques used, as well as differences in the patient populations studied.

Esophageal HPV Infection

Esophageal squamous papillomas (ESP) are the most common benign epithelial tumor of the esophagus. Although somewhat controversial, several studies employing molecular methods have shown a significant association with HPV infection (including types 6, 11, 16, and 18) in up to half of tested cases. Other etiologic factors may play a role as well, such as mucosal injury and repair due to reflux. With exceedingly rare exception, however, ESPs do not appear to progress to dysplasia and carcinoma.

Patients of all ages and both genders are affected. ESPs are usually asymptomatic, and found incidentally, but papillomas may cause epigastric pain, dysphagia, or signs of obstruction. Endoscopically, ESPs are discrete, sessile, or pedunculated white polyps with an exophytic or verrucoid appearance (Fig. 24.1). Endophytic growth patterns also have been described. They may be solitary or multiple and range in size from 0.3 to 5.0 cm, although most measure less than 1.0 cm. They are most commonly found at the gastroesophageal junction, but can be located anywhere in the esophagus. Microscopically, ESPs are multilobulated lesions with fibrovascular cores that extend outward from the center of the papilloma (Fig. 24.2). Nuclei may be slightly enlarged with surrounding clear halos, but the koilocytic

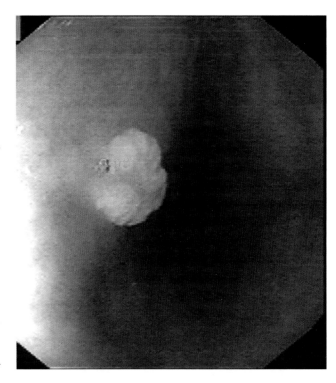

Fig. 24.1 Endoscopic photograph of a single, discrete, sessile white–pink esophageal squamous papilloma

atypia that typifies HPV infection of the cervix is often absent (Fig. 24.3). The basal zone is prominent, and some have a conspicuous granular cell layer. The epithelium matures at the surface, and parakeratosis is common (Fig. 24.4). Inflammation is variably present.

The main entities in the differential diagnosis are well-differentiated squamous cell carcinoma and verrucous carcinoma. ESPs lack significant epithelial atypia, an infiltrative growth pattern, and increased or atypical mitoses, but the differential diagnosis can be difficult to resolve in fragmented, poorly oriented biopsy specimens. Caution should be used if the biopsied lesion is large, destructive, recurrent, or shows extensive or circumferential involvement of the esophageal wall.

L.W. Lamps, *Surgical Pathology of the Gastrointestinal System: Bacterial, Fungal, Viral, and Parasitic Infections*,
DOI 10.1007/978-1-4419-0861-2_24, © Springer Science+Business Media, LLC 2009

Fig. 24.2 Low-power photomicrographs of esophageal squamous papillomas, showing papillary projections with fibrovascular cores extending outward from the center of the lesion (**a** and **b**). Note vascular congestion in **a**

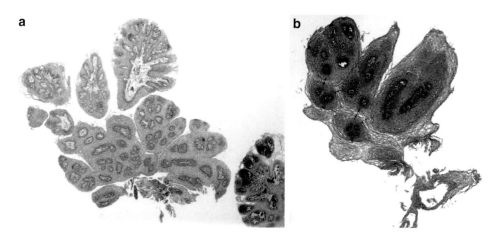

Esophageal squamous cell carcinoma. HPV infection has been implicated in the pathogenesis of esophageal squamous cell carcinoma, but this remains controversial. Although HPV may be a causative factor in some of these tumors, it is most likely important in only a small percentage of cases from high-risk geographical areas.

Anal HPV Infection

Condyloma acuminatum is the most common tumor of the anal and perianal region; similar to genital condylomas, it is caused by HPV infection. Anal condylomas may occur in conjunction with vulvar or penile warts, but also may be the sole site of infection, particularly in the male homosexual population. Grossly, condylomas are soft, fleshy, white to pink papillomatous lesions that can be single or multiple (Fig. 24.5). Large lesions may have a cauliflower-like appearance (Fig. 24.6). Microscopically, condylomas are papillary with acanthosis, surface maturation, and parakeratosis (Fig. 24.7). Koilocytic atypia is common, analogous to low-grade squamous epithelial lesions in the cervix, featuring enlarged, irregular, hyperchromatic nuclei with frequent binucleation and surrounding halos (Fig. 24.8). Mitototic figures confined to the lower third of the epithelium and dyskeratotic epithe-

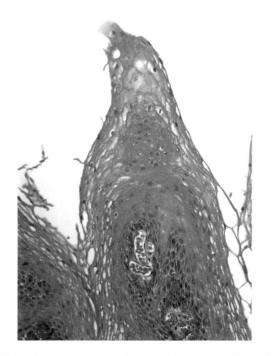

Fig. 24.3 Mature squamous epithelium at the surface of a papillary projection in an esophageal squamous papilloma. There are focal cells with clear halos, but well-developed koilocytic atypia is absent

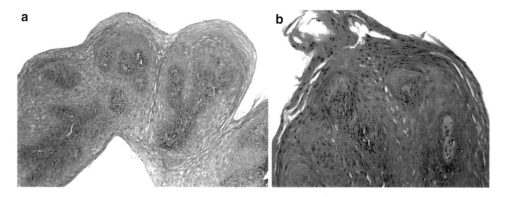

Fig. 24.4 Prominent basal zone, surface epithelial maturation, and parakeratosis in an esophageal squamous papilloma (**a** and **b**)

Fig. 24.5 Multiple fleshy pink-to-white perianal and anal condylomata. (**a** and **b**, courtesy Dr. George F. Gray, Jr.)

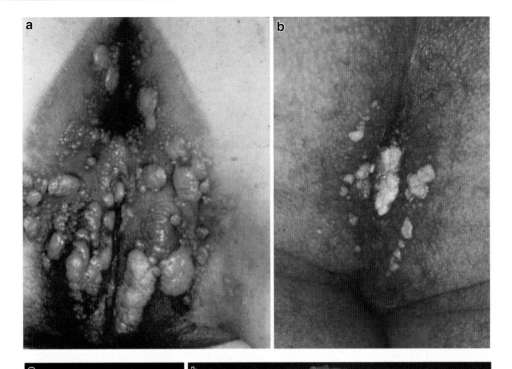

Fig. 24.6 External (**a**) and cut surfaces (**b**) of large cauliflower-like anal condylomata. Note that the papillary fronds can be appreciated grossly on the cut surface of the specimen (**b**). (Courtesy Dr. George F. Gray, Jr)

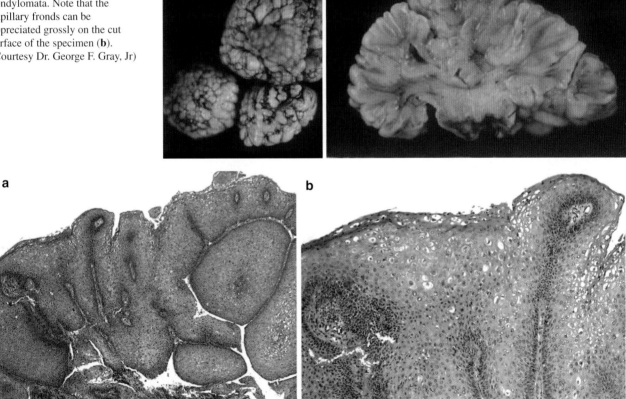

Fig. 24.7 Low-power lobulated, papillary configuration of an anal condyloma (**a**). Koilocytic atypia and parakeratosis are common (**b**)

lial cells may be seen as well. It is important to note that both condylomas and higher grade squamous intraepithelial lesions may be flat, and thus more difficult to detect on physical examination.

Anal squamous intraepithelial lesions and squamous cell carcinoma. Controversy remains regarding the risk of progression of anal condylomata to high-grade squamous intraepithelial lesions and carcinoma; as in the uterine cervix,

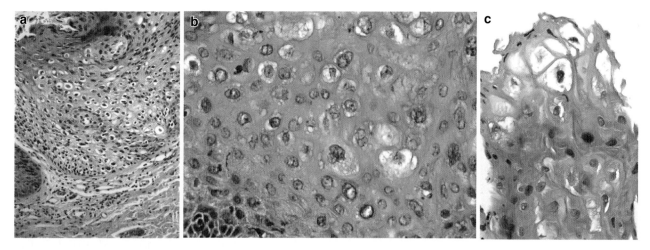

Fig. 24.8 Anal condyloma with prominent koilocytic atypia (**a**). Nuclei are enlarged, irregular, and hyperchromatic (**b**), with surrounding halos (**c**)

however, condylomas have frequently been reported in association with low- and high-grade squamous intraepithelial lesions (also known as anal intraepithelial neoplasia or AIN) and invasive squamous cell carcinoma. In addition, lower genital tract squamous dysplasia or neoplasia in women is a risk factor for anal disease, as is persistent high-risk HPV genotype infection, and anal and genital HPV-associated lesions often coexist. HIV-positive patients and renal and cardiac transplant patients appear to be at increased risk of progression of pre-invasive lesions to squamous cell carci-

noma. The progression of intraepithelial lesions/AIN to invasive carcinoma does appear to be less common than in the cervix, however. As HIV-positive patients live longer due to high activity anti-retroviral drug therapy, there likely will be an increase in high-grade squamous intraepithelial lesions and invasive carcinomas in this population due to latent HPV infection that would not have had time to manifest clinically if the patient succumbed earlier to complications of AIDS.

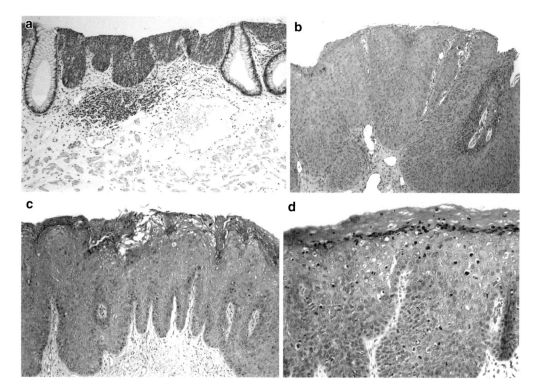

Fig. 24.9 High-grade squamous intraepithelial lesion/squamous cell carcinoma in situ is similar to its cervical counterpart. Dysplastic squamous epithelium completely lacking maturation extends into the rectal mucosa (**a**). Disorderly proliferation with lack of maturation, paraker-

atosis, and numerous mitoses (**b** and **c**). High-power view shows numerous mitoses, enlarged, hyperchromatic nuclei, dyskeratosis, and lack of maturation at the surface (**d**)

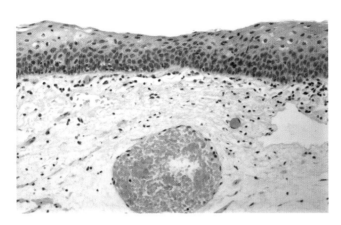

Fig. 24.10 Normal transitional-type mucosa in the anal canal must be distinguished from AIN

Squamous intraepithelial lesions/AIN are commonly found adjacent to invasive squamous cell carcinoma. The histologic features are similar to dysplasia of the uterine cervix (Fig. 24.9), featuring loss of orderly surface maturation, increased nuclear-to-cytoplasmic ratio, and increased mitotic figures with mitoses present in the upper half to one-third of the epithelium. Care must be taken to distinguish high-grade squamous intraepithelial lesions from the normal transitional epithelium of the anal canal (Fig. 24.10). In addition, both condylomas and squamous intraepithelial lesions/AIN are occasionally either mistaken for or found within resected hemorrhoids. The use of immunostains for p16 and Ki-67 may be useful in confirming the diagnosis of high-grade intraepithelial lesions, and in distinguishing AIN from transitional epithelium of the anal canal.

Many HPV types have been associated with anal condylomas, squamous intraepithelial lesions, and carcinomas, including high-risk types 16 and 18. Low-risk types 6 and 11 are most commonly associated with anal condylomas. In the uterine cervix, reflex HPV genotype testing following an atypical pap smear is a useful, widely employed screening strategy. Because the prevalence of high-risk HPV and the prognostic implications in the anal canal are not as well defined, the role of HPV DNA detection and genotyping is not currently clear. The presence or absence of detectable HPV in anal carcinomas does not appear to affect the prognosis of the tumor.

Selected References

Esophageal HPV Infection

1. Carr NJ, Bratthauer GL, Lichy JH, et al. Squamous cell papillomas of the esophagus: a study of 23 lesions for human papillomavirus by in situ hybridization and the polymerase chain reaction. Hum Pathol 25:536–40, 1994.

2. Chang F, Syrjanen S, Shen Q, et al. Human papillomavirus involvement in esophageal carcinogenesis in the high-incidence area of China: a study of 700 cases by screening and type-specific in situ hybridization. Scand J Gastroenterol 35:123–30, 2000.
3. Lavergne D, De Villiers E-M. Papillomavirus in esophageal papillomas and carcinomas. Int J Cancer 80:681–4, 1999.
4. Odze R, Antonioli D, Shocket D, et al. Esophageal squamous papillomas: a clinicopathologic study of 38 lesions and analysis for human papillomavirus by the polymerase chain reaction. Am J Surg Pathol 17:803–12, 1993.
5. Politoske EJ. Squamous papilloma of the esophagus associated with the human papillomavirus. Gastroenterol 102:668–73, 1992.
6. Poljak M, Cerar A, Seme K. Human Papillomavirus infection in esophageal carcinomas: a study of 121 lesions using multiple broad-spectrum polymerase chain reactions and literature review. Hum Pathol 29:266–71, 1998.
7. Syrjanen KJ. HPV infections and oesophageal cancer. J Clin Pathol 55:8, 2002.
8. Togawa K, Jaskiewicz K, Takahashi H, et al. Human papillomavirus DNA sequences in esophagus squamous cell carcinoma. Gastroenterol 107:128–36, 1994.
9. Waluga M, Hartleb M, Sliwinski ZK, et al. Esophageal squamous – cell papillomatosis complicated by carcinoma. Am J Gastroenterol 95:1592–3, 2000.

Anal HPV Infection

10. Bean SM, Eltoum I, Horton DK, et al. Immunohistochemical expression of p16 and Ki-67 correlates with degree of anal intraepithelial neoplasia. Am J Surg Pathol 31:555–61, 2007.
11. Frisch M, Fenger C, van den Brule AJC, et al. Variants of squamous cell carcinoma of the anal canal and perianal skin and their relation to human papillomaviruses. Can Res 59:753–7, 1999.
12. Haber MM. Histologic precursors of gastrointestinal tract malignancy. Gastroenterol Clin North Am 31:395–419, 2002.
13. Handley JM, Maw RD, Lawther H, et al. Human papillomavirus DNA detection in primary anogenital warts and cervical low-grade intraepithelial neoplasias in adults by in situ hybridization. Sex Transm Dis 19:225–9, 1992.
14. Longacre TA, Kong CS, Welton ML. Diagnostic problems in anal pathology. Adv Anat Pathol 15:263–78, 2008.
15. Luchtefeld MA. Perianal condylomata acuminata. Surg Clin North Am 74:1327–38, 1994.
16. Palefsky JM, Holly EA, Gonzales J, et al. Detection of human papillomavirus DNA in anal intraepithelial neoplasia and anal cancer. Can Res 51:1014–9, 1991.
17. Palmer JG, Scholefield JH, Coates PJ, et al. Anal cancer and human papillomaviruses. Dis Colon Rectum 32:1016–22, 1989.
18. Ramanujam PS, Venkatesh KS, Co Barnett T, Fietz MJ. Study of human papillomavirus infection in patients with anal squamous carcinoma. Dis Colon Rectum 39:37–9, 1996.
19. Ryan DP, Compton CC, Mayer RJ. Carcinoma of the anal canal. N Engl J Med 342:792–800, 2000.
20. Scholefield JH, Talbot IC, Whatrup C, et al. Anal and cervical intraepithelial neoplasia: possible parallel. Lancet 2(2):765–8, Sept 30, 1989.
21. Sobhani I, Vuagnat A, Walker F, et al. Prevalence of high-grade dysplasia and cancer in the anal canal in human papillomavirus-infected individuals. Gastroenterol 120:857–66, 2001.
22. Welton ML, Sharkey FE, Kahlenberg MS. The etiology and epidemiology of anal cancer. Surg Oncol Clin North Am 13:263–75, 2004.

Chapter 25

Human Immunodeficiency Virus

Keywords Human immunodeficiency virus • AIDS enteropathy • AIDS colopathy • Chronic HIV-associated esophageal ulcer

Gastrointestinal disease is an important cause of morbidity and mortality in patients infected with the human immunodeficiency virus (HIV) and those with the acquired immunodeficiency syndrome (AIDS). Although one or more opportunistic infections are often found in these patients, there is a subgroup in which no pathogens are found despite extensive clinical and pathological evaluation. The two major entities associated with HIV in the absence of other demonstrable pathogens, chronic idiopathic esophageal ulcers and AIDS enteropathy/colopathy, will be discussed here.

Chronic HIV-associated esophageal ulcers. Chronic idiopathic esophageal ulcers reportedly cause approximately 40–50% of ulcers found in HIV-infected patients. Evidence of HIV within the ulcerative lesions has been demonstrated by molecular, immunohistochemical, and ELISA assays, suggesting that HIV is capable of producing ulcers in the absence of other pathogens. The ability of HIV to directly cause these ulcers remains controversial, however, and details of the pathogenesis remain to be elucidated. Patients present with severe odynophagia, independent of food intake, chest pain, and weight loss. Massive, even fatal GI bleeding can occur if the ulcer erodes into vessels. Stricture formation as a complication of these ulcers has been reported rarely.

Pathologic features. The middle esophagus is the most common location, followed by the distal esophagus. Endoscopically, the ulcers consist of one or more well-circumscribed lesions of variable depth that can mimic ulcers caused by other infectious agents, particularly viral pathogens. They can be quite large (greater than 3.0 cm in greatest dimension), with irregular margins and overhanging, edematous edges (Fig. 25.1). They are often linear. Mucosal bridges and sinus tract formation may occur. Histologically, the ulcers contain granulation tissue with a mixed acute and chronic inflammatory infiltrate that often contains eosinophils (Fig. 25.2). The ulcers may extend into

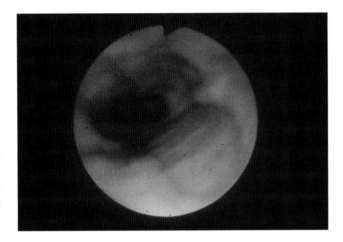

Fig. 25.1 Endoscopic photograph showing a large, irregular, somewhat linear chronic idiopathic esophageal ulcer in an AIDS patient. (Courtesy Dr. Audrey Lazenby)

the esophageal muscle layers. By definition, special histochemical stains and immunohistochemical stains for identifiable pathogens must be negative.

The diagnosis of idiopathic HIV-associated esophageal ulcers should be made only when other pathogens have been rigorously excluded, both clinically and histologically. This is especially important as these ulcers are sometimes treated with steroids.

AIDS (HIV) enteropathy/colopathy. This controversial entity has been loosely defined as the morphologic changes seen in the gut of patients with HIV/AIDS and chronic diarrhea, for which no other infectious cause has been identified. The controversy arises because asymptomatic patients may have similar morphologic findings on biopsy, and conversely severely symptomatic patients may have normal biopsies. In addition, there is always the added concern that a causative pathogen simply has been missed. Because HIV/AIDS patients do have severe impairments of gastrointestinal function including diarrhea, malabsorption, and weight loss, even in the absence of any demonstrable pathogen, some authors support using the term "AIDS enteropathy (or colopathy)" to describe the morphologic findings, provided that the bowel

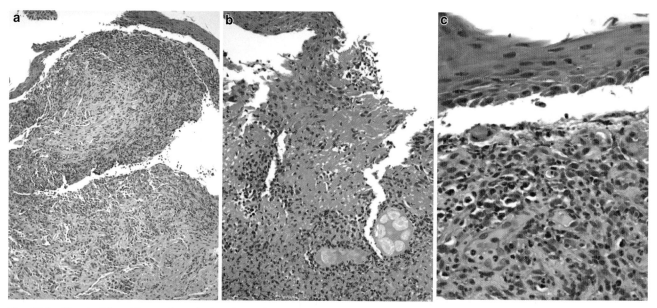

Fig. 25.2 Chronic idiopathic esophageal ulcer in an HIV-positive patient featuring acute and chronic inflammation with prominent granulation tissue formation and necrosis (**a–c**). Note extension of the ulcer into muscle (**a**) and eosinophils within the inflammatory exudate (**c**). (Courtesy Dr. Rhonda K. Yantiss)

has been adequately sampled and all other infectious causes have been excluded. Furthermore, it has been hypothesized that the effects of HIV on T-cells could explain the morphologic changes, or that HIV may selectively alter enterocyte function through a direct effect on the intracellular architecture of the epithelial cells. Other authorities believe that this is a poorly understood term that does not clearly represent a specific disease entity, and thus should be avoided. For the sake of completeness, the morphologic changes associated with the term AIDS/HIV enteropathy will be discussed here, although understanding of the clinicopathologic implications of this term obviously are still in evolution.

Endoscopy and colonoscopy are usually normal. In the small bowel, the histologic features include villous blunting and atrophy (Fig. 25.3), crypt hypertrophy

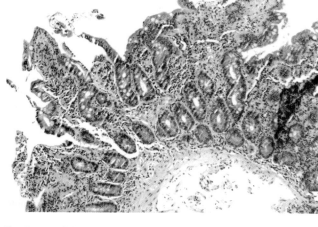

Fig. 25.4 Mild villous blunting and focal crypt hyperplasia in a case of HIV enteropathy. (Courtesy Dr. Joseph Misdraji)

(Fig. 25.4), increased intraepithelial lymphocytes, variably increased mononuclear cells in the lamina propria (Fig. 25.5), increased mitoses within glandular epithelial cells (Fig. 25.6), and increased numbers of apoptotic enterocytes at the surface and in the glands (Fig. 25.7). In the colon, inflammatory changes are similar (Fig. 25.8), but the most prominent change is increased apoptotic epithelial cells in the glandular epithelium (Fig. 25.9). The changes resemble those seen in mild graft-versus-host disease and chemotherapy-related mucosal injury. Other pathogens, particularly other viruses such as CMV and adenovirus that can produce similar histologic features, must be rigorously excluded.

Fig. 25.3 Mild villous blunting and an increase in plasma cells in the lamina propria in a case of HIV enteropathy. (Courtesy Dr. Joseph Misdraji)

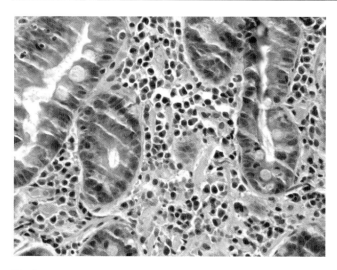

Fig. 25.5 Increased plasma cells in the lamina propria of the duodenum. (Courtesy Dr. Joseph Misdraji)

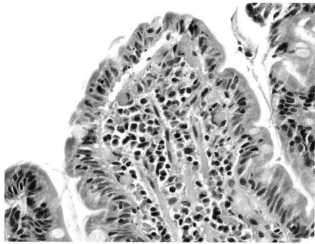

Fig. 25.7 Apoptotic enterocytes at the villous tips. (Courtesy Dr. Joseph Misdraji)

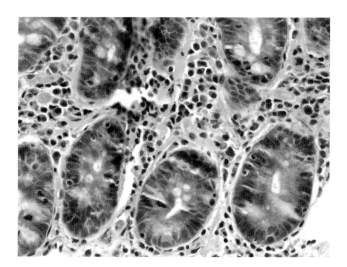

Fig. 25.6 Increased mitoses within duodenal glandular mucosa. (Courtesy Dr. Joseph Misdraji)

Selected References

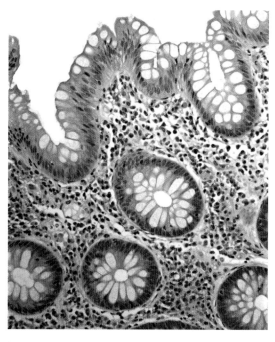

Fig. 25.8 A case of HIV colopathy shows intact architecture and an increase in plasma cells in the lamina propria, similar to the changes in the small bowel

1. Adeoti AG, Vega KJ, Dajani EZ, et al. Idiopathic esophageal ulceration in acquired immunodeficiency syndrome: successful treatment with misoprostol and viscous lidocaine. Am J Gastroenterol 93:2069–74, 1998.
2. Bartlett JG, Belitsos PC, Sears CL. AIDS enteropathy. Clin Infect Dis 15;726–35, 1992.
3. Borum M, Marks ZH. Esophageal stricture from idiopathic ulcers in an AIDS patient: a case report and review of the literature. J Clin Gastroenterol 28: 260–1, 1999.
4. Carlson S, Vokoo H, Craig RM. Small intestinal HIV-associated enteropathy: evidence for panintestinal enterocyte dysfunction. J Lab Clin Med 124:652–9, 1994.
5. Clayton F, Clayton CH. Gastrointestinal pathology in HIV-infected patients. Gastroenterol Clin North Am 26:191–240, 1997.
6. Delezay O, Yahi N, Tamalet C, et al. Direct effect of type 1 human immunodeficiency virus (HIV-1) on intestinal epithelial cell differentiation: relationship to HIV-1 enteropathy. Virology 238:231–42, 1997.
7. Dretler RH, Rausher DB. Giant esophageal ulcer healed with steroid therapy in an AIDS patient. Rev Infect Dis 11:768–9, 1989.
8. Ehrenpreis ED, Patterson BK, Brainer JA, et al. Histopathologic findings of duodenal biopsy specimens in HIV-infected patients with and without diarrhea and malabsorption. Am J Clin Pathol 97:21–8, 1992.
9. Greenson JK, Belitsos PC, Yardley JH, Bartlett JG. AIDS enteropathy: occult enteric infections and duodenal mucosal alterations in chronic diarrhea. Ann Intern Med 114:366–72, 1991.

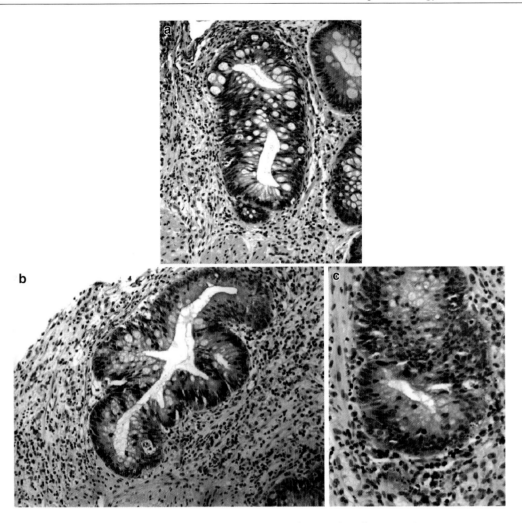

Fig. 25.9 Increased apoptotic epithelial cells in the colonic glands, similar to graft-versus-host disease (**a–c**)

10. Jalfon IM, Sitton JE, Hammer RA, et al. HIV-1 gp41 antigen demonstration in esophageal ulcers with acquired immunodeficiency syndrome. J Clin Gastroenterol 13:644–8, 1991.

11. Kotler DP, Reka S, Orenstein JM, Fox CH. Chronic idiopathic esophageal ulceration in the acquired immunodeficiency syndrome. J Clin Gastroenterol 15:284–90, 1992.

12. Pedro-Botet J, Miralles R, Sauleda J, Rubies-Prat J. Idiopathic ulcer of the esophagus in the AIDS syndrome: a potential life-threatening complication. Gastro Endos 35:470, 1989.

13. Rabeneck L. AIDS enteropathy: what's in a name? J Clin Gastroenterol 19:154–7, 1994.

14. Rabeneck L, Genta RM, Risser JMH, et al. Unceratin clinical significance of duodenal mucosal abnormalities in HIV-infected individuals. J Clin Gastroenterol 23: 11–4, 1996.

15. Rotterdam H, Tsang P. Gastrointestinal disease in the immuno-compromised host. Hum Pathol 25:1123–40, 1994.

16. Ullrich R, Zeitz M, Heise W, et al. Small intestinal structure and function in patients infected with human immunodeficinecy virus (HIV): evidence for HIV-induced enteropathy. Ann Intern Med 111:15–21, 1989.

17. Wilcox CM. Current concepts of gastrointestinal disease associated with human immunodeficiency virus infection. Clin Perspect Gastroenterol 3:9–17, Jan–Feb 2000.

18. Wilcox CM, Schwartz DA. Endoscopic characterization of idiopathic esophageal ulceration associated with human immunodeficiency virus infection. J Clin Gastroenterol 16:251–6, 1993.

19. Wilcox CM. Esophageal disease in the acquired immunodeficiency syndrome: etiology, diagnosis, and management. Am J Med 92:412–21, 1992.

Chapter 26

Miscellaneous Viral Infections

Keywords Measles • Rubeola • Herpes zoster • Chicken pox • Human herpesvirus-8 • Kaposi's sarcoma • Epstein–Barr virus • Adenocarcinoma • Lymphoepithelioma • Lymphoma

Measles (Rubeola virus). Although rare, measles infection produces a number of gastrointestinal manifestations, including appendicitis, enteritis, and mesenteric lymphadenitis. Histologic findings in measles-related appendicitis include lymphoid hyperplasia and multinucleate Warthin–Finkeldey giant cells (Fig. 26.1), predominantly within germinal centers; associated inflammation is variably present. Although the measles virus probably does not independently cause true appendicitis, the lymphoid hyperplasia may lead to obstruction, acute inflammation, and even gangrenous appendicitis. Patients often have a concomitant rash, although the gastrointestinal morphologic findings may precede the viral xanthem, and serologic findings and immunohistochemistry can help confirm the diagnosis. Measles rarely has been reported to cause viral gastritis and enteritis, with symptoms including abdominal pain, diarrhea, and malabsorption.

Herpes zoster/varicella. Herpes zoster/varicella can cause an ulcerative esophagitis, gastroenteritis, or enterocolitis. It is particularly important to be aware of this entity in the context of patients with shingles or chicken pox who have gastrointestinal complaints. Symptoms include fever, abdominal pain, vomiting, diarrhea (variably bloody), odynophagia, and weight loss. Patients often have stomatitis or the characteristic cutaneous findings of shingles or chicken pox; gastrointestinal involvement may precede skin involvement, however, or occur without skin involvement in some cases. Dissemination may occur in immunocompromised patients, and the infection may be fatal. Herpes zoster/varicella is also one of the many viruses implicated in intestinal pseudo-obstruction.

Gross and microscopic findings are similar to those in HSV infection, including erosions and ulcerations with associated vesicles. Lesions are often multiple, and intervening mucosa is often normal. The ulcers contain hemorrhage, necrotic debris, and a variable inflammatory infiltrate, and may extend into the submucosa. The viral inclusions are present at the edges of the ulcers and are indistinguishable

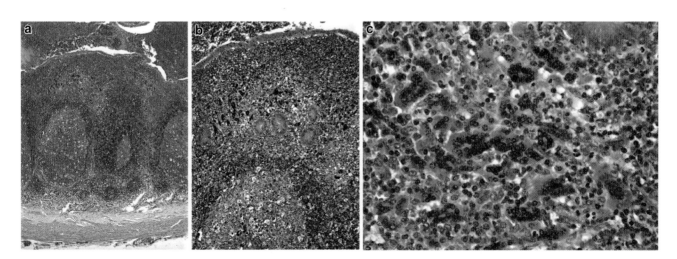

Fig. 26.1 Measles appendicitis. Marked lymphoid hyperplasia is visible at low power (**a** and **b**). Warthin-Finkeldey giant cells are present in the germinal centers of the hyperplastic lymphoid follicles, along with numerous tingible-body macrophages and abundant apoptotic debris (**b–c**). (Courtesy Dr. David Owen)

from HSV by light microscopy alone (Figs. 26.2 and 26.3). Immunohistochemistry and viral culture, along with molecular assays, can aid in distinguishing between HSV and herpes zoster/varicella infection (Fig. 26.4).

Human herpesvirus-8 (HHV-8). HHV-8, also known as Kaposi's sarcoma-associated herpesvirus, is strongly associated with Kaposi's sarcoma (KS). Gastrointestintal involve-

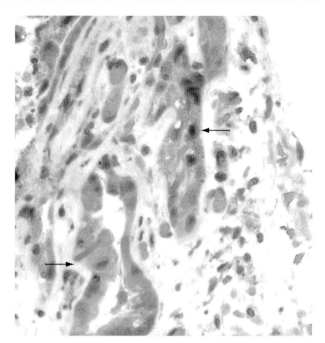

Fig. 26.4 In situ hybridization highlights the nuclear inclusions of herpes zoster/varicella and distinguishes them from herpes simplex virus. (Courtesy Dr. Joel K. Greenson)

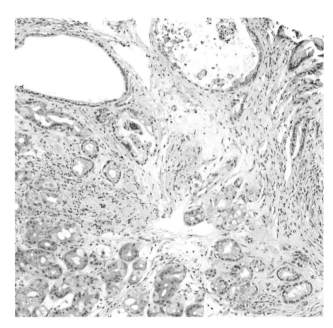

Fig. 26.2 Herpes zoster/varicella gastritis showing patchy acute inflammation with dilated gastric glands containing necrotic debris. Courtesy of Dr. Joel K. Greenson

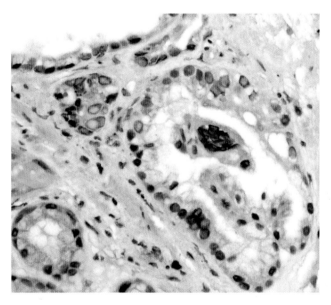

Fig. 26.3 High-power view of herpes zoster/varicella gastritis shows nuclear inclusions similar to herpes simplex virus within glandular epithelium. Focal multinucleate giant cells are seen as well. (Courtesy Dr. Joel K. Greenson)

ment by KS can be found in the majority of patients with cutaneous lesions. Gastrointestinal KS may ulcerate and bleed, but the bleeding is not usually severe, and the disease may be asymptomatic. Upper gastrointestinal involvement is more common than colonic disease. Lesions are often multifocal and consist of red to violet nodules, plaques, or polyps. Many lesions are submucosal, leading to difficulty in obtaining a satisfactory sample with endoscopic mucosal biopsy. Histologic features are similar regardless of site, and include a proliferation of capillaries with plump endothelial cells in early lesions. As the lesions progress, the capillary proliferation becomes more spindled with irregular, slit-like vascular spaces (Figs. 26.5, 26.6, and 26.7). Extravasated red cells and hemosiderin are variably present, and eosinophilic round cytoplasmac globular inclusions may be seen in some cases. The main entity in the differential diagnosis is *Bartonella*-associated bacillary angiomatosis; bacillary angiomatosis has more attendant inflammation and the bacteria can be detected on silver impregnation stains, with immunohistochemistry, and by molecular studies. Immunohistochemical stains for HHV-8 highlight the nuclei in KS as well (Fig. 26.8). HHV-8 also has been associated rarely with gastrointestinal lymphoma in HIV-positive patients.

Human herpesvirus-6 (HHV-6). HHV-6 is the causative agent in roseola, a common febrile disease of childhood. Transplant recipients (both solid organ and bone marrow) can develop asymptomatic reactivation as well as HHV-6 associated pneumonitis, hepatitis, and gastroenteritis. Symptoms

Fig. 26.5 Kaposi's sarcoma in the duodenum of an AIDS patient, featuring a spindled proliferation of small vessels with slit-like spaces, hemorrhage, and extravasated red blood cells (**a** and **b**)

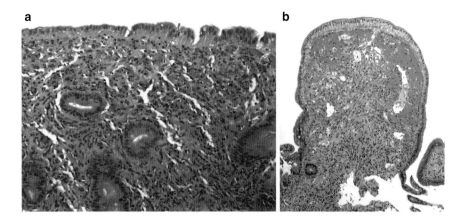

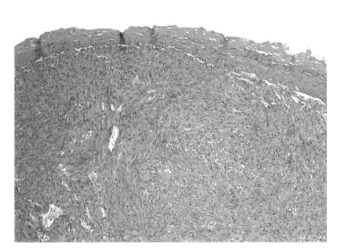

Fig. 26.6 Mesenteric lymph node involved by Kaposi's sarcoma

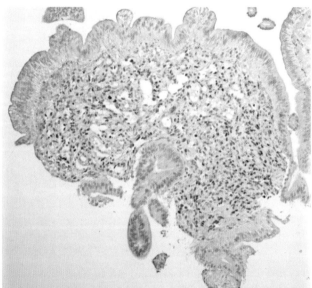

Fig. 26.8 Tumor cells show nuclear positivity with the HHV-8 immunostain

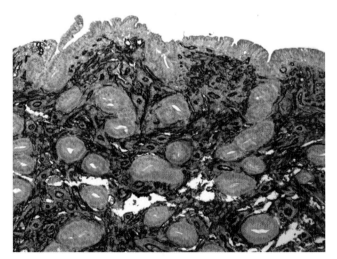

Fig. 26.7 CD31 immunostaining highlights the vascular proliferation in the small intestine

are usually mild, although severe gastroenteritis has been reported. The pathologic features of HHV-6 gastrointestinal infection have not been well studied, and the limited histologic studies available describe a mild gastritis. The virus has been detected by immunohistochemistry in the duodenal mucosa of both liver transplant patients and immunocompetent patients with dyspeptic symptoms.

Epstein–Barr virus (EBV). The importance of EBV in the gastrointestinal tract is primarily through its association with a wide variety of neoplasms, including numerous types of lymphoma, post-transplant lymphoproliferative disorders, and adenocarcinomas (both with and without lymphoepithelioma-like morphologic features) (Fig. 26.9). EBV-associated lymphomas and lymphoproliferative disorders are particularly important in HIV-infected and post-transplant patients. Very rarely, EBV has been reported to

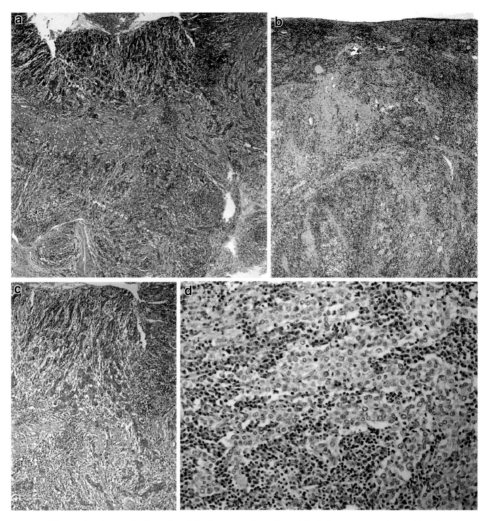

Fig. 26.9 PCR-proven EBV-associated gastric lymphoepithelioma-like adenocarcinoma. Ulcerated mucosa overlies infiltrative nests of poorly differentiated tumor cells with a prominent nodular lymphoid stroma (**a**). Low-power view showing ulcerated gastric mucosa, with underlying lymphocyte-rich neoplasm in which it is difficult to appre- ciate the epithelial component (**b**). Infiltrative nests of tumor cells with both intra- and extra-tumoral lymphocytes extend into the submucosa (**c**). High-power view shows nests of poorly differentiated epithelial cells with surrounding lymphocytic stroma

cause an ulcerative gastritis unassociated with malignancy. In addition, EBV has been implicated as an underlying cause of intestinal pseudoobstruction, along with many other DNA viruses, and it occasionally causes appendicitis during the course of infectious mononucleosis.

Selected References

Measles (Rubeola Virus)

1. Dossetor JF, Whittle HC. Protein-losing enteropathy and malabsorption in acute measles enteritis. Br Med J 2(5971):592–3, 1975.
2. Paik SY, Oh JT, Choi YJ, et al. Measles-related appendicitis. Arch Pathol Lab Med 126:82–4, 2002.
3. Pancharoen C, Ruttanamongkol P, Suwangool P, et al. Measles-associated appendicitis: two case reports and literature review. Scan J Infect Dis 33:632–3, 2001.
4. Vieth M, Dirschmid K, Oehler U, et al. Acute measles gastric infection. Am J Surg Pathol 25:259–62, 2001.
5. Whalen TV, Klos JR, Kovalcik PJ, Cross GH. Measles and appendicitis. Am Surg 46:412–3, 1980.

Herpes Zoster/Varicella Virus

6. Baker CJ, Gilsdorf JR, South MA, Singleton EB. Gastritis as a complication of varicella. South Med J 66:539–41, 1973.
7. Debinski HS, Kamm MA, Talbot IC, et al. DNA viruses in the pathogenesis of sporadic chronic idiopathic intestinal pseudo-obstruction. Gut 41:100–6, 1997.
8. Gill RA, Gebhard RL, Dozeman RL, Sumner HW. Shingles esophagitis: endoscopic diagnosis in two patients. Gastro Endos 30:26–7, 1984.
9. Mallet E, Maitre M, Mouterde O. Complications of the digestive tract in varicella infection including two cases of erosive gastritis. Eur J Pediatr 165:64–5, 2006.

10. Miliauskas JR, Webber BL. Disseminated Varicella at autopsy in children with cancer. Cancer 53:1518–25, 1984.
11. Pui JC, Furth EE, Minda J, Montone KT. Demonstration of Varicella-Zoster virus infection in the muscularis propria and myenteric plexi of the colon in an HIV-positive patient with Herpes Zoster and small bowel pseudo-obstruction (Ogilvie's syndrome). Am J Gastroenterol 96:1627–30, 2001.
12. Rivera P, Canelles P, Quiles F, et al. Gastrointestinal involvement in infections caused by Varicella virus. Endoscopy 30:S9, 1998.
13. Sherman RA, Silva J Jr., Gandour-Edwards R. Fatal varicella in an adult: case report and review of the literature. Rev Infect Dis 13:424–7, 1991.
14. Stemmer SM, Kinsman K, Tellschow S, Jones RB. Fatal noncutaneous visceral infection with Varicella-Zoster virus in a patient with lymphoma after autologous bone marrow transplantation. Clin Infect Dis 16:497–9, 1993.
15. Walsh TN, Lane D. Pseudo obstruction of the colon associated with varicella-zoster infection. Ir J Med Sci 151:318–9, 1982.
16. Wisloff F, Bull-Berg J, Myren J. Herpes Zoster of the stomach. Lancet 2(3):953, 1979.

Human Herpesvirus-8 (HHV-8)

17. Clayton F, Clayton CH. Gastrointestinal pathology in HIV-infected patients. Gastroenterol Clin North Am 26(2):191–240, 1997.
18. Depond W, Said JW, Tasaka T. Kaposi's sarcoma-associated herpesvirus and human herpesvirus 8 (KSHV/HHV8)-associated lymphoma of the bowel. Report of two cases in HIV-positive men with secondary effusion lymphomas. Am J Surg Pathol 23:992–4, 1997.
19. Dezube BJ. Acquired immunodeficiency syndrome-related Kaposi's sarcoma: clinical features, staging, and treatment. Semin Oncol 27:424–30, 2000.
20. Kahl P, Buettner R, Friedrichs N, et al. Kaposi's sarcoma of the gastrointestinal tract: report of two cases and review of the literature. Pathol Res Pract 203:227–31, 2007.

Human Herpesvirus-6 (HHV-6)

21. Breddemann A, Laer S, Schmidt KG, et al. Case report: severe gastrointestinal inflammation and persistent HHV-6B infection in a pediatric cancer patient. Herpes 14:41–4, 2007.
22. Durno C, Jones N, Hebert D, et al. Evidence linking human herpesvirus-6 (HHV-6) with disease in gastrointestinal transplantation. Transpl Proceed 32:1235–7, 2000.
23. Halme L, Arola J, Hockerstedt K, Lautenschlager I. Human herpesvirus 6 infection of the gastroduodenal mucosa. Clin Infect Dis 46:434–9, 2008.

Epstein-Barr Virus (EBV)

24. Bai M, Katsanos KH, Economou M, et al. Rectal Epstein-Barr virus-positive Hodgkin's lymphoma in a patient with Crohn's disease: case report and review of the literature. Scand J Gastroenterol 41:866–9, 2006.
25. Cao S, Cox K, Esquivel CO, et al. Posttransplant lymphoproliferative disorders and gastrointestinal manifestations of Epstein-Barr virus infection in children following liver transplantation. Transpl 66:851–6, 1998.
26. Chen ZM, shah R, Zuckerman GR, Wang HL. Epstein-Barr virus gastritis: an underrecognized form of severe gastritis simulating gastric lymphoma. Am J Surg Pathol 31:1446–51, 2007.
27. Herath CHP, Chetty R. Epstein-Barr virus-associated lymphoepithelioma-like gastric carcinoma. Arch Pathol Lab Med 132:706–9, 2008.
28. Ioachim HL, Antonescu C, Giancotti F, et al. EBV-associated anorectal lymphomas in patients with acquired immune deficiency syndrome. Am J Surg Pathol 21:997–1006, 1997.
29. Lai YC, Ni YH, Jou ST, et al. Post-transplant lymphoproliferative disorders localizing to the gastrointestinal tract after liver transplantation: report of five pediatric cases. Pediatr Transplant 10:390–4, 2006.
30. Lopez-Navidad A, Domingo P, Cadafalch J, et al. Acute appendicitis complicating infectious mononucleosis: case report and review. Rev Infect Dis 12:297–302, 1997.
31. Takada K. Epstein-Barr virus and gastric carcinoma. J Clin Pathol 53:255–61, 2000.
32. Wu MS, Shun CT, Wu, CC, et al. Epstein-Barr virus-associated gastric carcinomas: relation to H. pylori infection and genetic alterations. Gastroenterol 118:1031–8, 2000.

Chapter 27

Miscellaneous Protozoal Infections

Keywords Protozoa • Amoebae • Flagellates • Coccidians • Ciliates • *Blastocystis hominis* • Entamoeba species • *Endolimax nana* • *Iodamoeba butschlii* • Amoeba of low pathogenicity • *Dientameba fragilis* • Commensal • *Balantidium coli*

Protozoa are prevalent pathogens in tropical and subtropical countries, although they also cause some of the most common intestinal infections in North America. Immigration, increasing numbers of immunocompromised patients, use of institutional child-care facilities, and the development of improved diagnostic techniques for stool collection, handling, and examination have enhanced our understanding and recognition of protozoa. A summary of protozoa affecting the gastrointestinal tract is given in Table 27.1, and selected protozoan infections are discussed below and in subsequent chapters.

Table 27.1 Selected protozoa affecting the gastrointestinal tract

Amoebae	Flagellates	Coccidians	Ciliates	Uncertain
Entamoeba histolytica	*Trypanosoma cruzi*	Microsporidia	*Balantidium coli*	*Blastocystis hominis*
Entamoeba coli	*Leishmania donovanii* and related species	Cyclospora		
Entamoeba hartmani				
Entamoeba polecki				
Endolimax nana	*Giardia lamblia*	Cryptosporidium		
Iodamoeba butschlii	*Dientamoeba fragilis*	*Isospora belli*		
		Toxoplasma gondii		

Non-pathogenic amoebae or amoebae of "low pathogenicity." These amoebae are referred to as non-pathogenic amoeba or amoeba of low pathogenicity, and this group includes *Entamoeba hartmani, Entamoeba coli, Iodamoeba buetschlii, Endolimax nana,* and *Entamoeba polecki.* Isolation of supposedly "non-pathogenic" parasites in a patient with an undiagnosed diarrheal illness, particularly an immunocompromised individual, is an increasingly common clinical problem. In some series, non-pathogenic protozoa have been reported in up to 50% of HIV-infected patients, but their presence did not correlate with gastrointestinal symptoms. Few carefully conducted clinical studies of these organisms exist. Anecdotal studies of supposedly symptomatic infections that responded to directed therapy are difficult to interpret, for it is difficult to know if patients responded to therapy because the therapy actually eradicated an identified organism of "low pathogenicity," or if therapy eradicated an undetected true pathogen. In addition, many patients from whom non-pathogenic amoebae are recovered also harbor other pathogens. Some authorities, however, do believe that these organisms are capable of causing symptomatic gastrointestinal disease in rare instances.

Entamoeba polecki is generally thought to be non-pathogenic, as discussed above, but it does appear to cause diarrhea and abdominal pain in rare patients. Infection is more common in areas where humans live in close contact with pigs. Most reported infections in humans have been from New Guinea, and it has been rarely reported in Venezuela and parts of Southeast Asia. Most cases in the Western hemisphere are seen in immigrants. These organisms may be difficult to distinguish from other similar parasites, particularly *E. histolytica.* Detailed comparison of cyst forms can distinguish *E. polecki* from other amoeba in stool smears, however, as it has a consistently uninucleate cyst.

Dientameba fragilis is a parasite of low pathogenicity that occasionally causes symptomatic infection. Its exact classification is controversial, and it has been classified as both an amoeba and as a flagellate; most recently, it has been grouped as an "atypical" flagellate similar to trichomonads. Children are most often affected, and there is a higher incidence in Native Americans in South Dakota and Arizona, institutionalized patients, foreign travelers, and communities with poor hygienic practices. Symptoms include diarrhea, abdominal pain, flatulence, bloating, vomiting, fatigue, and weight loss, and symptoms may persist for months. Peripheral eosinophilia is variably present, especially in children. Transmission is believed to be predominantly person-to-person, rather than water- or food-borne, and some suggest that *D. fragilis* may be transmitted via the egg of the pinworm *Enterobius vermicularis*. In fact, some authorities recommend that if *D. fragilis* is found, it is imperative to search for *E. vermicularis* infection as well. *D. fragilis* exists only in trophozoite form. The trophozoite is usually binucleate, but may contain up to four nuclei, which often contain large granules. Although the trophozoites apparently attach to the crypts of the large bowel, usually in the right colon, they are not believed to cause actual tissue damage. *D. fragilis* is best diagnosed in fresh, recently passed stool specimens that are fixed and permanently stained (Fig. 27.1).

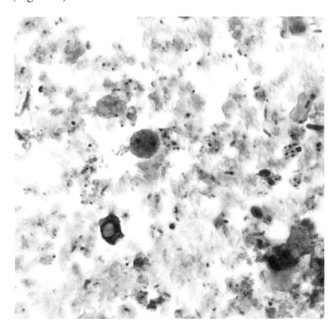

Fig. 27.1 Trichrome-stained stool smear showing trophozoite of *D. fragilis*, with two nuclei and somewhat granular cytoplasm. (Courtesy Dr. Stephan Juretschko)

Blastocystis hominis, another organism of low pathogenicity, is a frequent commensal inhabitant of the human gastrointestinal tract. Its exact taxonomic position remains uncertain, but it is usually classified as a protozoan. Its ability to cause symptomatic enteric disease remains controversial. Since organisms have been recovered from patients with diarrhea in the absence of any other pathogen, some believe that it does cause symptoms (including abdominal pain, diarrhea, flatulence, and vomiting) when present in large numbers, particularly in immunocompromised patients and children.

Most of the protozoa discussed above are diagnosed in stool samples, and multiple stool samples that are quickly examined after collection increase the yield. Protozoa of low pathogenicity are occasionally found in tissue sections; however, their presence does not automatically imply that they are responsible for symptomatic infection, and alternative causes of gastrointestinal disease still should be considered.

Balantidium coli. B. coli has the dual distinction of being both the largest protozoan and the only ciliate capable of causing disease in humans. It is rarely found in temperate zones, but is common in the tropics, especially the Philippines. It is most often a parasite of pigs and other domestic and wild animals. Human infections are commonly linked to close contact with pigs, water contaminated with pig excreta, and butchering; person-to-person transmission is also believed possible. Although most human infections are asymptomatic, this ciliate may produce a spectrum of clinical and pathologic changes similar to that of *E. histolytica*. It infects the terminal ileum and colon, particularly the rectosigmoid, and pathologic features include mucosal ulceration, edema, hemorrhage, and necrosis (Fig. 27.2). The inflammatory infiltrate is often predominantly mononuclear, and inflammation and necrosis may be transmural (Fig. 27.3). Bowel perforation, peritonitis, and widespread dissemination have been reported rarely. Other rare manifestations include appendicitis and superinfection of patients with chronic idiopathic inflammatory bowel disease.

Balantidium coli are distinguished from amoebae by their large size (50–200 μm in length by 40–70 μm in diameter),

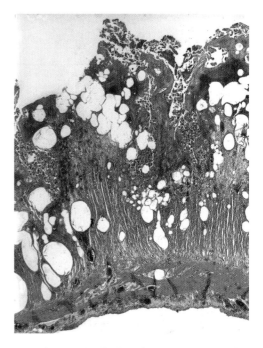

Fig. 27.2 Invasive *B. coli* infection with transmural necrosis and hemorrhage, along with organisms invading into the submucosa and superficial muscularis propria. (Courtesy Dr. David Owen)

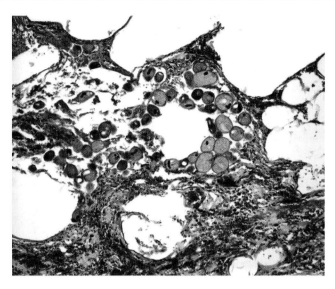

Fig. 27.3 Many large *B. coli* are present within the necroinflammatory infiltrate and hemorrhage. (Courtesy Dr. David Owen)

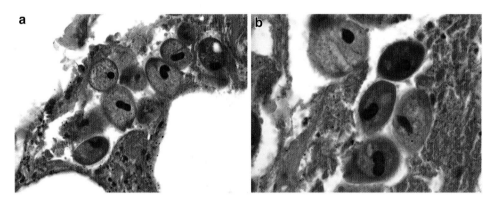

Fig. 27.4 *B. coli* are easily identified in tissue sections by their large size, large kidney bean-shaped macronucleus, and numerous cilia (**a** and **b**, courtesy Dr. David Owen)

prominent kidney bean-shaped macronucleus and smaller round micronucleus, and of course, the presence of hundreds of cilia that beat in coordinated rhythm. They are easily identified in tissue sections (Fig. 27.4).

men who have sex with men from Sydney, Australia. Am J Trop Med Hyg 76:549–52, 2007.

Selected References

General

1. Juckett G. Intestinal protozoa. Am Fam Physician 53:2507–16, 1996.
2. Peters CS, Sable R, Janda WM, et al. Prevalence of enteric parasites in homosexual patients attending an outpatient clinic. J Clin Microbiol 24:684–5, 1986.
3. Stark D, Fotedar R, van Hal S, et al. Prevalence of enteric protozoa in human immunodeficiency virus (HIV)-positive and HIV-negative

Amoebae

4. Aucott JN, Ravdin JI. Amebiasis and "nonpathogenic" intestinal protozoa. Infect Dis Clin North Am 7(3):467–83, 1993.
5. Chacin-Bonilla L. *Entamoeba polecki*: human infections in Venezuela. Trans Roy Soc Trop Med Hyg 86:634, 1992.
6. Gay JD, Abell TL, Thompson JH Jr., Loth V. *Entamoeba polecki* infection in southeast Asian refugees: multiple cases of a rarely reported parasite. Mayo Clin Proc 60:523–30, 1985.
7. Lawless DK, Knight V. Human infection with *Entamoeba polecki*: report of four cases. Am J Trop Med Hyg 15:701–4, 1966.
8. Levin RL, Armstrong DE. Human infection with *Entamoeba polecki*. Am J Clin Pathol 54:611–14, 1970.

Dientamoeba fragilis

9. Butler WP. *Dientamoeba fragilis*: an unusual intestinal pathogen. Dig Dis Sci 41:1811–13, 1996.
10. Grendon JH, Digiacomo RF, Frost FJ. Descriptive features of *Diemtamoeba fragilis* infections. J Trop Med Hyg 98:309–15, 1995.
11. Johnson EH, Windsor JJ, Clark CG. Emerging from obscurity: biological, clinical, and diagnostic aspects of *Dientamoeba fragilis*. Clin Microbiol Rev 17:553–70, 2004.
12. Millet V, Spencer MJ, Chapin M, et al. *Dientamoeba fragilis*, a protozoan parasite in adult members of a semicommunal group. Dig Dis Sci 28:335–9, 1983.
13. Spencer MJ, Chapin MR, Garcia LS. *Dientamoeba fragilis*: a gastrointestinal protozoan infection in adults. Am J Gastroenterol 77:565–9, 1982.
14. Stark DJ, Beebe N, Marriott D, et al. Dientamoebiasis: clinical importance and recent advances. Trends Parasitol 22:92–6, 2006.

Blastocystis hominis

15. Albrecht H, Stellbrink HJ, Koperski K, Greten H. *Blastocystis hominis* in human immunodeficiency-related diarrhea. Scand J Gastroenterol 30:909–14, 1995.
16. Markell EK, Udkow MP. *Blastocystis hominis*: pathogen or fellow traveler? Am J Trop Med Hyg 35:1023–6, 1986.
17. O'Gorman MA, Orenstein SR, Proujanski R, et al. Prevalence and characteristics of *Blastocystis hominis* infection in children. Clin Pediatr 32:91–6, 1993.
18. Sun T, Katz S, Tanenbaum B, Schenone C. Questionable clinical significance of *Blastocystis hominis* infection. Am J Gastroenterol 84:1543–7, 1989.
19. Tan, KSW. Blastocystis in humans and animals: new insights using modern methodologies. Vet Parasitol 126:121–44, 2004.
20. Tungtrongchitr A, Manatsathit S, Kositchaiwat C, et al. *Blastocystis hominis* infection in irritable bowel syndrome. Southeast Asian J Trop Med Public Health 35:705–10, 2004.
21. Zaki M, Daoud AS, Pugh RNH, et al. Clinical report of *Blastocystis hominis* infection in children. J Trop Med Hyg 94:118–22, 1991.

Balantidium coli

22. Ferry T, Bouhour D, De Monbrison F, et al. Severe peritonitis due to *Balantidium coli* acquired in France. Eur J Clin Microbiol Infect Dis 23:393–5, 2004.
23. Ladas SD, Savva S, Frydas A, et al. Invasive balantidiasis presented as chronic colitis and lung involvement. Dig Dis Sci 34:1621–3, 1989.
24. Schwartz DA, Mixon JP. Balantidiasis. In Connor DH, Chandler FW et al. (eds): Pathology of Infectious Diseases, Stamford, CT: Appleton and Lange, 1997, pp. 1141–1145.
25. Walzer PD, Judson FN, Murphy KB, et al. Balantidiasis outbreak in Truk. Am J Trop Med Hyg 22:33–41, 1973.

Chapter 28

Entamoeba histolytica

Keywords *Entamoeba* species • Amebic dysentery • Amebiasis

Entamoeba histolytica is a motile protozoan that infects approximately 10% of the world's population, predominantly in tropical and subtropical regions. In the United States, this infection is most often seen in immigrants, overseas travelers, male homosexuals, and institutionalized persons. Infection is usually acquired through contaminated water or food and can be spread by the fecal–oral route. Sexual transmission has been reported occasionally. Risk factors for symptomatic infection include pediatric age group, malnutrition, pregnancy, immunosuppression, and steroids.

Many infected patients are asymptomatic or have only vague, non-specific gastrointestinal complaints that may mimic irritable bowel syndrome. Symptomatic patients most commonly have diarrhea, abdominal cramps, and variable right lower quadrant tenderness; this may be referred to as "non-dysenteric" amebiasis. Invasive disease, most often manifested as amoebic dysentery or liver abscess, reportedly occurs in less than 10% of infected persons. Amebic dysentery presents suddenly, approximately 1–3 weeks after exposure, with severe abdominal cramps, tenesmus, fever, and diarrhea (which may be mucoid and/or bloody).

Complications of intestinal amoebiasis include bleeding; perforation; dissemination to other sites, particularly the liver; fistula formation between the intestine and the skin, peritoneum, and urogenital tract; and toxic megacolon. The latter complication is often associated with corticosteroid use.

Entamoeba histolytica is occasionally found in the appendix, generally in association with heavy infection of the right colon. The organism is usually present in the lumen and does not invade. Patients presenting with signs and symptoms of acute appendicitis, who are found to have mucosal ulceration and acute inflammation of the appendix at appendectomy, have been described rarely.

Pathologic features. The cecum is the most common site of involvement, followed by the right colon, rectum, sigmoid, and appendix. Colonoscopy may be normal in asymptomatic patients or those with mild disease. When patients do have macroscopic findings, small ulcers are initially seen, which may coalesce to form large, irregular geographic or serpiginous ulcers (Fig. 28.1). Ulcers may undermine adjacent mucosa to produce the classic "flask-shaped" lesions, and there may be inflammatory polyps as well. The intervening mucosa is often grossly normal. Unusual macroscopic findings include fulminant colitis resembling ulcerative colitis, pseudomembrane formation mimicking *C. difficile*-related pseudomembranous colitis, and large inflammatory masses consisting of organisms and granulation tissue (amoebomas).

Histologically, early lesions may show a mild neutrophilic infiltrate (Fig. 28.2), but in some cases numerous organisms are present at the luminal surface with little associated inflammation. In more advanced disease, ulcers are often deep, extending into the submucosa (Fig. 28.3), with undermining of adjacent mucosa (Fig. 28.4). The adjacent mucosa may be histologically normal or may show gland distortion

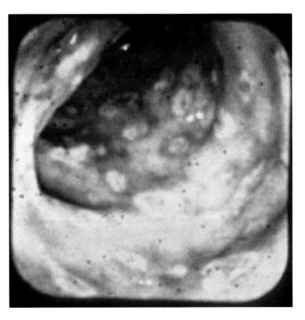

Fig. 28.1 Colonoscopic photograph of confluent ulcers in amoebiasis. (Courtesy Dr. Margie Scott)

L.W. Lamps, *Surgical Pathology of the Gastrointestinal System: Bacterial, Fungal, Viral, and Parasitic Infections*, DOI 10.1007/978-1-4419-0861-2_28, © Springer Science+Business Media, LLC 2009

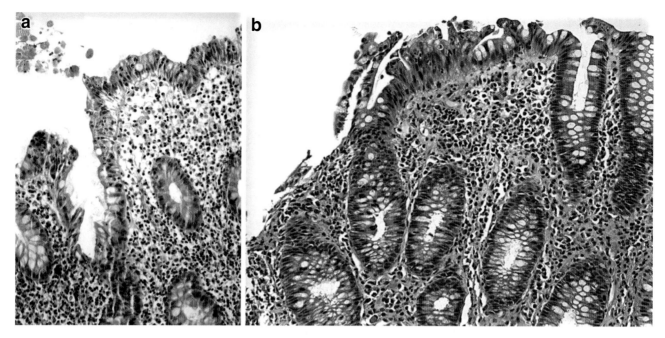

Fig. 28.2 Early lesions of non-invasive *E. histolytica* show superficial neutrophilic inflammation, along with a mixed inflammatory infiltrate in the lamina propria. Note cluster of amoebae at the top left (**a**). Higher power view showing early superficial neutrophilic infiltrate (**b**)

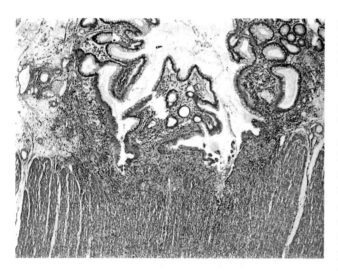

Fig. 28.3 Deep, punched-out ulcer extending into the muscular wall in a case of invasive amoebiasis

and inflammation that can mimic chronic idiopathic inflammatory bowel disease. There is usually abundant amorphous eosinophilic necrotic material containing nuclear debris (Fig. 28.5). In early lesions, the organisms are concentrated at the luminal surface (Fig. 28.6), and then later in ulcer beds, usually within the necrotic material. Invasive amoebae may be detected occasionally within the bowel wall (Fig. 28.7). In many cases, the abundant necrotic debris greatly exceeds the amount of associated inflammation that is present.

In asymptomatic patients or those with only mild symptoms, histologic findings may range from normal to a heavy mixed inflammatory infiltrate. Organisms may be particularly difficult (if not impossible) to detect in these patients. Histologic evidence of invasive amebiasis is not generally seen in patients who have only mild, or absent, symptoms.

*Morphologic features of the organism.*Trophozoites have distinct cell membranes with foamy cytoplasm (Fig. 28.8). The nuclei are round and eccentrically located, with peripheral margination of chromatin and a central karyosome (Figs. 28.8 and 28.9). The presence of ingested red blood cells is essentially pathognomonic of *E. histolytica* and helps to distinguish it from other amoebae (see below) (Figs. 28.8, 28.9, and 28.10). Distinction of trophozoites from macrophages within inflammatory exudates may be difficult, particularly in poorly fixed tissue sections. Amoebae are trichrome and PAS positive (Fig. 28.11); in addition, their nuclei are usually more rounded, smaller, paler, and have a more open nuclear chromatin pattern than those of macrophages. Macrophages stain with CD68, alpha-1-antitrypsin, and chymotrypsin, whereas amoebae do not.

Differential diagnosis. *Balantidium coli* may mimic *E. histolytica* histologically, but it is much larger, has a kidney-bean shaped macronucleus, and is ciliated. *E. histolytica* may be distinguished from most other amoebae by the presence of ingested red blood cells.

Two other species of amoeba, *E. dispar* and *E. moshkovskii*, which are histologically indistinguishable from *E. histolytica*, have recently received attention because they have been recovered from the stool of patients with gastrointestinal symptoms. To date, there is no convincing evidence that *E. dispar* causes symptomatic gastrointestinal disease,

Fig. 28.4 Classic "flask-shaped" ulcer with undermining of adjacent intact mucosa in a case of invasive amoebiasis (**a** and **b**; **a**, courtesy Dr. David Owen). The latter patient was clinically believed to have Crohn's disease and given steroids, leading to fulminant amoebic colitis

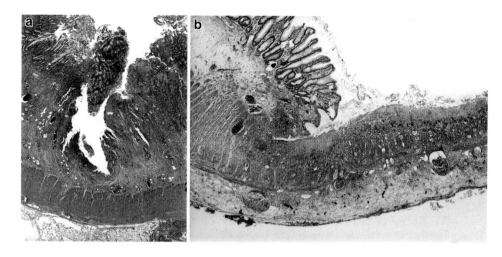

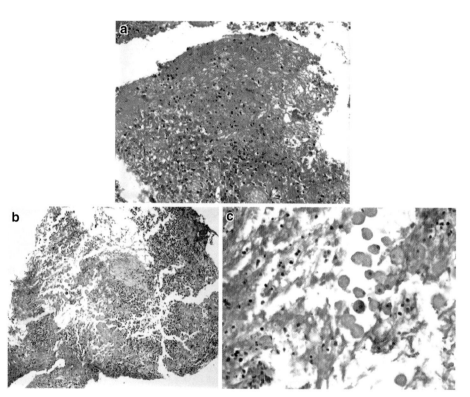

Fig. 28.5 Amorphous eosinophilic debris typical of *E. histolytica* infection, containing necrotic material and nuclear debris, but few intact neutrophils (**a**). The amount of debris may greatly exceed the number of organisms (**b** and **c**)

and many studies are confounded by co-infection with *E. histolytica* and other gastrointestinal pathogens. Some authorities, however, do currently refer to the organism as *E. histolytica–E. dispar* complex, due to the high rate of coinfection. There are rare reports of symptomatic infection with *E. moshkovskii,* although many of these are also confounded by co-infection with *E. histolytica* and other pathogens, and thus the true pathogenicity of this species remains controversial. In the context of a patient with symptomatic amebiasis and the microscopic identification of organisms with an accompanying tissue reaction, however, distinction between these species is rarely important for clinical management purposes. If speciation is absolutely necessary, serologic tests

and PCR assays exist that can distinguish between the three organisms.

The differential diagnosis of amebiasis also includes Crohn's disease, ulcerative colitis, ischemic colitis, *C. difficile*-related pseudomembranous colitis, and other types of infectious colitis. Many of the characteristic features of Crohn's disease are absent in amoebiasis, including transmural lymphoid aggregates, mural fibrosis, granulomas, and neural hyperplasia. Although amoebiasis can cause architectural distortion, the cryptitis, crypt abscesses, marked basal lymphoplasmacytosis, diffuse architectural distortion, and disease distribution typical of ulcerative colitis are not usually present in amoebiasis. A careful search for trophozoites

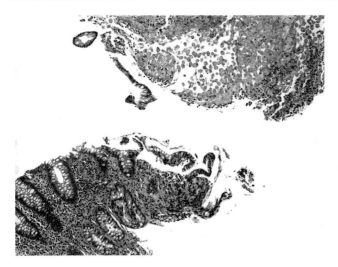

Fig. 28.6 Colon biopsy from non-invasive amoebiasis, showing clusters of amoeba within necrotic material at the luminal surface of the right colon

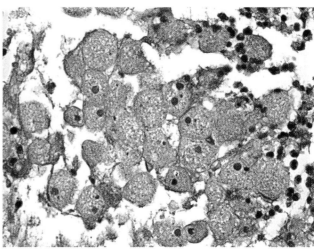

Fig. 28.8 Amoebae have distinct cell membranes and foamy cytoplasm

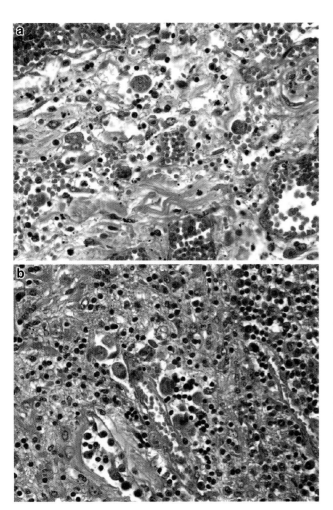

Fig. 28.7 Amoebae in the bowel wall in a case of invasive amoebiasis (**a** and **b**, courtesy Dr. David Owen). Lymphovascular invasion is occasionally seen (**b**)

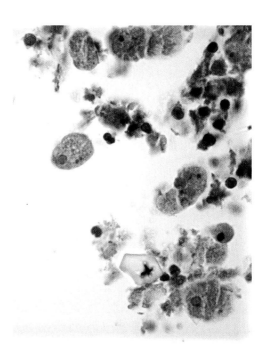

Fig. 28.9 The nuclei of amoeba are eccentrically placed and pale, with peripheral chromatin margination and a central karyosome

in unusual cases of inflammatory bowel disease or those from patients from endemic regions is warranted, however, as steroid administration can cause life-threatening complications if the diagnosis of amoebiasis is missed. Amoebomas can mimic colonic adenocarcinoma grossly and radiographically, and are often diagnosed only after biopsy or resection with tissue examination. Useful diagnostic tests for *E. histolytica* include stool examination for cysts and trophozoites, stool culture, serologic tests, and PCR assays, although the latter are not widely available.

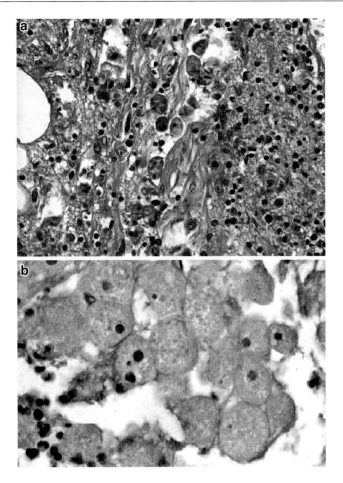

Fig. 28.10 Ingestion of red blood cells is pathognomonic of *E. histolytica* (**a** and **b**; **a**, courtesy Dr. David Owen)

Selected References

1. Brandt H, Tamayo P. Pathology of human amebiasis. Hum Pathol 1:351–85, 1970.
2. Braunstein H, Connor DH. Amebiasis-infection by *Entamoeba histolytica*. In: Connor DH, Chandler FW et al. (eds): Pathology of Infectious Diseases, Stamford, CT: Appleton and Lange, 1997, pp. 1127–33.
3. Gonin P, Trudel L. Detection and differentiation of Entamoeba histolytica and Entamoeba dispar isolates in clinical samples by PCR and enzyme-linked immunosorbent assay. J Clin Microbiol 41:237–41, 2003.
4. Fotedar R, Star, D, Beebe N, et al. Laboratory diagnostic techniques for *Entamoeba* species. Clin Microbiol Rev 20:511–32, 2007.
5. Gotohda N, Itano S, Okada Y, et al. Acute appendicitis caused by amoebiasis. J gastroenterol 135:861–3, 2000.
6. Hardin RE, Ferzli GS, Zenilman ME, et al. Invasive amebiasis and ameboma formation presenting as a rectal mass: an uncommon case of malignant masquerade at a western medical center. World J Gastroenterol 13:5659–61, 2007.
7. Juckett GJ. Intestinal protozoa. Am Fam Physician 53:2507–16, 1996.
8. Lewthwaite P, Gill GV, Hart CA, Beeching NJ. Gastrointestinal parasites in the immunocompromised. Curr Opin Infect Dis 18:427–35, 2005.
9. Lebbad M, Svard SG. PCR differentiation of *Entamoeba histolytica* and *Entamoeba dispar* from patients with amoeba infection initially diagnosed by microscopy. Scand J Infect Dis 37:680–85, 2005.
10. Li E, Stanley SL. Protozoa: Amebiasis. Gastroenterol Clin North Am 25(3):471–92, 1996.
11. Nadler S, Cappell MS, Bhatt B, et al. Appendiceal infection by *Entamoeba histolytica* and *Strongyloides stercoralis* presenting like acute appendicitis. Dig Dis Sci 35:603–8, 1990.
12. Ng DCK, Kwok SY, Cheng Y, et al. Colonic amebic abscess mimicking carcinoma of the colon. Hong Kong Med J 12:71–3, 2006.
13. Okamoto M, Kawabe T, Ohata K, et al. Amebic colitis in asymptomatic subjects with positive fecal occult blood test results: clinical features different from symptomatic cases. Am J Trop Med Hyg 73:934–5, 2005.
14. Panosian CB. Parasitic diarrhea. Infect Dis Clin North Am 2(3):685–703, 1988.
15. Pillai DR, Keystone JS, Sheppard DC, et al. *Entamoeba histolytica* and *Entamoeba dispar*: epidemiology and comparison of diagnostic methods in a setting of nonendemicity. Clin Infect Dis 29:1315–18, 1999.
16. Ravdin JI. Amebiasis. Clin Infect Dis 20:1453–66, 1995.

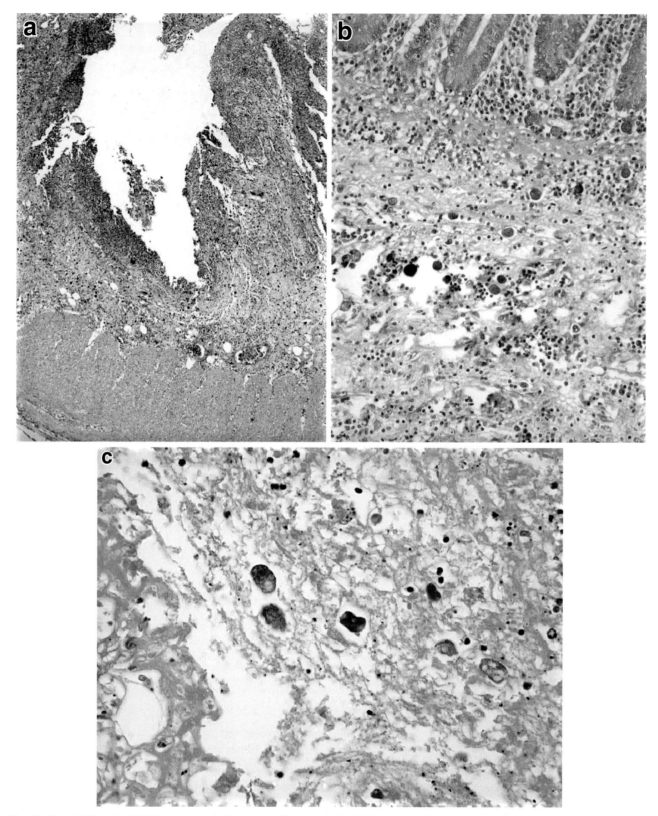

Fig. 28.11 A PAS stain highlights the amoeba in a case of invasive amoebiasis. Low-power photomicrograph shows a characteristic flask-shaped ulcer (**a**). The PAS stain highlights parasites in the submucosa (**b**). High-power photomicrograph of PAS-stained amoebae within the bowel wall (**c**). (Courtesy Dr. David Owen)

17. Reed SL: Amebiasis: an update. Clin Infect Dis 14:385–93, 1992.
18. Stanley Jr. SL. Amoebiasis. Lancet 361(9362):1025–34, 2003.
19. Variyam EP, Gogate P, Hassan M, et al. Nondysenteric intestinal amebiasis: colonic morphology and search for *Entamoeba histolytic*a adherence and invasion. Dig Dis Sci 34:732–40, 1989.
20. Wiwanitkit V. Intestinal parasite infection in HIV infected patients. Curr HIV Res 4:87–96, 2006.
21. Yildirim S, Nursal T, Tarim A, et al. A rare cause of acute appendicitis: parasitic infection. Scand J Infect Dis 37:757–9,2005.

Chapter 29

Intestinal Flagellates

Keywords Flagellate • *Giardia lamblia* • Diarrhea • *Leishmania donovani* • Leishmaniasis • Kala-azar • *Trypanosoma cruzi* • Chagas disease • Megaesophagus • Megacolon

Giardia lamblia. Anton Van Leeuwenhoek first identified *Giardia* in 1681, when he examined one of his own stools with a home-made lens. It took over 200 years, however, for scientists to demonstrate that *Giardia* is a true enteric pathogen rather than a commensal organism. Giardiasis occurs throughout temperate and tropical regions worldwide, and is one of the most common human protozoal enteric pathogens. It is the most clinically significant protozoan pathogen in the United States. The overall prevalence rate is 2–7%, but reaches up to 35% within day-care centers. Risk factors for infection include pediatric age group, travel to foreign countries, use of drinking and recreational water from untreated sources, institutional settings (including day-care centers), living with an infected child, and immune compromise, particularly common variable immunodeficiency.

Transmission is through contaminated water or food, and person-to-person transmission via the fecal–oral route is common. Transmission via oral–anal sexual practices has also been well documented. The cyst, which is the infective form, is extremely hardy, chlorine-resistant, and may survive in water for several months. The mechanism by which these organisms cause gastrointestinal illness remains poorly understood. Postulated mechanisms include production of a physical barrier to absorption by coating of the small bowel by the trophozoites, actual mucosal injury by trophozoites, associated bacterial overgrowth and bile salt deconjugation, and reduction in small bowel enzyme activity.

Many infections are asymptomatic. Acute giardiasis presents as diarrhea and weight loss, which may be accompanied by abdominal pain and distension, nausea, vomiting, flatulence, signs of malabsorption, and extreme fatigue. The diarrhea is often explosive, foul-smelling, and watery. The infection may resolve spontaneously, but often persists for weeks or months if left untreated. A significant percentage of patients go on to develop chronic giardiasis, featuring diarrhea often accompanied by marked weight loss, signs of malabsorption, and anemia. Complications include dehydration, especially in children, and failure to thrive among infants and small children. Extraintestinal manifestations are rare, but include urticaria, cholecystitis, pancreatitis, peripheral eosinophilia, reactive arthritis, and inflammatory ocular findings.

Pathologic features. *Giardia* is found primarily in the proximal small bowel, although they are detected rarely in the stomach and colon. Endoscopic examination is generally unremarkable. Small intestinal biopsies usually show no tissue reaction to the organism (Fig. 29.1). A minority of cases shows mild to moderate villous blunting, crypt hyperplasia, and increased lamina propria inflammatory cells including plasma cells, lymphocytes, and neutrophils.

Trophozoites are present at the luminal surface, including the surface of intervillous spaces, and tissue invasion

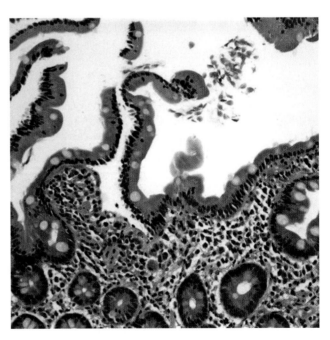

Fig. 29.1 Duodenal biopsy showing no increase in inflammation within either the lamina propria or the epithelium. A cluster of *Giardia* is present at the surface. (Courtesy Dr. Rick Ryals)

L.W. Lamps, *Surgical Pathology of the Gastrointestinal System: Bacterial, Fungal, Viral, and Parasitic Infections,*
DOI 10.1007/978-1-4419-0861-2_29, © Springer Science+Business Media, LLC 2009

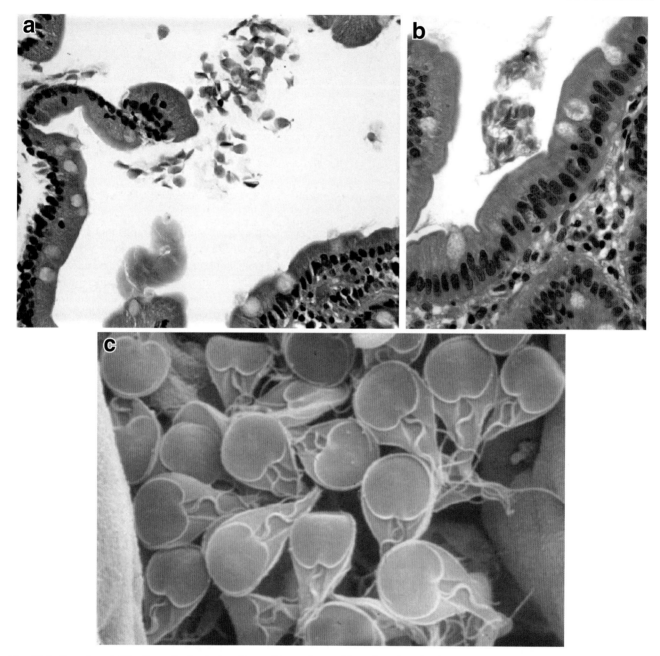

Fig. 29.2 Pear-shaped *Giardia* at the luminal surface, with no tissue invasion or increase in inflammation (**a**, courtesy Dr. Rick Ryals). Higher power view of a cluster of *Giardia* present at the luminal surface, with no tissue invasion (**b**, courtesy Drs. Rodger C. Haggitt and Mary P. Bronner). Scanning electron micrograph of *Giardia* coating the luminal surface of the duodenum (**c**, courtesy Dr. George F. Gray, Jr.)

is not a feature of this infection (Fig. 29.2). The flagellated trophozoites resemble pears that are cut lengthwise, and contain two ovoid nuclei with a central karyosome (Fig. 29.3). The somewhat scattered distribution of the parasite at the luminal surface has been referred to as "falling leaves" (Fig. 29.4). Absence, or a marked decrease, of plasma cells in the lamina propria in a patient with giardiasis should alert the pathologist to the possibility of an underlying immunodeficiency disorder such as common variable immunodeficiency (Fig. 29.5).

Differential diagnosis. The differential diagnosis is primarily with normal small bowel. Since the distribution of organisms can be quite focal, examination of multiple levels is often necessary to establish the diagnosis. Complementary diagnostic tests include examination of recently passed stool specimens, endoscopic brush or touch cytology, and duodenal fluid aspiration. In fact, touch cytology (imprint from endoscopic biopsy specimens performed before the tissue is placed in formalin) may significantly increase diagnostic

Fig. 29.3 The trophozoites of *Giardia* resemble pears cut lengthwise, with two prominent nuclei (**a**, courtesy Dr. Eric Rosenbaum). Cross-sectional view of a cluster of *Giardia*, showing the two prominent nuclei (**b**, courtesy Drs. Rodger C. Haggitt and Mary P. Bronner)

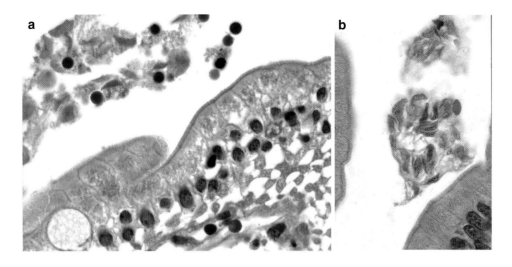

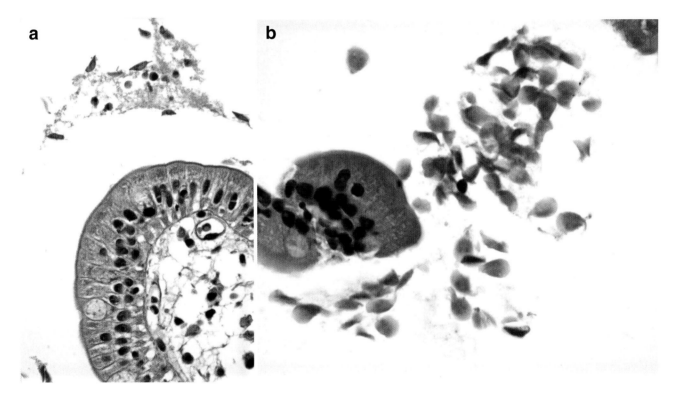

Fig. 29.4 The haphazard arrangement of *Giardia* at the luminal surface have been compared to "falling leaves." (**a**, courtesy Dr. Eric Rosenbaum; **b**, courtesy Dr. Rick Ryals)

yield, since many of the luminal trophozoites may be washed away during processing of the tissue.

Leishmania donovani and related species. Leishmaniasis, caused by an obligate intracellular protozoan transmitted by sandfly bites, is endemic in over 80 countries in Africa, Asia, south and central America, and Europe. The infection may remain localized at the site of the bite or may disseminate widely via the reticuloendothelial system. Visceral leishmaniasis (or kala-azar) is emerging as an important opportunistic infection among HIV-infected patients, particularly in

southwestern Europe. In endemic areas, it often affects children and young adults.

Most infections are asymptomatic. When progression to symptomatic visceral infection occurs, the average incubation period is 3–8 months, but may last for years. Gastrointestinal involvement is rare, and involvement is generally part of widely disseminated disease. Any level of the gastrointestinal tract may be affected. Patients with gastrointestinal involvement have variable presentations depending on the site of involvement, including fever, abdominal pain,

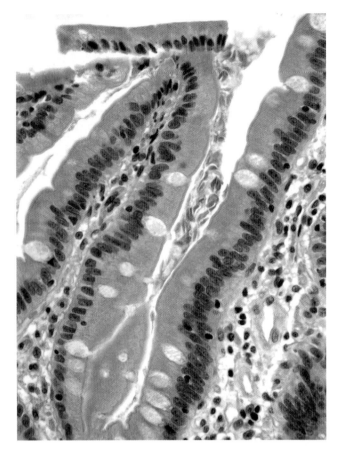

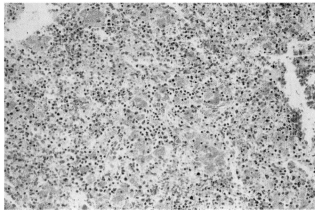

Fig. 29.6 Macrophages distended by amastigotes in a case of visceral leishmaniasis (kala-azar). (Courtesy Dr. George F. Gray, Jr)

Fig. 29.5 Giardiasis in a patient with common variable immuno-deficiency; note lack of plasma cells in the lamina propria. (Courtesy Drs. Rodger C. Haggitt and Mary P. Bronner)

diarrhea, dysphagia, malabsorption, and weight loss. Many patients have hepatosplenomegaly. Laboratory abnormalities include pancytopenia, polyclonal hypergammaglobulinemia, hypoalbuminemia, and elevated erythrocyte sedimentation rate and C-reactive protein.

Pathologic features. The spectrum of endoscopic findings may include normal mucosa, focal ulceration, or mucosal changes of enteritis. Amastigotes are most often seen in duo-

denal or gastric biopsies, but may also be found in the large bowel. Histologically, amastigote-containing macrophages are seen within the lamina propria (Fig. 29.6). When present in large numbers, macrophages may distend and blunt small intestinal villi. A significant associated inflammatory infiltrate is usually absent. The amastigotes are rounded, 2–4-µ basophilic organisms with a round to oval central nucleus and a thin external membrane (Fig. 29.7). The kinetoplast lies tangentially or at right angles to the nucleus, producing a characteristic "double-knot" configuration. They are highlighted by Giemsa staining.

Differential diagnosis. The differential diagnosis primarily includes other parasitic and fungal infections. *Leishmania* may be confused with organisms such as *Histoplasma* and *T. cruzi*. *Leishmania* are GMS negative, which distinguishes them from fungi, and are present in the macrophages of the lamina propria rather than surrounding the myenteric plexus (as opposed to Chagas disease). The kinetoplast of *Leishmania* distinguishes it from *Toxoplasma* species, which may also stain with Giemsa. Serologic studies, tissue culture, and immunohistochemistry may aid in the diagnosis.

Fig. 29.7 Macrophages containing numerous *Leishmania* amastigotes. The amastigotes are rounded, 2–4-µm basophilic organisms with a round to oval central nucleus and a thin external membrane. (**a**, courtesy Drs. Joe Misdraji and Richard Kradin; **b**, courtesy Dr. Bruce Smoller)

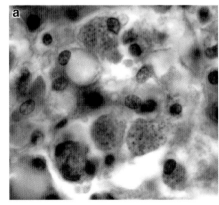

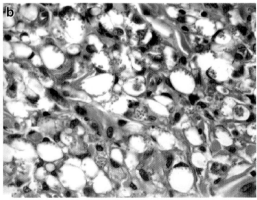

Fig. 29.8 Elongated and markedly dilated esophagus ("megaesophagus") secondary to Chagas disease (**a** and **b**). (Courtesy Dr. Dennis Baroni-Cruz)

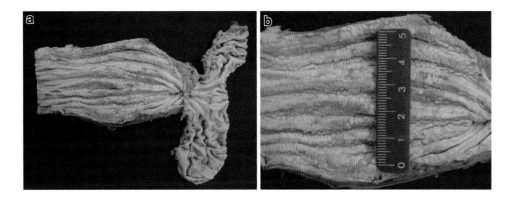

Trypanosoma cruzi (*Chagas disease*). Chagas disease is one of the most serious public health problems in South America. The prevalence in the United States is unknown, and most infections diagnosed in the USA have been in immigrants from endemic areas. Most acute infections are unrecognized. Infected persons then enter the chronic phase, which in the absence of effective therapy lasts for a lifetime. Gastrointestinal dysfunction is the second most common manifestation of chronic Chagas disease (after cardiac involvement), and parasitic involvement of the enteric nervous system most frequently causes an achalasia-like megaesophagus (Fig. 29.8) and/or a megacolon. The stomach and small bowel are more rarely affected.

Gastrointestinal involvement is seen almost exclusively in patients from Argentina, Bolivia, Chile, Paraguay, southern Peru, Uruguay, and parts of Brazil, but very rarely in northern South America, central America, and Mexico. This geographical pattern is thought to be linked to differences in strains of the parasite.

Gastrointestinal disease results from damage to intramural neurons. Upper gastrointestinal symptoms include dysphagia, odynophagia, reflux, aspiration, weight loss, cough, and regurgitation. Imaging studies may show a range of appearances from mild achalasia to megaesophagus. Lower gastrointestinal symptoms include constipation, stool impaction, and abdominal pain; imaging studies reveal a markedly dilated and elongated megacolon. Patients with colonic involvement are at increased risk for volvulus, stercoral ulceration, and ischemia due to stool impaction.

Pathologic features. Histologically, there is inflammatory destruction of the myenteric plexus, with eventual loss of the great majority of neurons. The inflammatory infiltrate is primarily lymphocytic (Fig. 29.9), with inflammation of the nerve fibers and ganglion cells that extends into the muscular wall. Accompanying findings include degenerative neuronal changes, loss of nerve fibers and ganglion cells, and fibrosis. However, the parasite is rarely visible in the myenteric plexi. When seen, the amastigotes are spherical and 2–3 μm in

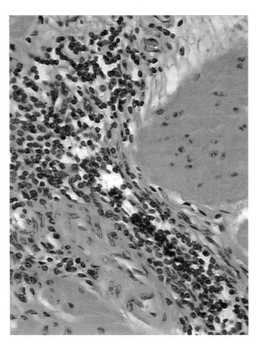

Fig. 29.9 Lymphocytic infiltrate surrounding the nerve fibers in the myenteric plexus. (Courtesy Dr. A.B.M. da Silveira)

diameter, with elongated, rod-shaped, darkly staining kinetoplasts and lightly stained spherical nuclei.

Differential diagnosis. The differential diagnosis includes idiopathic primary achalasia as well as other visceral neuropathies. In contrast, many of these latter disorders lack inflammation of the myenteric plexus. Unlike primary achalasia, Chagas disease usually involves other organ systems (especially the heart) or other areas of the GI tract such as the colon. Nevertheless, often the differential is resolved only clinically. Helpful laboratory tests include PCR assays, serologic studies, and culture. Negative laboratory tests do not exclude infection, however, given the frequently low levels of parasitemia.

Selected References

Giardiasis

1. Debongnie JC, Mairesse J, Donnay M, Dekoninck X. Touch cytology: a quick, simple, sensitive screening test in the diagnosis of infections of the gastrointestinal mucosa. Arch Pathol Lab Med 118:1115–8, 1994.
2. Farthing MJG. Giardiasis. Gastroenterol Clin North Amer 25(3):493–515, 1996.
3. Juckett G. Intestinal protozoa. Am Fam Physician 53:2507–16, 1996.
4. Katelaris PH, Farthing MJG. Diarrhoea and malabsorption in giardiasis: a multifactorial process? Gut 33:295–7, 1992.
5. Lengerich EJ, Addiss DG, Juranek DD. Severe giardiasis in the United States. Clin Infect Dis 18:760–3, 1994.
6. Oberhuber G, Kaster N, Stolte M.. Giardiasis: a histologic analysis of 567 cases. Scand J Gastroenterol 32:48–51, 1997.
7. Ortega YR and Adam RD. Giardia: overview and update. Clin Infect Dis 25:545–50, 1997.
8. Oksenhendler F, Gerard L, Fieschi C, et al. Infections in 252 patients with common variable immunodeficiency. Clin Infect Dis 46:1547–54, 2008.
9. Panosian C. Parasitic diarrhea. Infect Dis Clin North Am 2(3):685–703, 1988.
10. Schwartz DA, Mixon JP, Owen RL. Giardiasis. In: Connor DH, Chandler FW et al. (eds): Pathology of Infectious Diseases, Stamford, CT: Appleton and Lange, 1997, pp. 1177–83.
11. Washington K, Stenzel TT, Buckley RH, Gottfried MR. Gastrointestinal pathology in patients with common variable immunodeficiency and X-lined agammaglobulinemia. Am J Surg Pathol 20:1240–52, 1996.

Leishmaniasis

12. Alvarez-Nebreda ML, Alvarez-Fernandez E, Rada S, et al. Unusual duodenal presentation of leishmaniasis. J Clin Pathol 58:1321–2, 2005.
13. Baba CS, Makharia GK, Mathur P, et al. Chronic diarrhea and malabsoprtion caused by *Leishmania donovani*. Ind J Gastroenterol 25:309–10, 2006.
14. Berenguer J, Moreno S, Cercenado E, et al. Visceral leishmaniasis in patients infected with human immunodeficiency virus (HIV). Ann Intern Med 111:129–32, 1989.
15. Daneshbod K. Visceral leishmaniasis (kala-azar) in Iran: a pathologic and electron microscopic study. Am J Clin Pathol 57:156–66, 1972.

16. DeNigris EC, Garvin DF, Grogl M, Cotelingam JD. Leishmaniasis. In: Connor DH, Chandler FW et al. (eds): Pathology of Infectious Diseases, Stamford, CT: Appleton and Lange, 1997, pp. 1191–1204.
17. Ellul P, Piscopo T, Vassallo M. Visceral leishmaniasis diagnosed on duodenal biopsy. Clin Gastroenterol Hepatol 5:A26, 2007.
18. Fernandez-Guerrero ML, Aguado JM, Buzon L, et al. Visceral leishmaniasis in immunocompromised hosts. Am J Med 83:1098–1102, 1987.
19. Hofman V, Marty P, Perrin C, et al. The histological spectrum of visceral leishmaniasis caused by *Leishmania infantum* MON-1 in acquired immune deficiency syndrome. Hum Pathol 31:75–84, 2000.
20. Mofredj A, Guerin JM, Leibinger F, Masmoudi R. Viscera leishmaniasis with pericarditis in an HIV-infected patient. Scand J Infect Dis 34:151–3, 2002.
21. Sendino A, Barbado J, Mostaza JM, et al. Visceral leishmaniasis with malabsorption syndrome in a patient with acquired immunodeficiency syndrome. Am J Med 89:673–5, 1990.
22. Wilson ME, Streit JA. Visceral leishmaniasis. Gastroenterol Clin North Am 25(3):535–51, 1996.
23. Zimmer G, Guillous L, Gauthier T, et al. Digestive leishmaniasis in acquired immunodeficiency syndrome; a light and electron microscopic study of two cases. Mod Pathol 9:966–9, 1996.

Trypanosoma cruzi

24. Bern C, Montgomery SP, Herwaldt BL, et al. Evaluation and treatment of Chagas disease in the United States: a systematic review. JAMA 298:2171–81, 2007.
25. Corbett CEP, Ribeiro Jr. U, das Gracas Prianti, M, et al. Cell-mediated immune response in megacolon from patients with chronic Chagas' disease. Dis Colon Rectum 44:993–8, 2001.
26. Da Silveira ABM, Lemos EM, Adad SJ, et al. Megacolon in Chagas disease: a study of inflammatory cells, enteric nerves, and glial cells. Hum Pathol 38:1256–64, 2007.
27. de Oliveira RB, Troncon LEA, Dantas RO, Meneghelli UG. Gastrointestinal manifestations of Chagas' disease. Am J Gastroenterol 93:884–9, 1998.
28. Kirchhoff LV. American trypanosomiasis (Chagas' disease). Gastroenterol Clin N Amer 25(3):517–33, 1996.
29. Krishnamurthy S, Schuffler MD. Pathology of neuromuscular disorders of the colon. Gastroenterol 93:610–639, 1987.
30. Lack EE, Filie A. American trypanosomiasis. In: Connor DH, Chandler FW et al. (eds): Pathology of Infectious Diseases, Stamford, CT: Appleton and Lange, 1997, pp. 1297–1304.

Chapter 30

Coccidians

Keywords Coccidian • Immunocompromise • *Cryptosporidium* sp. • *Cyclospora cayetanensis* • Diarrhea • *Microsporidia* sp. • *Isospora belli* • *Toxoplasma gondii*

Coccidial infection is particularly important when considering the differential diagnosis of diarrhea in patients with AIDS. With the possible exception of *Microsporidia,* however, all coccidians are capable of causing diarrhea (often prolonged) in otherwise healthy patients, especially infants and young children, travelers to developing nations, and individuals who are institutionalized.

Transmission is normally via the fecal–oral route, either directly or through contaminated food and water. Many coccidial infections are asymptomatic. Symptomatic patients most often present with diarrhea, which may be accompanied by fever, weight loss, abdominal pain, and malaise. Stool does not usually contain red blood cells or leukocytes. In immunocompetent persons, infection is usually self-limited, but immunocompromised patients are at risk for chronic, severe diarrhea, with malabsorption, dehydration, and eventual death.

Endoscopic findings are usually absent or mild. Although electron microscopy was once considered the "gold standard" for diagnosis, it is expensive, time-consuming, and not widely used. Examination of stool specimens may be very

helpful, although coccidians are easily missed without the use of special stains. Analysis of mucosal biopsy specimens is more sensitive, however. ELISA techniques, immunohistochemistry, and PCR studies are also available for diagnosing these parasites. A comparison of the morphologic features in tissue sections of the most important gastrointestinal coccidians is given in Table 30.1, and they are discussed in detail below.

Cryptosporidium. *Cryptosporidium* has a worldwide distribution and causes intestinal infection in both humans and animals. Species most commonly infecting humans include *C. parvum, C. hominis,* and *C. meleagridis. Cryptosporidium* can infect healthy infants, children, and adults, as well as immunocompromised patients. High-risk groups include children in day-care centers, patients in mental institutions, travelers to developing countries, immigrants, and immunocompromised patients. Transmission is through contaminated food and water, and person-to-person spread via the fecal–oral route is common. The oocyst is very hardy and is both chlorine and ozone resistant.

Patients present with non-bloody, watery diarrhea that may be mucoid. Diarrhea is often protracted and associated with dehydration. Abdominal cramps, malaise, nausea, vomiting, weight loss, and fever may also occur, particularly in immunocompromised patients. Dissemination may occur as well. Infection is often self-limited in immunocompetent

Table 30.1 A comparison of the morphologic features of enteric coccidians in tissue sections

Feature	Microsporidia	Cryptosporidia	Cyclospora	Isospora
Size	2–3 μm spores (smallest coccidian)	2–5 μm	2–3 μm schizonts 5–6 μm merozoites	15–20 μm (largest coccidian)
Location	Epithelial cells; rarely macrophages	Apical surface	Upper third of epithelial cell	Epithelial cells and macrophages
Staining properties	Modified trichrome, Giemsa, Gram, Warthin–Starry positive	Giemsa, Gram stain positive	Acid-fast, auramine positive; GMS, PAS, Giemsa negative	Giemsa, Gram, PAS positive
Other	May be birefringent under polarized light	Organism bulges out of luminal surface of enterocyte apex	Parasitophorous vacuole	Parasitophorous vacuole Eosinophilic infiltrate

patients, although symptoms may be prolonged and some require supportive care. This organism is most common in the small bowel, but may infect any segment of the GI tract. *Cryptosporidium* rarely infects the pancreaticobiliary tree, causing sclerosing cholangitis, pancreatitis, or acalculous cholecystitis.

Pathologic features. Endoscopy is usually normal, although mucosal atrophy or small erosions may be seen. The characteristic appearance of *Cryptosporidium* is that of a 2–5 μm, basophilic spherical body that protrudes or bulges from the apex of the enterocyte at the luminal surface (Fig. 30.1). The organisms have been referred to as "blue beads" in H&E sections (Fig. 30.2). They may be found in crypts (Fig. 30.3) or in surface epithelium. Associated mucosal changes include villous atrophy (occasionally severe), crypt hyperplasia, mixed lamina propria inflammation, and rarely cryptitis (Fig. 30.4). Surface epithelial cells may show degenerative changes and disarray. Giemsa

and Gram stains highlight the organisms, but are not necessary for diagnosis, and immunohistochemical antibodies are available. *Cryptosporidium* may be distinguished from most other coccidians by their size and unique apical location (see Table 30.1).

Cyclospora cayetanensis. Cyclospora is the most recently discovered enteric coccidian. It has a worldwide distribution, and transmission is through the fecal–oral route or ingestion of contaminated water or food. Infection may be asymptomatic; symptomatic patients present with diarrhea, nausea, weight loss, abdominal pain, bloating, and extreme fatigue. *Cyclospora* can infect immunocompromised or immunocompetent patients.

Pathologic features. This organism most commonly infects the small bowel. Histologic changes in mucosal biopsies are similar to other coccidians, including mild villous blunting, patchy lamina propria inflammation (Fig. 30.5), and surface epithelial disarray. There are few detailed light

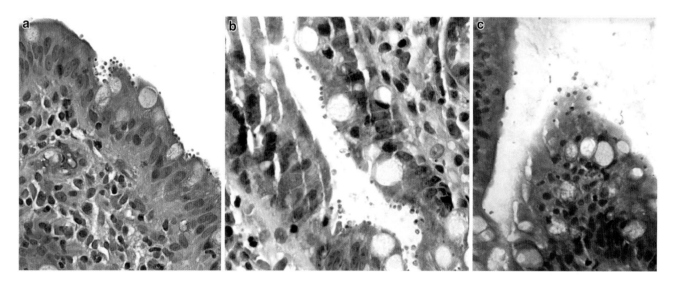

Fig. 30.1 *Cryptosporidium* at the luminal surface of small bowel biopsies. Note surface epithelial disarray and a predominantly mononuclear cell infiltrate in the lamina propria with rare eosinophils (**a**, courtesy Dr. Joel K. Greenson). Higher power view of 2–5-μm, basophilic organisms protruding from the apex of the enterocytes (**b** and **c**)

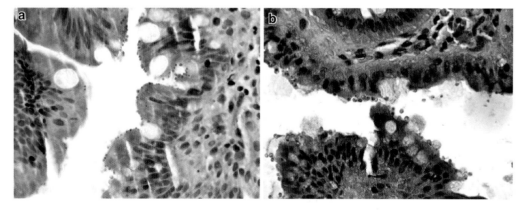

Fig. 30.2 *Cryptosporidia* have been referred to as "blue beads" in H&E sections (**a** and **b**)

Fig. 30.3 Parasites may be found in crypts as well as surface epithelium, as illustrated by this colon biopsy

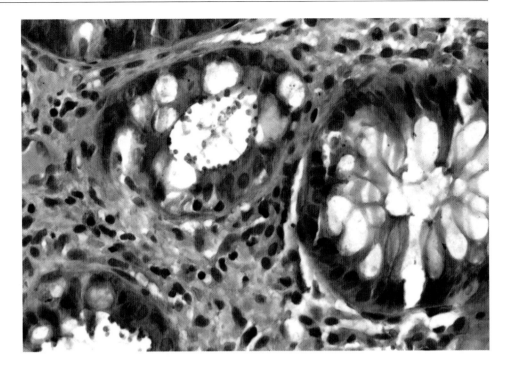

microscopic descriptions of this parasite, and there is still some disagreement regarding the spectrum of morphologic features in tissue sections. It was originally thought that although larger, *Cyclospora* could mimic the apical location of *Cryptosporidia*; this is no longer thought to be true, however. Intracellular forms of *Cyclospora* include 2–3-μm schizonts and 5–6-μm banana-shaped merozoites located within enterocytes (Fig. 30.6). Organisms are often located within the upper third of the enterocyte, within a parasitophorous vacuole (Fig. 30.7). The organisms are acid-fast with modified Kinyoun or similar stains and are also positive with auramine. However, they are GMS, PAS, Gram, and trichrome negative.

Differential diagnosis. The major differential diagnosis is with *Isospora* and *Cryptosporidium*. *Cyclospora* organisms are much larger than *Cryptosporidium* and lack the apical location. In addition, *Cyclospora* autofluoresce under ultraviolet light on unstained or iodine-stained stool preps or duodenal aspirates. When crescent-shaped, *Cyclospora* may be confused with *Isospora*, which are generally larger; in addtion, *Isospora* are PAS positive. It is important to differentiate cyclosporiasis from cryptosporidiosis, as *Cyclospora* can be effectively treated with antibiotics, whereas cryptosporidiosis is not antibiotic-susceptible and is treated with supportive care only.

Isospora belli and related species. *Isospora* has a worldwide distribution, but is more common in tropical and subtropical regions than temperate climates. It causes infection in both humans and animals. It is transmitted by ingestion of food or water contaminated with oocysts. Patients present with chronic diarrhea, dehydration, weight loss, anorexia,

malaise, and abdominal pain, along with signs of malabsorption. Patients with isosporiasis are more likely to have peripheral eosinophilia than those infected by other coccidians. Infection may be severe and debilitating in immunocompromised patients. Widespread dissemination has been reported rarely.

Isospora has an extremely complex life cycle, which contributes to the variety of appearances that the organism can manifest in tissue sections. Sporocysts are ingested, followed by release of sporozoites. Free sporozoites invade enterocytes, which then develop into trophozoites. Asexual reproduction results in schizonts containing several merozoites; mature merozoites, which can infect new cells, are released into the bowel lumen. Merozoites can undergo either asexual or sexual reproduction. The latter produces female macrogamonts and male microgametes. Fertilization results in oocysts that are released into the lumen and excreted.

Pathologic features. The small bowel is most commonly involved, although the colon and biliary tree also may be affected. Endoscopy is usually normal, but mild mucosal eryethema and granularity may be seen. Histologic changes include villous blunting, which may be severe; villous fusion; crypt hyperplasia; mixed inflammation in the lamina propria, often with prominent eosinophils (Fig. 30.8); and in chronic infections, fibrosis of the lamina propria. Surface nuclear disorganization is a prominent feature as well (Fig. 30.9). Tissue reaction may be minimal, however.

Isospora is the largest coccidian (15–20 μm). Intraepithelial inclusions are present in all stages of infection (Fig. 30.10), and can be found within both epithelial cells

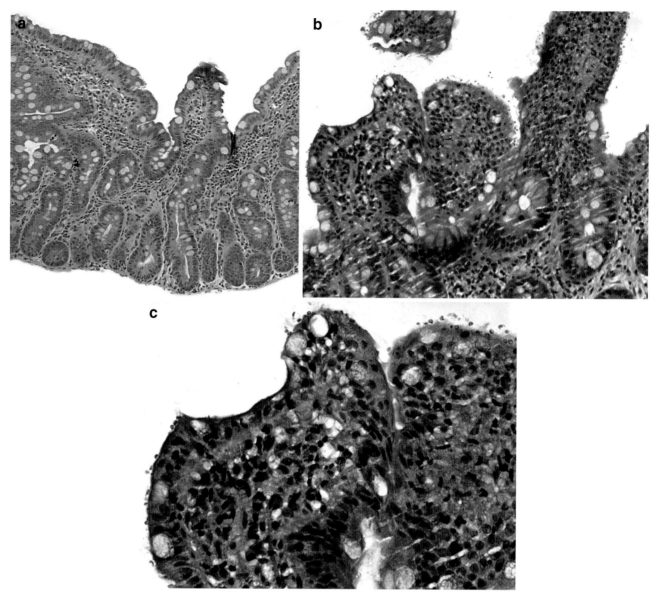

Fig. 30.4 Associated small bowel mucosal changes in cryptosporidiosis. Low-power view illustrates include villous atrophy, crypt hyperplasia, and a mononuclear cell infiltrate in the lamina propria (**a**, courtesy Dr. Joel K. Greenson). Villous blunting, surface epithelial cell disarray, and a mixed infiltrate in the lamina propria with mononuclear cells as well as eosinophils (**b**, courtesy Dr. Michelle Riddick-Nelson). Higher power view showing surface epithelial cell disarray and numerous eosinophils in the lamina propria (**c**, courtesy Dr. Michelle Riddick-Nelson)

and macrophages in the lamina propria. Inclusions are both perinuclear and subnuclear. Schizonts and merozoites (the asexual forms) are crescent or banana shaped; sexual forms are round with a prominent nucleus. The organisms often have an associated loose parsitophorpous vacuole. GMS and Giemsa stains are useful to highlight the organism. Although *Isospora* are PAS positive, they may be easily confused with goblet cells. The differential diagnosis includes other coccidians (see above and Table 30.1).

Microsporidia. Microsporidia have a worldwide distribution. They are present in many environmental water sources and have many animal hosts as well. Human-to-human transmission and fecal/oral spread are also common. *Enterocytozoon bieneusi* and *Encephalitozoon intestinalis* are the most common human pathogens in this group. Patients present with chronic, non-bloody, non-mucoid diarrhea, with associated dehydration, weight loss, and signs of malabsorption. Symptoms are often worse with food. Disseminated infection may occur, especially with *E. intestinalis* infection. Microsporidia is the coccidian least likely to infect immunocompetent persons.

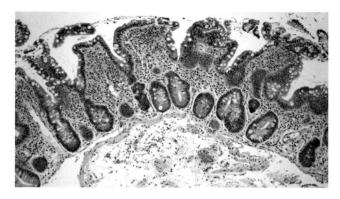

Fig. 30.5 Small bowel biopsy in cyclosporiasis, showing mild villous blunting and a patchy mononuclear cell infiltrate in the lamina propria. (Courtesy Dr. Rhonda Yantiss)

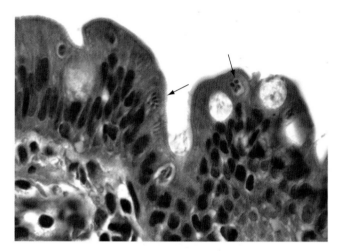

Fig. 30.6 Both crescent-shaped merozoites and round schizonts are located within the surface enterocytes. (Courtesy Dr. Rhonda Yantiss)

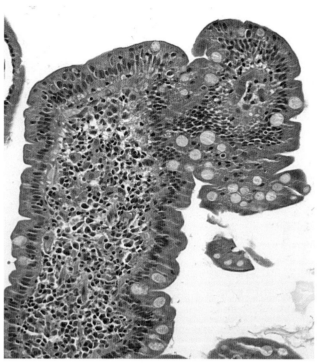

Fig. 30.8 Small bowel villus with surface epithelial disarray and mixed inflammatory infiltrate in the lamina propria. *Isospora*, the largest coccidian, is visible even at low power. (Courtesy Dr. Joel K. Greenson)

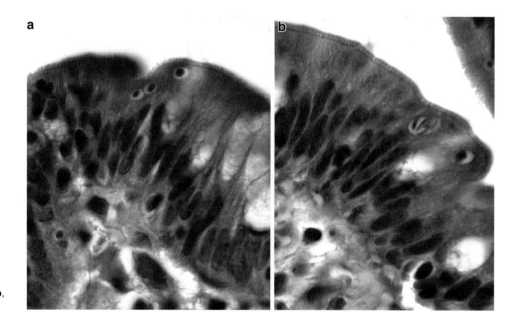

Fig. 30.7 Organisms are often located within the upper third of the enterocyte, within a parasitophorous vacuole (**a** and **b**, courtesy Dr. Rhonda Yantiss)

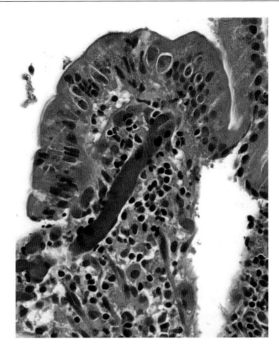

Fig. 30.9 High-power view of surface disarray and mixed inflammatory infiltrate in the lamina propria, along with crescent-shaped asexual forms and ovoid sexual forms of *Isospora* within the surface epithelium. (Courtesy Dr. Joel K. Greenson)

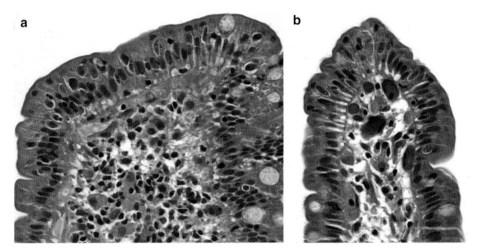

Fig. 30.10 Organisms are often present within a loose parasitophorous vacuole. Inclusions are both perinuclear and subnuclear. Asexual forms are crescent or banana shaped, and the sexual forms are ovoid to round with a more prominent nucleus (**a** and **b**, courtesy Dr. Joel K. Greenson)

Pathologic features. Any level of the gastrointestinal tract may be affected, including the biliary tree, but the small bowel is the most common site of infection. Endoscopy is usually normal. Histologic findings include focal mild villous blunting, a patchy lamina propria lymphoplasmacytic infiltrate, variably increased surface intraepithelial lymphocytes, vacuolization of the surface epithelium, and surface epithelial cell disarray (Fig. 30.11). There may be minimal to no tissue reaction, however. The organisms are present as small spores, 2–3 μm in size (Fig. 30.12), as well as large plasmodia that are located within the supranuclear cytoplasm of epithelial cells (Fig. 30.13) or occasionally lamina propria macrophages (most common with *E. intestinalis*). Associated vacuoles may cup or flatten the enterocyte nucleus.

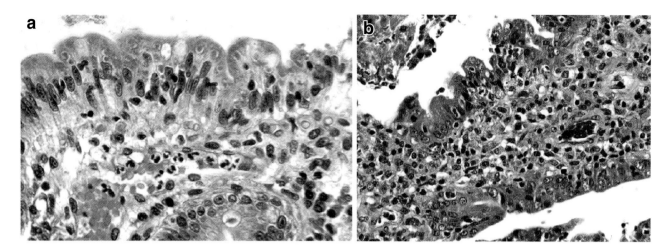

Fig. 30.11 Small bowel biopsy in microsporidiosis (**a**). Numerous round plasmodial forms are present in the apical cytoplasm; note surface epithelial disarray and numerous intraepithelial lymphocytes (courtesy Dr. Joel K. Greenson). Similar changes are seen in the gallbladder (**b**), including surface epithelial disarray, cytoplasmic vacuolization, intraepithelial lymphocytosis, and numerous plasmodial forms and spores present within the surface epithelium

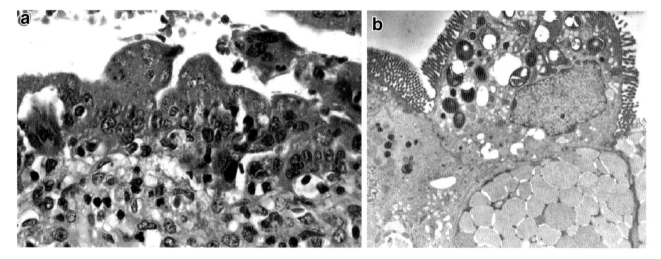

Fig. 30.12 Higher power view showing surface epithelial disarray; small spores and plasmodia are faintly visible on H&E sections (**a**). Electron micrograph shows spores within the apical cytoplasm (**b**, courtesy Dr. Joel K. Greenson)

Microsporidia are difficult to detect in routine H&E stained sections. A modified trichrome stain can aid greatly in the diagnosis (Fig. 30.14), and the organisms also stain with Warthin–Starry, Giemsa, and Gram stains (Fig. 30.15). Occasionally, *Microsporidia* polarize within biopsy specimens, since the chitin-rich internal polar filament of the organism is birefringent under polarized light. However, this method is unreliable, due to unpredictability of spore birefringence and variability depending on the type of microscope and light source used. Distinction of *Microsporidia* from other enteric coccidians is detailed in Table 30.1.

Toxoplasma gondii. Gastrointestinal toxoplasmosis is primarily a disease of immunocompromised hosts, and usually presents in patients with concomitant ocular, central nervous system, cardiac, or pulmonary disease. Patients with gastrointestinal involvement generally present with diarrhea, abdominal pain, vomiting, fever, and weight loss. Gastric and colonic involvement are most common, followed by the small bowel; esophageal involvement is rare. Ulcers

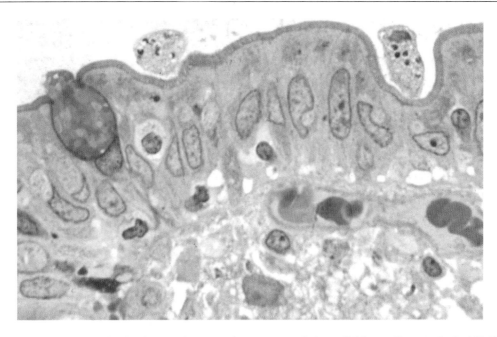

Fig. 30.13 Plastic-embedded thick section for electron microscopy shows spores and plasmodial forms. (Courtesy Dr. Joel K. Greenson)

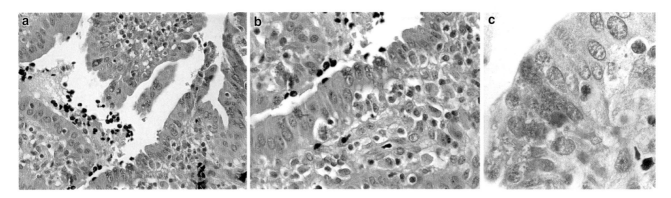

Fig. 30.14 The modified trichrome stain aids greatly in the diagnosis of microsporidiosis. Spores are visible at low power, staining bright red in a gray background (**a** and **b**). Spores are present in the supranuclear cytoplasm, and associated vacuoles may cup or flatten the nucleus (**b** and **c**)

have been described grossly, with organisms usually located within the ulcer base (Fig. 30.16). Both crescent-shaped tachyzoites as well as tissue cysts containing brady-zoites may be present within tissue sections (Fig. 30.17). Associated lymphadenopathy may be present, featuring reactive lymphoid hyperplasia with clusters of epithelioid histiocytes (Fig. 30.18). Cysts may be found in nodes rarely (Fig. 30.19). Immunohistochemistry and PCR assays, as well as serologic tests, are useful diagnostic aids; however, serologies may be unreliable in severely immunocompromised patients.

Selected References

Enteric Coccidians

1. Brandborg LL, Goldberg B, Breidenbach WC. Human coccidiosis – a possible cause of malabsorption. N Eng J Med 283:1306–13, 1970.
2. Cama VA, Ross JM, Crawford S, et al. Differences in clinical manifestations among *Cryptosporidium* species and subtypes in HIV-infected persons. J Infect Dis 196:684–91, 2007.

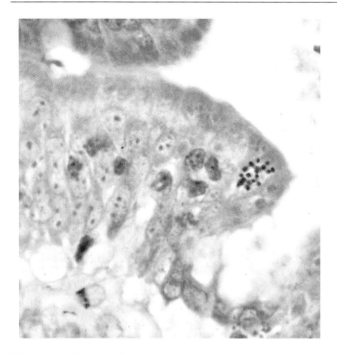

Fig. 30.15 *Microsporidia* also stain red to purple with tissue Gram stain. (Courtesy Dr. Joel K. Greenson)

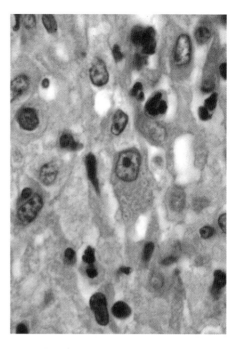

Fig. 30.17 *Toxoplasma* organisms are present within a macrophage within the submucosal inflammatory infiltrate. (Courtesy Dr. Rodger C. Haggitt and Dr. Mary P. Bronner)

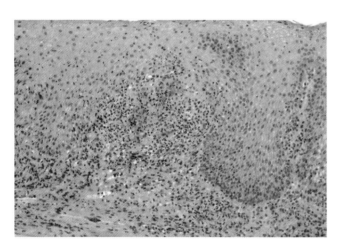

Fig. 30.16 Esophageal biopsy in a case of gastrointestinal toxoplasmosis, showing marked neutrophilic inflammation in the submucosa. (Courtesy Dr. Rodger C. Haggitt and Dr. Mary P. Bronner)

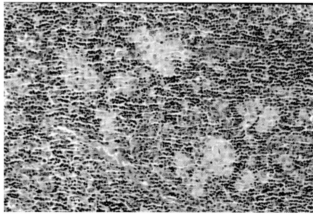

Fig. 30.18 Associated lymphadenopathy may be present, featuring reactive lymphoid hyperplasia with clusters of epithelioid histiocytes. (Courtesy Dr. George F. Gray, Jr)

3. Carlson JR, Helton CL, Munn RJ, et al. Disseminated microsporidiosis in a pancreas/kidney transplant recipient. Arch Pathol Lab Med 128:e41–3, 2004.
4. Clayton F, Heller T, Kotler DP. Variation in the enteric distribution of *Crytosporidia* in acquired immunodeficiency syndrome. Am J Clin Pathol 102:420–5, 1994.
5. Connor BA, Reidy J, Soave R. Cyclosporiasis: clinical and histopathologic correlates. Clin Infect Dis 28:1216–21, 1999.
6. Curry A, Smith HV. Emerging pathogens: *Isospora, Cyclospora*, and *Microsporidia*. Parasitology 117:S143–59, 1998.
7. Eberhard ML, Pieniazek NJ, Arrowood MJ. Laboratory diagnosis of *Cyclospora* infections. Arch Pathol Lab Med 121:792–7, 1997.
8. Franzen C, et al. *Cryptosporidia* and *Microsporidia*-waterborne diseases in the immunocompromised host. Diagn Microbiol Infect Dis 34:245–62, 1999.
9. Goodgame R. Understanding intestinal spore-forming protozoa: *Cryptosporidia, Microsporidia, Isospora*, and *Cyclospora*. Ann Intern Med 124:429–41, 1996.
10. Huang DV, Chappell C, Okhuysen PC. Cryptosporidiosis in children. Sem Pediatr Infect Dis 15:253–9, 2004.

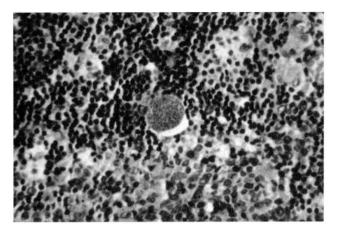

Fig. 30.19 *Toxoplasma* cysts are found in lymph nodes very rarely. (Courtesy Dr. Margie A. Scott)

11. Kotler DP, Giang TT, Garro ML, et al. Light microscopic diagnosis of microsporidiosis in patients with AIDS. Am J Gastroenterol 89:540–4, 1994.

12. Lamps LW, Bronner MP, Vnencak-Jones CL, Tham KT, Mertz HR, Scott MA. Optimal screening and diagnosis of *Microsporida* in tissue sections. Am J Clin Pathol 109:404–10, 1998.

13. Ma P, et al. *Isospora belli* diarrheal infection in homosexual men. AIDS Res 1:327–38, 1983–1984.

14. Marcial-Seoane MA, Serrano-Olmo J. Intestinal infection with *Isospora belli*. PRHSJ 14:137–40, 1995.

15. Orenstein JM. Cryptosporidiosis. In: Connor DH, Chandler FW et al. (eds): Pathology of Infectious Diseases, Stamford, CT: Appleton and Lange, 1997, pp. 1147–58.

16. Orenstein JM. Isosporiasis. In: Connor DH, Chandler FW et al. (eds): Pathology of Infectious Diseases, Stamford, CT: Appleton and Lange, 1997, pp. 1185–90.

17. Panosian CB. Parasitic diarrhea. Infect Dis Clin North Am 2(3):685–703, 1988.

18. Pinge-Suttor V, Douglas C, Wettstein A. *Cyclospora* infection masquerading as celiac disease. Med J Australia 180:295–6, 2004.

19. Rivasi F, et al. Gastric cryptosporidiosis: correlation between intensity of infection and histological alterations. Histopathol 34:405–9, 1999.

20. Sun T. *Cyclospora* infection. In: Connor DH, Chandler FW et al. (eds): Pathology of Infectious Diseases, Stamford, CT: Appleton and Lange, 1997, pp. 1159–62.

21. Sun T, Ilardi CF, Asnis D, et al. Light and electron microscopic identification of *Cyclospora* species in small intestine: evidence of the presence of asexual life cycle in the human host. Am J Clin Pathol 105:216–20, 1996.

22. Velasquez JN, Carnevale S, Mariano M, et al. Isosporiasis and unizoite tissue cysts in patients with acquired immunodeficiency syndrome. Hum Pathol 32:500–5, 2001. Al-Kassab AK, Habte-Gabr E, Mueller WF, Azher Q. Fulminant disseminated toxoplasmosis in an HIV patient. Scand J Infect Dis 27:183–5, 1995.

23. Wichro E, Hoelzl D, Krause R, et al. Microsporidiosis in travel-associated diarrhea in immune-competent patients. Am J Trop Med Hyg 73:285–7, 2005.

Toxoplasma gondii

24. Al-Kassab AK, Habte-Gabr E, Mueller WF, Azher Q. Fulminant disseminated toxoplasmosis in an HIV patient. Scand J Infect Dis 27:183–5, 1995.

25. Bertoli F, Espino M, Arosemena JR, et al. A spectrum in the pathology of toxoplasmosis in patients with acquired immunodeficiency syndrome. Arch Path Lab Med 119:214–24, 1995.

26. Bonacini M, Kanel G, Alamy M. Duodenal and hepatic toxoplasmosis in a patient with HIV infection: review of the literature. Am J Gastroenterol 91:1838–40, 1996.

27. Ganji M, Tan A, Maitar MI, et al. Gastric toxoplasmosis in a patient with acquired immunodeficiency syndrome. A case report and review of the literature. Arch Pathol Lab Med 127:732–4, 2003.

28. Merzianu M, Gorelick SM, Paje V, et al. Gastric toxoplasmosis as the presentation of acquired immunodeficiency syndrome. Arch Pathol Lab Med 129: e87–90, 2005.

Chapter 31

Miscellaneous Helminthic Infections

Keywords Helminth • Trematode • Fluke • Cestode • Tapeworm • Nematode • Roundworm • *Fasciolopsis buski* • *Echinostoma* sp. • *Heterophyes* sp. • *Taenia* sp. • *Hymenolepsis nana* • *Ascaris* sp. • Hookworms • *Necator* sp. • *Ancyclostoma* sp. • Anemia • Malabsorption • Obstruction • Whipworm • *Trichuris trichiura* • *Capillaria* sp. • *Angiostrongylus costaricensis* • *Trichinella* sp.

The parasitic helminthes include trematodes (flukes), cestodes (tapeworms), and nematodes (roundworms) (Table 31.1). Although the most common method of diagnosing gastrointestinal helminthic infections is examination of stool for ova and parasites, these organisms are occasionally detected in biopsy or resection specimens. In addition, worms are increasingly frequently visualized endoscopically. Gastrointestinal helminths have a worldwide distribution, but their clinical importance varies with geographic region. They are more often a cause of serious disease in nations with deficient sanitation systems, poor socio-economic status, and hot, humid climates. Helminthic infections may be encountered in immigrants, however, as well as patients who travel to endemic areas, and they are an increasingly important problem in immunocompromised hosts. Helminths can cause severe and life-threatening nutritional problems, especially in children. The most common site of anatomic infection is the small bowel, although the stomach and large bowel may be involved. Hookworms, roundworms (both *Ascaris* and *Enterobius*), and whipworms are the most common helminthic infections in humans. A more detailed discussion of selected helminthic gastrointestinal infections is given below.

Intestinal flukes (*Fasciolopsis buski*, *Echinostoma* species, *Heterophyes* species). Food-borne trematodiasis remains a worldwide public health problem and is most common in Asia and the Pacific. Over 50 species of intestinal flukes have been described in humans, but most clinically significant infections are due to *F. buski*, *Echinostoma* species, and *Heterophyes* species. They are ingested along with aquatic plants, fish, shellfish, or amphibians. Flukes are

Table 31.1 General classification of medically important parasitic helminths

	Trematodes (flukes)	Cestodes (tapeworms)	Nematodes (roundworms)
Examples	*Fasciola* (liver fluke) *Fasciolopsis* (giant intestinal fluke) *Echinostoma* (intestinal fluke) *Schistosoma* *Clonorchis, Opisthorchis* (Asian liver fluke, biliary fluke) *Heterophyes* *Paragonimus*	*Diphyllobothrium* (fish tapeworm) *Taenia* (pork and beef tapeworm) *Echinococcus* *Hymenolepsis* (dwarf tapeworm)	*Trichuris* (whipworm) *Capillaria* *Trichinella* *Strongyloides* *Ancylostoma* (hookworm) *Ascaris* (roundworm) *Toxocara* (visceral larva migrans) *Anisakis* *Angiostrongylus* *Oesophagostoma* *Enterobius* (pinworm, threadworm)
Important characteristics	– Fish are principal hosts – Flat, sometimes leaf-shaped bodies with oral and ventral sucker – Incomplete digestive tract	– Have scolex and proglottids – No digestive tract	One of the largest and most widespread groups of multicellular animals Affect virtually all plants and animals Elongated, cylindrical bodies Complete digestive tract

L.W. Lamps, *Surgical Pathology of the Gastrointestinal System: Bacterial, Fungal, Viral, and Parasitic Infections*, DOI 10.1007/978-1-4419-0861-2_31, © Springer Science+Business Media, LLC 2009

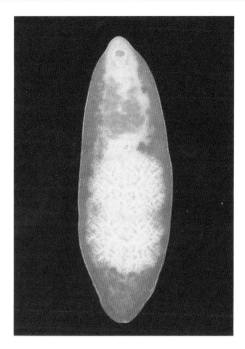

Fig. 31.1 *Fasciolopsis buski* is a flat, fleshy, ovoid fluke measuring up to 8 cm in length. (courtesy ARP Press, Fig. 5.1, from Meyers, WE et al. Pathology of Infectious Diseases: Vol. 1 – Helminthiases. American Registry of Pathology, Washington, DC 2000)

ovoid to flat, fleshy worms ranging in size from 1.0 mm (*Heterophyes*) to 7.5 cm (*Fasciolopsis*) in length; they may be seen endoscopically (Fig. 31.1). After maturation, the adult worm attaches to the proximal small bowel mucosa or rarely to the stomach, ileum, or colon. The majority of infections are asymptomatic. Symptoms usually occur as a result of heavy infection, and include diarrhea, often alternating with constipation, abdominal pain, anorexia, nausea, vomiting, and malabsorption. Mild anemia and eosinophilia are common. Ileus, obstruction, and GI bleeding have been described as well. Mucosal ulceration, inflammation, hemorrhage, edema, and abscess formation may occur at sites of tissue attachment, and *Heterophyes* species can actually penetrate the wall of the intestine, with associated ulceration and inflammation.

Cestodes. Taenia saginata (beef tapeworm), *Taenia solium* (pork tapeworm), and *Hymenolepis nana* (dwarf tapeworm) occasionally cause gastrointestinal disease in humans. These worms are flat and segmented, consisting of a head (scolex) and multiple segments (proglottids), but no true body cavity (Fig. 31.2). Cestodes range in size from 2.5 mm (*Hymenolepis*) to 30 m (*T. saginata*); the latter can live for up to 20 years.

Taenia saginata is endemic in Latin America and Africa, with moderate prevalence in Europe, Japan, and South Asia. The distribution reflects cattle farming in areas with poor sanitation. Infection is acquired through eating undercooked beef. *T. solium* has a worldwide distribution that correlates with pig farming and poor sanitation. It is endemic in Southeast Asia, Central and South America, Mexico, the Philippines, Africa, India, Eastern Europe, and Micronesia. Infection is acquired through ingestion of raw or undercooked pork. Most patients with taeniasis are asymptomatic, although many pass proglottids and/or eggs in the stool. Some patients have nausea and epigastric pain, and rarely patients report vomiting, diarrhea, or obstruction. Appendicitis due to proglottids lodged in the appendix has been reported. Malabsorption and weight loss are rare. Histologically, there is mild mucosal inflammation at the attachment site.

Diphyllobothrium (fish tapeworm) is common in northern Europe and Scandinavia, as well as the Great Lakes region and Alaska in North America. Infection is acquired through eating raw fish. The majority of infections are asymptomatic even though the worm can achieve a length of over 20 m (Fig. 31.3). The adult worm lives in the small bowel. Symptoms including diarrhea, fatigue, dizziness, paresthesias, and increased hunger are sometimes reported, and fish tapeworm is also a rare cause of B12 deficiency. There are no reported associated histologic changes in the gastrointestinal tract.

Hymenolepis nana (dwarf tapeworm) is the most common cestode infection in humans. It has a worldwide distribution, and is more common in warm climates and in areas of poor sanitation. It is the smallest adult tapeworm, measuring 2.5–5 mm by 1.0 mm. Most infections are

Fig. 31.2 Coiled adult *T. saginata* measuring many meters, with a tiny scolex at the loose end (**a**). Higher power gross photograph illustrating that the worm is composed of many flat segments or proglottids (**b**). (courtesy ARP Press, Figs. 7.1 and 7.2, from Meyers, WE et al. Pathology of Infectious Diseases: Vol. 1 – Helminthiases. American Registry of Pathology, Washington, DC 2000)

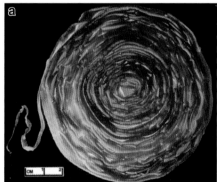
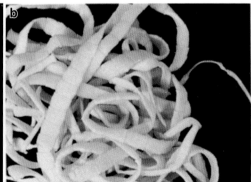

Fig. 31.3 *D. latum* has a narrow anterior end and a very wide posterior end (**a**). The proglottids of the adult are usually broader than they are long (**b**). (courtesy ARP Press, Figs. 10.2 and 10.3, from Meyers, WE et al. Pathology of Infectious Diseases: Vol. 1 – Helminthiases. American Registry of Pathology, Washington, DC 2000)

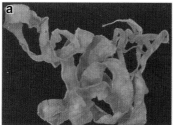
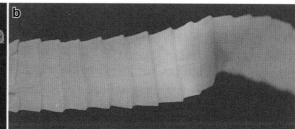

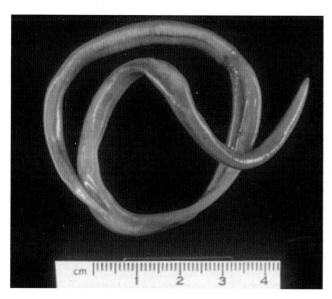

Fig. 31.4 Ascarids measure up to 30 cm in length and 6 mm in diameter, with a cylindrical, unsegmented body (**a**). (Courtesy Dr. George F. Gray, Jr)

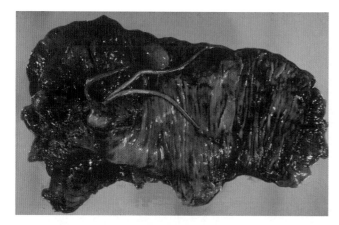

Fig. 31.5 *Ascaris* incidentally found within a segment of colon resected for colon cancer. (Courtesy Dr. George F. Gray, Jr)

although heavy infections may cause villous blunting and inflammation.

Nematodes. Ascaris lumbricoides (roundworm) is the largest helminth and one of the most common parasites in humans. Children are most often affected. It has a worldwide distribution, but is most common in Asia, Africa, and Latin America, and in areas of poor sanitation. The worms are ingested from exposure to contaminated food, water, or soil. Ascarids measure up to 30 cm in length and 6 mm in diameter, with a cylindrical, unsegmented body (Figs. 31.4 and 31.5). The pulmonary phase of infection occurs first, as the larvae migrate through the lungs. In the intestinal phase, worms may be present anywhere from the stomach to the ileocecal valve, but are most common in the jejunum. Infection is usually asymptomatic. Heavy infection or worm migration (as noted by Wasadikar and Kulkarni, ascarids have "a tendency to explore orifices and ducts," often provoked by fever, medications, anesthesia, or change in diet) can cause abdominal pain and distension, nausea, vomiting, and diarrhea. Patients may pass worms in either stool or vomit. Serious complications, particularly common in children, usually arise when enough worms are present to form a mass; these include obstruction (Fig. 31.6), volvulus, intussusception, pancreaticobiliary obstruction, and

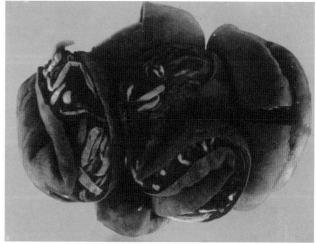

Fig. 31.6 Segment of small bowel obstructed by numerous ascarids. (Courtesy Dr. George F. Gray, Jr)

asymptomatic, although heavy infection may cause diarrhea, abdominal cramps, and anorexia. Immunocompromised patients may be susceptible to very heavy worm burdens, and dissemination has been reported rarely. The worms inhabit the upper ileum, and histologic findings are usually absent,

appendicitis. Heavy worm burdens can also cause malnutrition and growth retardation, often complicated by the fact that children in endemic areas often have a poor diet in addition to parasitic infection. Although most patients can be managed medically, those with obstruction may require surgical intervention. The worms may be found endoscopically or in resection specimens, and tissue damage occurs primarily at anatomic sites of attachment. Patients with obstruction may have associated ischemic bowel.

Hookworms (*Necator americanus* and *Ancylostoma duodenale*) are common parasites in all tropical and subtropical countries. Infection may occur through penetration of the skin, or through direct ingestion. The worms attach to the small intestinal wall and withdraw blood from villous cap-

illaries, resulting in anemia; children and women of reproductive age are particularly susceptible. Other clinical signs and symptoms include abdominal pain, diarrhea, malnutrition, significant childhood growth retardation, hypoproteinemia, and cough with eosinophilia when the worms migrate. Pica is also associated with hookworm infection. Any level of the GI tract may be involved. Endoscopically, the worms (measuring about 1 cm in length) are visible to the naked eye and are white, red-brown, or gray, depending on the amount of ingested blood or hemosiderin deposition (Fig. 31.7). The worms lacerate the mucosa of the bowel as they attach, causing focal hemorrhage, and previous bite marks may appear as pigmented spots (Fig. 31.8). Histologic changes are often minimal, but may include villous blunting and an

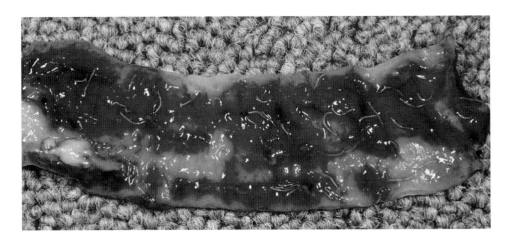

Fig. 31.7 Numerous hookworms attached to small bowel. The worms lacerate the mucosa of the bowel as they attach, causing focal hemorrhage. (Courtesy Drs. James Britt and Jason Doss)

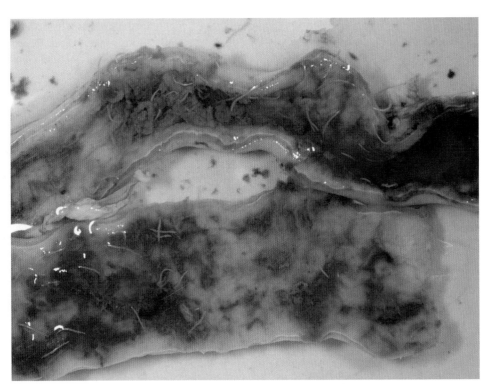

Fig. 31.8 Underwater photograph of bowel specimen with hookworms, highlighting shallow ulcerations and pigmented spots at areas of attachment. (Courtesy Drs. James Britt and Jason Doss)

eosinophilic infiltrate. Pieces of worm may, occasionally, be detected in biopsy specimens.

Trichuris trichiura (whipworm) is a soil helminth with a worldwide distribution; it is most common in tropical climates. In the United States, it is most often seen in immigrants and in the rural Southeast. Infection is acquired by ingesting contaminated water or food. The worms measure 3–5 mm in length and may be seen endoscopically; male worms have the characteristic coiled, whip-like tail (Figs. 31.9 and 31.10). Most infections are asymptomatic, especially if only a few worms are present. Patients with heavier infection may develop diarrhea, gastrointestinal bleeding, malabsorption, anemia, and appendicitis. Unusual clinical manifestations include an ulcerative inflammatory process similar to Crohn's disease and rectal prolapse. The worms can live anywhere in the intestine, but are most commonly found in the right colon and ileum. They thread their anterior end under the epithelium, which may cause mucosal edema, erythema, hemorrhage, and ulceration at the attachment site. Histologically, enterocyte atrophy with an associated mixed inflammatory infiltrate (sometimes rich in eosinophils) and occasional crypt abscesses may be seen.

Capillaria infection (intestinal capillariasis) is most common in the Philippines, Thailand, and other parts of Asia, although cases have been reported in non-endemic areas. The worms are ingested with infected raw fish. Clinical symptoms include diarrhea and abdominal pain, along with signs of malabsorption that may be severe and life-threatening.

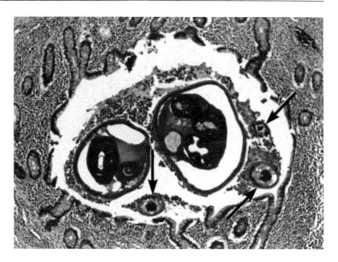

Fig. 31.10 Cross section of whipworm in the lumen of the appendix. Note the cross sections through both the thick posterior and thin (*arrow*) anterior segments. (courtesy ARP Press, Fig. 31.21, from Meyers, WE et al. Pathology of Infectious Diseases: Vol. 1 – Helminthiases. American Registry of Pathology, Washington, DC 2000)

The worms measure 2–4 cm in length (Fig. 31.11) and are most commonly found in the crypts of the small bowel, but they may also invade the lamina propria. There is usually no associated inflammatory reaction, although villous blunting, mucosal sloughing, and mild inflammatory changes have been described.

Angiostrongylus costaricensis, a Central and South American nematode endemic in Costa Rica, may cause dra-

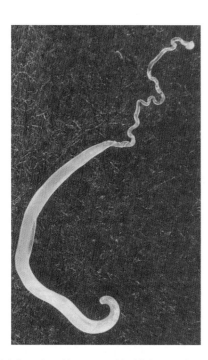

Fig. 31.9 Adult male whipworm with thick posterior end and thin (whip-like) anterior end. (courtesy ARP Press, Fig. 31.1, from Meyers, WE et al. Pathology of Infectious Diseases: Vol. 1 – Helminthiases. American Registry of Pathology, Washington, DC 2000)

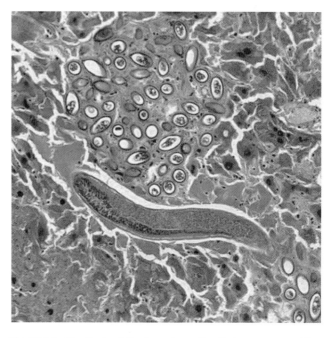

Fig. 31.11 *Capillaria philippinesnsis* are tiny, 2–4 mm worms with a smooth cuticle. The eggs have bipolar plugs. (Courtesy Dr. John Watts)

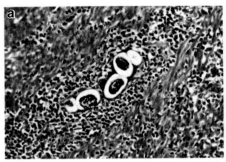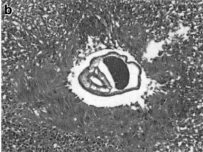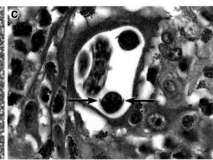

Fig. 31.12 *A. costaricensis* eggs in a vessel, with surrounding eosinophilic inflammation (**a**). Cross section of a worm within an artery, with marked surrounding eosinophilic inflammation (**b**). High-power view of larva within egg in the wall of the cecum (**c**). (courtesy ARP Press, Figs. 25.7, 25.21, and 25.17, from Meyers, WE et al. Pathology of Infectious Diseases: Vol. 1 – Helminthiases. American Registry of Pathology, Washington, DC 2000)

matic, even fatal, ileocecal infection characterized by the presence of large obstructive inflammatory masses with perforation and mesenteric vessel thrombosis. Typical clinical findings also include right upper quadrant pain, painful rectal examination, leukocytosis, and eosinophilia. Histologic findings include a massive eosinophilic infiltrate (Fig. 31.12), granulomatous inflammation, and an eosinophilic vasculitis. Worms may be present within arteries.

Trichinella spiralis, the causative agent of trichinosis, is also a rare cause of diarrhea. Esophagostomiasis (infection by *Oesophagostomum* species), a parasitic disease generally seen in non-human primates, may form deep inflammatory masses, predominantly in the right colon and appendix.

The differential diagnosis of helminthic infections usually involves differentiation between the various types of worms. Other entities to be considered, particularly when the worm is not readily found, include causes of ulcerative inflammation, eosinophilic infiltration, and granulomatous inflammation, such as tuberculosis, amebiasis, allergic enteritis, and chronic idiopathic inflammatory bowel disease.

Selected References

General

1. Bruckner DA. Helminthic food-borne infections. Clin Lab Med 19(3):639–60, 1999.
2. Cook GC. The clinical significance of gastrointestinal helminths – a review. Trans Roy Soc Trop Med Hyg 80:675–85, 1986.

Trematodes

3. Chai JY, Darwin MK, Lymbery AJ. Fish-borne parasitic zoonoses: status and issues. Int J Parastiol 35:1233–54, 2005.
4. Fried B, Gracyk Tk, Tamang L. Food-borne intestinal trematodiases in humans. Parasitol Res 93:159–70, 2004.
5. Liu LX and Harinasuta KT. Liver and intestinal flukes. Gastroenterol Clin North Am 25:627–36, 1996.
6. Marty AM, Anderson EM. Fasciolopsiasis and other intestinal trematodiases. In: Meyers WM, Neafie RC, Marty AM, Wear DJ. (eds): Pathology of Infectious Diseases: Vol. 1, Helminthiases. Washington, DC: AFIP Press, 2000, pp. 93–106.
7. Plaut AG, Kampanart-Sanyakorn C, Manning GS. A clinical study of Fasciolopsis buski infection in Thailand. Trans Roy Soc Trop Med Hyg 63:470–8, 1969.

Cestodes

8. Barry M, Cappello M. Cestodes. In: Blaser MJ, Smith PD, Ravdin JI, et al. Infections of the Gastrointestinal Tract. New York: Raven Press, 1995, pp. 1155–66.
9. Marty AM, Neafie RC. Hymenolepiasis and miscellaneous cyclophyllidiases. In: Meyers WM, Neafie RC, Marty AM, Wear DJ. (eds): Pathology of Infectious Diseases: Vol. 1, Helminthiases. Washington, DC: AFIP Press, 2000, pp.197–214.
10. Neafie RC, Marty AM, Johnson AM. Taeniasis and cysticercosis. In: Meyers WM, Neafie RC, Marty AM, Wear DJ. (eds): Pathology of Infectious Diseases: Vol. 1, Helminthiases. Washington, DC: AFIP Press, 2000, pp. 117–36.
11. Rausch RL, Scott EM, Rausch VR. Helminths in Eskimos in western Alaska, with particular reference to Diphyllobothrium infection and anaemia. Trans Roy Soc Trop Med Hyg 61:351–7, 1967.
12. Sanchez AL, Lindback J, Schantz PM, et al. A population-based, case-control study of Taenia solium taeniasis and cysticercosis. Ann Trop Med Parasit 93:247–58, 1999.

Nematodes

13. Akgun Y. Intestinal obstruction caused by Ascaris lumbricoides. Dis Colon Rectum 39:1159–63, 1996.
14. Bitar M, Strauchen JA, Sequeira RJ, Wu M. A case of lower gastrointestinal bleeding and small bowel tumorous masses. Arch Pathol Lab Med 129:800–2, 2005.

15. Chandra B, Long JD. Diagnosis of Trichuris trichiura (whipworm) by colonoscopic extraction. J Clin Gastroenterol 27:152–7, 1998.

16. Cooper ES, Whyte-Alleng CAM, Finzi-Smith JS, MacDonald TT. Intestinal nematode infections in children: the pathophysiological price paid. Parasitol 104:S91–103, 1992.

17. Despommier DD. *Trichinella spiralis*. In: Blaser MJ, Smith PD, Ravdin JI, et al. Infections of the Gastrointestinal Tract. New York: Raven Press, 1995, pp. 1179–88.

18. Dronda F, Chaves F, Sanz A, Lopez-Velez R. Human intestinal capillariasis in an area of nonendemicity: case report and review. Clin Infect Dis 17:909–12, 1993.

19. Elsayed S, Yilmaz A, Hershfield N. *Trichuris trichiura* worm infection. Gastro Endosc 60:990–1, 2004.

20. Gopinath R, Keystone JS. Ascariasis, Trichuriasis, and Enterobiasis. In: Blaser MJ, Smith PD, Ravdin JI, et al. (eds): Infections of the Gastrointestinal Tract. New York: Raven Press, 1995, pp. 1167–77.

21. Grencis RK, Hons BSc, Cooper ES. Enterobius, Trichuris, Capillaria, and Hookworm including Ancyclostoma caninum. Gastroenterol Clin North Am 25(3):579–97, 1996.

22. Hotez PJ. Hookworm infections. In: Blaser MJ, Smith PD, Ravdin JI, et al. Infections of the Gastrointestinal Tract. New York: Raven Press, 1995, pp. 1189–96.

23. Kenney M, Yermakov V. Infection of man with *Trichuris vulpis*, the whipworm of dogs. Am J Trop Med Hyg 29:1205–8, 1980.

24. Loria-Cortes R, Lobo-Sanahuja JF. Clinical abdominal angiostrongylosis: a study of 116 children with intestinal eosinophilic granuloma caused by *Angiostrongylus costaricensis*. Am J Trop Med Hyg 29:538–44, 1980.

25. Kramer MH, Greer GJ, Quinonez JF, et al. First reported outbreak of abdominal angiostrongyliasis. Clin Infect Dis 26:365–72, 1998.

26. Meyers WM, Marty AM, Neafie RC. Ancylostomiasis. In: Meyers WM, Neafie RC, Marty AM, Wear DJ. (eds): Pathology of Infectious Diseases: Vol. 1, Helminthiases. Washington, DC: AFIP Press, 2000, pp. 353–65.

27. Morera P, Neafie RC, Marty AM. Angiostrongyliasis costaricensis. In: Meyers WM, Neafie RC, Marty AM, Wear DJ. (eds): Pathology of Infectious Diseases: Vol. 1, Helminthiases. Washington, DC: AFIP Press, 2000, pp. 385–96.

28. Ochoa B. Surgical complications of ascarisis. World J Surg 15:222–7, 1991.

29. Prociv P, Croese J. Human eosinophilic enteritis caused by dog hookworm Ancylostoma caninum. Lancet 335(2):1299–303, 1990.

30. Sandler M. Whipworm infestation in the colon and rectum simulating Crohn's colitis. Lancet July 25, p. 210, 1981.

31. Sinniah B: Trichuriasis: In: Connor DH, Chandler FW et al. (eds): Pathology of Infectious Diseases, Stamford, CT: Appleton and Lange, 1997, pp. 1585–8.

32. Surendran N, Paulose MO. Intestinal complications of round worms in children. J Pediatr Surg 23:931–5, 1988.

33. Walden J. Other roundworms: Trichuris, Hookworm, and Strongyloides. Prim Care 18: 53–74, 1991.

34. Wasadikar PP, Kulkarni AB. Intestinal obstruction due to ascariasis. Br J Surg 84:410–2, 1997.

35. Wiersma R, Hadley GR. Small bowel volvulus complicating intestinal ascariasis in children. Br J Surg 75:86–7, 1988.

Chapter 32

Enterobius vermicularis (Pinworms)

Keywords *Enterobius vermicularis* • Pinworm • Appendicitis • Granuloma • Ova

Pinworms are one of the most common human parasites. Prevalence is highest among children aged 5–10, and it has been reported that pinworm infections of the GI tract affect 4–28% of children worldwide. These nematodes have a worldwide distribution, but are more common in cold or temperate climates and in developed countries. They are extremely common in the United States and Northwestern Europe. The infective egg resides in dust and soil, and transmission is believed to be via the fecal–oral route. Pinworms are known as *Oxyuris vermicularis* in the older literature.

The worms live and reproduce in the ileum, cecum, proximal colon, and appendix, and the female migrates to the anus to deposit eggs and die. The perianal eggs and worms produce the characteristic symptoms of pruritis ani, which often leads to perianal scratching and insomnia. Although many infections are asymptomatic, appendicitis, colitis, vulvovaginitis, and peritoneal involvement have all been described. Heavy infections may cause abdominal pain, nausea, and vomiting.

The etiologic role of *Enterobius* in appendicitis and colitis remains controversial. Although pinworms are detected in approximately 0.6–13% of resected appendices (Fig. 32.1), they are usually not invasive, and their ability to cause mucosal damage has been a subject of intense debate. The relationship between pinworm infection and the symptoms of acute appendicitis also remains unclear. Some authorities believe that the lack of inflammation surrounding invasive pinworms indicates that the organism invades only after the appendix has been removed in order to escape the decrease in oxygen tension. However, invasion has been documented occasionally, with associated mucosal ulceration and inflammation, and it has been suggested that if additional sections were submitted from appendices containing lumenal pinworms, more cases of invasive enterobiasis would be found. In addition, both worms and ova may obstruct the appendiceal lumen and cause inflammation similar to that caused by fecaliths.

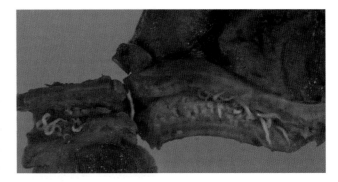

Fig. 32.1 Pinworms present within the lumen of a resected appendix. The worms are 2–5 mm in length, white or ivory, and pointed at both ends; the posterior end is curved. (Courtesy Dr. George F. Gray, Jr)

Pathologic findings. In the appendix, the mucosa usually appears normal, and pinworms are most often found in the appendiceal lumen (Fig. 32.2). Even invasive pinworms incite little, or no, inflammatory reaction, but rarely an inflammatory infiltrate composed of neutrophils and eosinophils may occur, along with hemorrhage and ulceration (Fig. 32.3). In the colon affected by enterobiasis, the mucosa is usually normal as well, although rare cases of severe eosinophilic colitis associated with heavy pinworm infections have been reported. Granulomas, sometimes with necrosis, may develop as a reaction to degenerating worms or eggs; granulomas have been described in the liver, omentum, and peritoneum, as well as the appendix, anus, and colon in rare cases.

The worms are 2–5 mm in length, white or ivory, and pointed at both ends; the posterior end is curved (Fig. 32.1). They may be seen with the naked eye or endoscope (Fig. 32.4). Morphologically, pinworms have prominent lateral alae with easily visible internal organs (Fig. 32.5); eggs are ovoid with one flat side and a bilayered refractile shell (Fig. 32.6).

Differential diagnosis. The morphologic features of the worm, described above, are characteristic of enterobiasis. Primary *Enterobius* infection may be difficult to distinguish from infection complicating a pre-existing inflammatory

L.W. Lamps, *Surgical Pathology of the Gastrointestinal System: Bacterial, Fungal, Viral, and Parasitic Infections,* DOI 10.1007/978-1-4419-0861-2_32, © Springer Science+Business Media, LLC 2009

Fig. 32.2 Several non-invasive pinworms are present in the lumen of an appendix that lacks significant inflammation (**a**). Even at low power, the lateral alae and internal organs are easily visible (**b**). (Courtesy Dr. Amy Hudson)

Fig. 32.3 Low-power view of invasive pinworms (**a**). Note associated mucosal ulceration and neutrophilic inflammation (**b**)

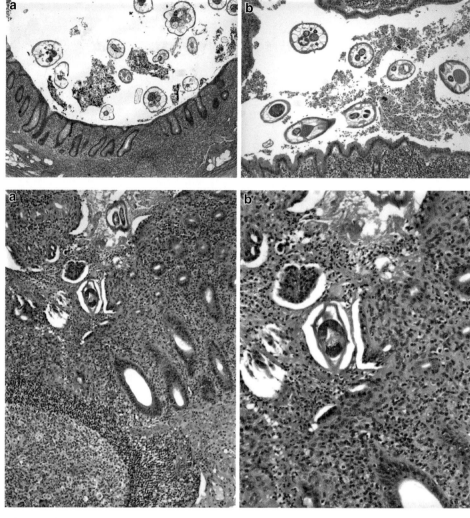

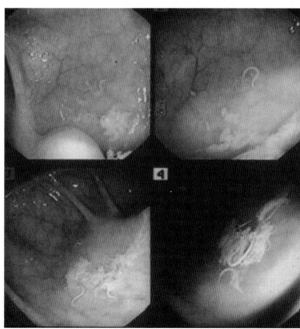

Fig. 32.4 Endoscopically visible pinworms in the right colon

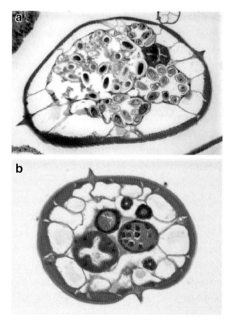

Fig. 32.5 In cross section, pinworms have easily visible lateral alae and internal organs (**a** and **b**). Gravid females contain eggs (**a**)

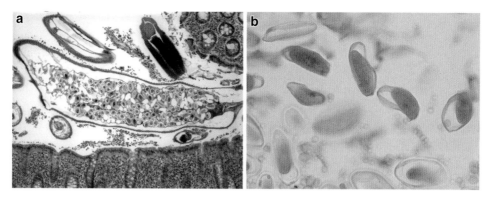

Fig. 32.6 Longitudinal section of a gravid female containing numerous eggs (**a**, courtesy Dr. Amy Hudson). Eggs are ovoid with one flat side and a bilayered refractile shell (**b**)

disorder, such as an inflamed anal fissure. In addition, it may be difficult to distinguish between primary *Enterobius* infection and the presence of worms complicating or existing within the context of pre-existing acute appendicitis. Ova are rare in feces, but the legendary scotch tape test, ideally performed first thing in the morning, may be a useful adjunct to diagnosis.

Selected References

1. Arca MJ, Gates RL, Groner JI, et al. Clinical manifestations of appendiceal pinworms in children: an institutional experience and a review of the literature. Pediatr Surg Int 20:372–5, 2004.
2. Budd JS, Armstrong C. Role of *Enterobius vermicularis* in the aetiology of appendicitis. Br J Surg 74:748–9, 1987.
3. Cook GC. The clinical significance of gastrointestinal helminths – a review. Trans Roy Soc Trop Med Hyg. 80:675–85, 1986.
4. Cooper ES, Whyte-Alleng CAM, Finzi-Smith JS, MacDonald TT. Intestinal nematode infections in children: the pathophysiological price paid. Parasitol 104 suppl:S91–103, 1992.
5. Grencis RK, Hons BSc, Cooper ES. *Enterobius, Trichuris, Capillaria*, and Hookworm including *Ancyclostoma caninum*. Gastroenterol Clin North Am 25(3):579–97, 1996.
6. Lamps LW. Appendicitis and infections of the appendix. Semin Diagn Pathol 21:86–97, 2004.
7. Liu LX, Chi J, Upton MP, Ash LR. Eosinophilic colitis associated with larvae of the pinworm *Enterobius vermicularis*. Lancet 346(1):410–2, 1995.
8. Mogensen K, Pahle E, Kowalski K. *Enterobius vermicularis* and acute appendicitis. Acta Chir Scand 151:705–7, 1985.
9. Sinniah B, Leopairut RC, Connor DH. Voge. M. Enterobiasis: a histopathological study of 259 patients. Ann Trop Med Parasitol 85:625–35, 1991.
10. Sinniah B. Enterobiasis. In: Connor DH, Chandler FW, et al (eds): Pathology of Infectious Diseases, Stamford, CT: Appleton and Lange, 1997, pp. 1415–8.
11. Wiebe BM. Appendicitis and *Enterobius vermicularis*. Scan J Gastroenterol. 26:336–8, 1991.
12. Williams DJ, Dixon MF. Sex, *Enterobius vermicularis* and the appendix. Br J Surg 75:1225–6, 1988.
13. Yildirim S, Nursal TZ, Tarim A, et al. A rare cause of acute appendicitis: parasitic infection. Scand J Infect Dis 37:757–9, 2005.

Chapter 33

Strongyloides stercoralis

Keywords *Strongyloides stercoralis* • Corticosteroid • Larva

The nematode *Strongyloide stercoralis* has a worldwide distribution. It is endemic in tropical climates; in the United States, it is endemic in the southeast, urban areas with large immigrant populations, and mental institutions. Stronglyoidiasis occurs primarily in adults, many of whom are hospitalized, suffer from chronic illnesses, or are immunocompromised. Corticosteroids and HTLV-1 viral infection are also associated with strongyloidiasis.

S. stercoralis is contracted from soil containing the organism. It penetrates the skin, enters the venous system, travels to the lungs, and then migrates up the respiratory tree and down the esophagus to reach the small intestine. The female lives in the small intestine and lays eggs there that hatch into rhabditiform larvae, which are excreted. An extremely important feature of the *Strongyloides* life cycle is that rhabditiform larvae can mature into infective filariform larvae within the host, via molting. This autoinfective (also known as hyperinfective) capability allows the organism to infect the host and cause illness for long periods of time, sometimes upwards of 30 years. In addition, widespread dissemination (defined as migration of the organism to organs beyond the lung and gastrointestinal tract) may occur in immunocompromised patients, causing severe and even fatal illness. Interestingly, AIDS patients do not appear to be unusually susceptible to strongyloidiasis. Corticosteroids appear to be responsible for the conversion of chronic, low-grade strongyloidiasis into fulminant disseminated infection in many cases. Although the mechanism is incompletely understood, possible mechanisms include the ability of steroids to deplete eosinophils, as well as the possibility that steroids may trigger larval molting. Fulminant

strongyloidiasis is also associated with disseminated bacterial infections, apparently because the worms carry enteric bacteria with them as they invade the intestinal wall and migrate to other sites.

Many patients are asymptomatic. When patients are symptomatic, symptoms are quite variable and include diarrhea, abdominal pain and tenderness, nausea, vomiting, weight loss, and GI bleeding. Gastrointestinal manifestations may be accompanied by mesenteric adenopathy, rash, urticaria, pruritis, mild anemia, peripheral eosinophilia and leukocytosis, and concomitant pulmonary symptoms. Rarely, severe or chronic infection may lead to bowel obstruction and stenosis.

Pathologic features. Lesions may be seen in the stomach (Fig. 33.1), small bowel, and colon (Fig. 33.2). Endoscopically, findings include hypertrophic mucosal folds, edema, petechial hemorrhage and erythema, and ulcers. Raised polypoid lesions of the small and large bowel have been reported, sometimes with associated xanthoma-like changes.

In mild infection, histologic features include mucosal congestion and an increased mononuclear infiltrate in the lamina propria. In more severe infections, there is edema, villous blunting (Fig. 33.3), cryptitis (Fig. 33.4), and a dense eosinophilic and neutrophilic infiltrate in the lamina propria (Fig. 33.5). Ulceration may be seen in severe infections and is most often seen in hyperinfections. Ulceration may be accompanied by fibrosis and stenosis. Perforation has been described rarely. Granulomas are occasionally present as well. Both adult worms and larvae may be found in the crypts (Figs. 33.6, 33.7, and 33.8), but they may be difficult to detect. Worms typically have sharply pointed tails that may be curved (Figs. 33.9 and 33.10). In severe infections, larvae may be seen transmurally and in lymphatics and small vessels. Rarely, larvae may be found within

Fig. 33.1 Gastric biopsy from a patient in the southeastern United States on long-term chemotherapy. Numerous organisms are present within the glands, without a significant associated inflammatory infiltrate

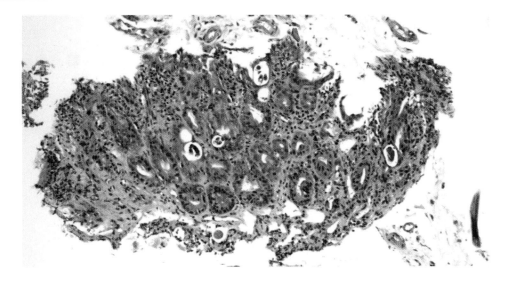

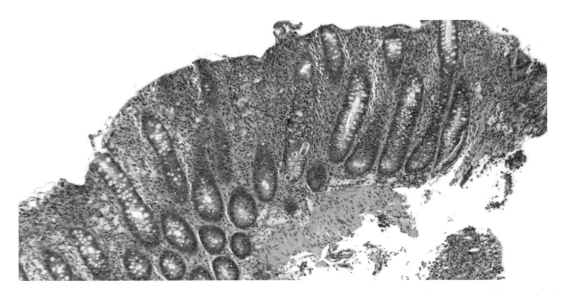

Fig. 33.2 Low-power view of a colon biopsy showing intraglandular organisms, visible even at low power, with associated cryptitis. (Courtesy Dr. Lucas Campbell)

mesenteric lymph nodes, with an accompanying eosinophilic infiltrate.

S. sterocoralis is also a rare cause of appendicitis (Fig. 33.11). Patients may have symptoms that are clinically indistinguishable from acute non-specific appendicitis, and the diagnosis of strongyloidiasis is almost always made post-surgically. Affected appendices typically show organisms within the appendiceal crypts, with a marked transmural eosinophilic infiltrate and variably present granulomas.

Differential diagnosis. The presence of larvae with sharply pointed, sometimes curved tails within the glands of the gastrointestinal mucosa is essentially diagnostic of strongyloidiasis. In the proper clinical and geographic setting, however, *Capillaria* infection is also in the differential diagnosis. Rarely, fulminant intestinal strongyloidiasis may mimic chronic idiopathic inflammatory bowel disease. Ancillary diagnostic tests include stool examination for larvae, worms, or eggs, and serologic tests.

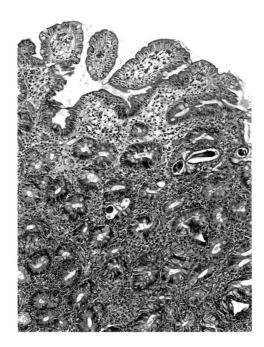

Fig. 33.3 Duodenal biopsy showing edema and mild villous blunting, along with a mixed inflammatory infiltrate in the lamina propria. Organisms are seen in the glands. (Courtesy Dr. Kari Caradine)

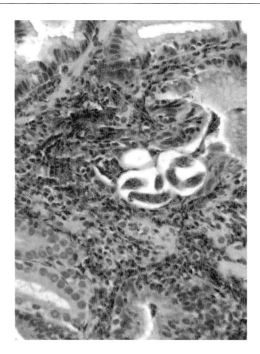

Fig. 33.5 Larvae may be accompanied by a dense eosinophilic infiltrate

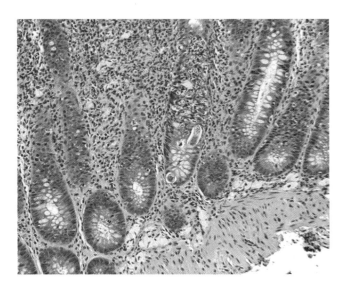

Fig. 33.4 *S. stercoralis* larvae are present in the colonic glands, with associated neutrophilic cryptitis. (Courtesy Dr. Lucas Campbell)

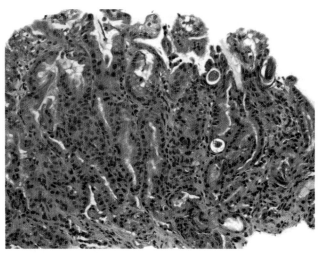

Fig. 33.6 Cross-sections of *Strongyloides* are seen within the gastric glands

Selected References

1. Al-Hasan MN, McCormick M, Ribes JA. Invasive enteric infections in hospitalized patients with underlying strongyloidiasis. Am J Clin Pathol 128:622–7, 2007.

2. Berry AJ, Long EG, Smith JH, et al. Chronic relapsing colitis due to *Strongyloides stercoralis*. Am J Trop Med Hyg 32:1289–93, 1983.

3. Concha R, Harrington W Jr., Rogers AI. Intestinal strongyloidiasis: recognition, management, and determinants of outcome. J Clin Gastroenterol 39:203–11, 2005.

4. Genta RM, Haque AK. Strongyloidiasis. In: Connor DH, Chandler FW et al. (eds): Pathology of Infectious Diseases, Stamford, CT: Appleton and Lange, 1997, pp. 1567–76.

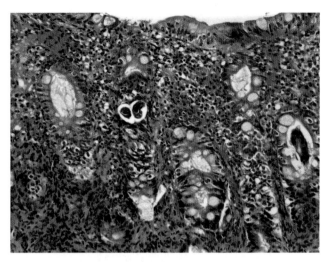

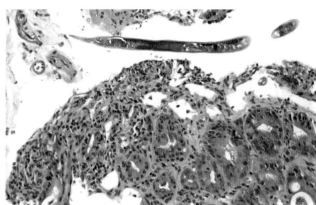

Fig. 33.9 Longitudinal view of *S. stercoralis* floating above the gastric epithelium. Note sharply pointed tail

Fig. 33.7 Cross-sections of larvae within the colonic glands, with associated cryptitis and a dense mixed inflammatory infiltrate in the lamina propria that is rich in eosinophils and neutrophils. (Courtesy Dr. Kari Caradine)

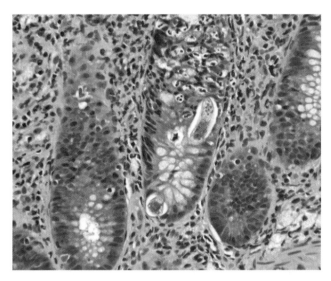

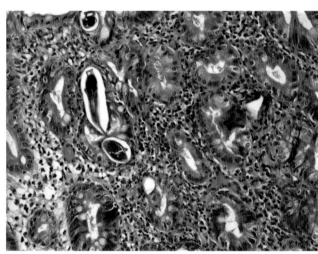

Fig. 33.8 High-power view of organism within the colonic glands, with associated cryptitis. (Courtesy Dr. Lucas Campbell)

Fig. 33.10 High-power view of organisms within colonic glands; note curved, sharply pointed tail

5. Gutierrez Y, Bhatia P, Garbadawala ST, et al. Strongyloides stercoralis eosinophilic granulomatous enterocolitis. Am J Surg Pathol 20:603–12, 1996.
6. Heyworth MF. Parasitic diseases in immunocompromised hosts. Cryptosporidiosis, Isosporiasis, and Strongyloidiasis. Gastroenterol Clin North Am 25(3):691–707, 1996.
7. Kishimoto K, Hokama A, Hirata T, et al. Endoscopic and histopathological study on the duodenum of *Strongyloides stercoralis* hyperinfection. World J Gastroenterol 14:1768–73, 2008.
8. Keiser PB, Nutman TB. *Strongyloides stercoralis* in the immunocompromised population. Clin Microbiol Rev 17:208–17, 2004.
9. Lamps LW. Appendicitis and infections of the appendix. Semin Diagn Pathol 21:86–97, 2004.
10. Lessnau KD, Can S, Talavera W. Disseminated *Strongyloides stercoralis* in human immunodeficiency virus-infected patients. Treatment failure and a review of the literature. Chest 104:119–22, 1993.
11. Meyers WM, Neafie RC, Marty AM. Strongyloidiasis. In: Meyers WM, Neafie RC, Marty AM, Wear DJ. (eds): Pathology of Infectious Diseases: Vol. 1, Helminthiases. Washington, DC: AFIP Press, 2000, pp.341–52.
12. Milder JE, Walzer PD, Kilgore GK, et al. Clinical features of *Strongyloides stercoralis* infection in an endemic area of the United States. Gastroenterology 80:1481–8, 1981.
13. Nadler S, Cappell MS, Bhatt B, et al. Appendiceal infection by *Entamoeba histolytica* and *Strongyloides stercoralis* presenting like acute appendicitis. Dig Dis Sci 35:603–8, 1990.

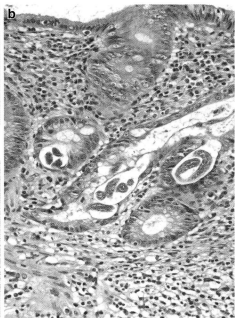

Fig. 33.11 *S. stercoralis* are seen within the appendiceal glands, while *Enterobius vermicularis* are within the overlying luminal debris (**a**). Higher power view of larvae within the appendiceal glands, with a mixed inflammatory infiltrate in the lamina propria (**b**). (Courtesy Dr. Dennis Baroni-Cruz)

14. Noodleman JS. Eosinophilic appendicitis: demonstration of *Strongyloides stercoralis* as a causative agent. Arch Pathol Lab Med 105:148–9, 1981.
15. Ramdial PK, Hlatshwayo NH, Singh B. *Strongyloides stercoralis* mesenteric lymphadenopathy: clue to the etiopathogenesis of intestinal pseudo-obstruction in HIV-infected patients. Annals Diagn Pathol 10:209–14, 2006.
16. Rivasi F, Pampiglione S, Boldorini R, Cardinale L. Histopathology of gastric and duodenal *Strongyloides stercoralis* locations in fifteen immunocompromised subjects. Arch Pathol Lab Med 130:1792–8, 2006.
17. Al Samman M, Haque S, Long JD. Strongyloidiasis colitis: a case report and review of the literature. J Clin Gastroenterol 28:77–80, 1999.
18. Thompson BF, Fry LC, Wells CD, et al. The spectrum of GI strongyloidiasis: an endoscopic-pathologic study. Gastro Endosc 59:906–10, 2004.
19. Weight SC, Barrie WW. Colonic strongyloides infection masquerading as ulcerative colitis. J R Coll Surg Edinb 42:202–3, 1997.

Chapter 34

Anisakis Simplex and Related Nematodes

Keywords Anisakiasis simplex • Larva • Sushi • Anisakiasis • Eosinophil

This disease involves the penetration of the wall of the gastrointestinal tract by the larvae of *Anisakis simplex* or related species. *Anisakis simplex* is the most well known of these worms; related species that infect humans include *Pseudoterranova* (*Phocanema*) *decipiens, Anasakis* type II, and *Contracaecum* species. *A. simplex* and *P. decipiens* are responsible for most human infections. These nematodes parasitize fish and sea mammals, and thus humans ingest them by eating raw, pickled, or smoked fish. The potential for transmission to humans is greater in areas where eating raw or inadequately cooked fish is common, and thus the number of cases in the United States has increased in recent years with the popularity of sushi, sashimi, and ceviche. Even skilled chefs and consumers may have difficulty detecting the parasite in fish, although adequate cooking and freezing both kill the parasite.

The most common clinical manifestations are those of acute gastric anisakiasis, characterized by epigastric pain, chills, nausea, and vomiting within 12–24 h of ingestion of parasitized food. The allergenic potential of *Anisakis* species is well recognized, and thus some patients with acute gastric anisakiasis also manifest hypersensitivity symptoms such as urticaria, angioedema, peripheral eosinophilia, and anaphylaxis. Patients with chronic infection may be asymptomatic; symptomatic patients generally have mild nausea, dyspepsia, and abdominal pain, and some have peripheral eosinophilia. Patients with intestinal anisakiasis (rather than gastric) may have abdominal pain, nausea, vomiting, diarrhea, and melena. Threadlike filling defects can be seen if patients undergo an upper GI radiographic series.

Occasionally, larvae may be identified and removed endoscopically. Symptoms usually disappear rapidly after removal of the larvae. If the larvae cannot be removed, symptoms will persist until it dies in the wall of the gut. Obstruction (secondary to the marked edema and inflammation) along with perforation and peritonitis has been reported rarely in association with the *Anisakis* larvae.

Pathologic features. The stomach is the most frequent site of involvement, although the small bowel, colon (usually right colon), and appendix also may be involved. Endoscopic findings include mucosal edema, thickened mucosal folds, hemorrhage, erosions, and ulcers. Polypoid masses may be present associated with larvae. Inflammatory changes usually surround the organism (Fig. 34.1), and histologic

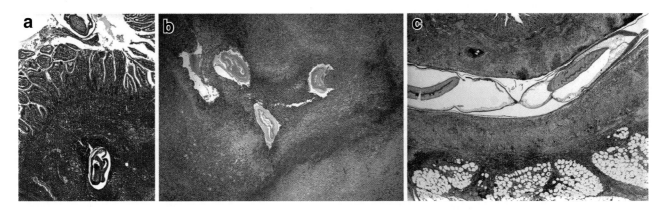

Fig. 34.1 Areas of geographic necrosis and an inflammatory infiltrate rich in neutrophils and eosinophils surround *Anisakis* larvae in intestinal anisakiasis (**a** and **b**). Note transmural eosinophilic infiltrate extending into subserosal fat (**c**). (**a** and **c**, courtesy Dr. David Owen; **b**, courtesy Drs. A. Morgan Wright and Melissa Upton)

L.W. Lamps, *Surgical Pathology of the Gastrointestinal System: Bacterial, Fungal, Viral, and Parasitic Infections*,
DOI 10.1007/978-1-4419-0861-2_34, © Springer Science+Business Media, LLC 2009

Fig. 34.2 Necrotic debris and an inflammatory infiltrate rich in eosinophils surround larva in cross section (**a**) and longitudinal section (**b**) in anisakiasis. (Courtesy Dr. David Owen)

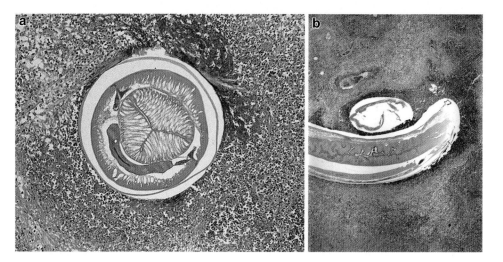

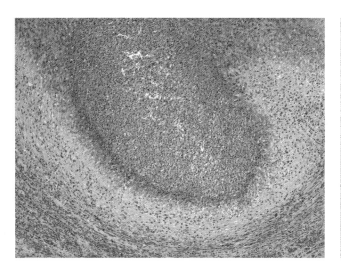

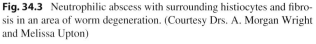

Fig. 34.3 Neutrophilic abscess with surrounding histiocytes and fibrosis in an area of worm degeneration. (Courtesy Drs. A. Morgan Wright and Melissa Upton)

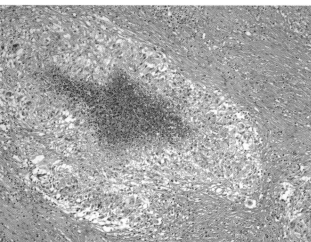

Fig. 34.4 Granuloma with central necrosis and eosinophilic infiltrate in an area of worm degeneration. (Courtesy Drs. A. Morgan Wright and Melissa Upton)

findings include an inflammatory infiltrate rich in eosinophils and neutrophils, which may form areas of "geographic" necrosis (Figs. 34.1 and 34.2) that can extend transmurally into serosal and mesenteric tissues. Eosinophilic abscesses, granulomas, and giant cells may be present, particularly as the larvae die and degenerate (Figs. 34.3 and 34.4).

Larvae (ranging from 0.5 to 5.0 cm in length) are cream to white and occasionally seen in tissue sections, particularly resection specimens. They have distinctive Y-shaped lateral chords, prominent multilayered cuticles, and numerous muscle cells (Fig. 34.5); they lack lateral alae or wings extending from the cuticles.

Differential diagnosis. The symptoms may mimic peptic ulcer disease, appendicitis, Crohn's disease, or an acute abdomen. Diagnosis may be challenging, as anisakids do not usually produce eggs or larvae in humans. Larvae are only rarely seen in stool samples, but they may be recovered from sputum or vomitus. Serologic tests exist, but are not widely available, and patients with infection by some species of *Ascaris* may show cross-reactivity. In addition, antibodies may remain elevated for months after infection and worm removal.

Fig. 34.5 *Anisakis* larvae have a prominent multilayered cuticle that lacks lateral alae or wings (**a**, courtesy Drs. A. Morgan Wright and Melissa Upton) and distinctive Y-shaped lateral chords (**b**, courtesy Dr. David Owen)

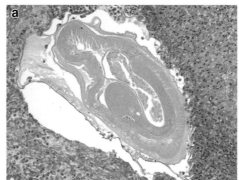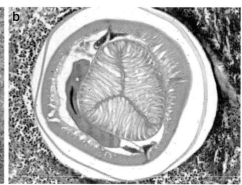

Selected References

1. Andersen EM, Lichtenfels JR. Anisakiasis. In: Meyers WM, Neafie RC, Marty AM, Wear DJ. Pathology of Infectious Diseases: Vol. 1, Helminthiases. Washington, DC: AFIP Press, 2000, pp. 423–31.
2. Bruckner DA. Helminthic food-borne infections. Clin Lab Med 19:639–60, 1999.
3. Couture C, Measures L, Gagnon J, Desbiens C. Human intestinal anisakiosis due to consumption of raw salmon. Am J Surg Pathol 27:1167–72, 2003.
4. Daschner A, Alonso-Gomez A, Cabanas R, et al. Gastroallergic anisakiasis: borderline between food allergy and parasitic disease – clinical and allergologic evaluation of 20 patients with confirmed acute parasitism. J All Clin Imm 105:176–81, 2000.
5. Deardorff TL, Fukumura T, Raybourne RB. Invasive anisakiasis. Gastroenterol 90:1047–50, 1986.
6. Gomez B, Tabar AI, Tunon T, et al. Eosinophilic gastroenteritis and *Anisaki*s. Allergy 53:1148–54, 1998.
7. Ikeda K, Kumashiro R, Kifune T. Nine cases of acute gastric anisakiasis. Gastro Endosc 35:304–8, 1989.
8. Matsumoto T, Iida M, Kimura Y, et al. Anisakiasis of the colon: radiologic and endoscopic features in six patients. Radiol 183: 97–9, 1992.
9. Kliks MM. Anisakiasis in the western United States: four new case reports from California. Am J Trop Med Hyg 32:526–32, 1983.
10. Sakanari JA, Loinaz HM, Deardorff TL, et al. Intestinal anisakiasis: a case diagnosed by morphologic and immunologic methods. Am J Clin Pathol 90:107–13, 1988.
11. Schuster R, Petrini JL, Choi R. Anisakiasis of the colon presenting as bowel obstruction. Am Surg 69:350–2, 2003.
12. Sugimachi K, Inokuchi K, Ooiwa T, et al. Acute gastric anisakiasis: analysis of 178 cases. JAMA 253:1012–3, 1985.

Chapter 35

Schistosomiasis

Keywords Schistosomiasis • *Schistosoma* sp • Ova • Granuloma • Acid-fast • Spine

Schistosomiasis is one of the most common diseases in the world; it is also known as bilharziasis, after its discovery by Sir Theodore Bilharz in Egypt in 1851. All species of *Schistosoma* that infect humans have the capability to cause significant gastrointestinal disease, but the gut is a target organ in *S. mansoni, S. japonicum, S. mekongi,* and *S. intercalatum* infections. These trematodes are endemic in Africa, Asia, and parts of the Americas. In the United States, infected patients are often immigrants, travelers, or persons who have worked abroad. Humans become infected by exposure to contaminated water.

The severity of the disease and the likelihood of significant sequelae are related to the intensity and duration of the infection. In addition, egg deposition is seemingly random and non-uniform. Acute symptomatic infection most often occurs in immunologically naïve adults infected for the first time; this is rarely seen in inhabitants of endemic areas. Most patients in endemic areas have chronic schistosomiasis and are asymptomatic or have only mild chronic complaints. Patients with symptomatic gastrointestinal infection generally present with diarrhea (often bloody), accompanied by anemia, weight loss, and protein-losing enteropathy. More dramatic gastrointestinal presentations have been described, such as a profound dysentery-like illness, obstruction, perforation, intussusception, rectal prolapse, fistulae, and perianal abscesses.

Schistosomes (most frequently *S. haematobium*) occasionally cause appendicitis. Patients often present with typical signs and symptoms of acute appendicitis, although some may present with inflammatory masses. Similar to *E. vermicularis*, the ability of schistosomes to actually cause appendicitis has been debated. It has been demonstrated in at least some cases, however, that schistosomes do cause acute appendicitis, either by inducing granulomatous inflammation or by causing such marked fibrosis that luminal obstruction leads to signs and symptoms of acute appendicitis.

Pathologic findings. Any level of the GI tract may be affected. The histologic findings in schistosomiasis result from inflammation and fibrosis in reaction to the eggs deposited in tissue; the worms themselves cause little damage. In general, there is an active phase of infection, characterized by more intense inflammation, and an inactive phase, characterized by decreasing inflammation and increasing fibrosis and calcification of ova.

Endoscopically, schistosomes may cause inflammatory polyposis (most commonly in the distal colon and rectum) with associated mucosal granularity, friability, punctate ulcers, and hemorrhages (Fig. 35.1). Inflammatory polyps and mucosal ulcers are common earlier in infection, and histologically there is granulomatous inflammation and an inflammatory infiltrate that may be rich in eosinophils associated with the ova (Fig. 35.2). Eggs or parts of eggs may be detected within granulomas. There may be an associated Splendore–Hoeppli reaction. As lesions progress, there is increased fibrosis, as well as an increase in macrophages and multinucleated giant cells (Fig. 35.3); remote lesions may show only fibrosis and calcified eggs, with virtually no inflammatory reaction (Fig. 35.4). The marked fibrosis may lead to luminal narrowing and obstruction of the bowel.

In the appendix, early lesions feature transmural inflammation rich in eosinophils, often with a granulomatous reaction to ova. Older lesions may be fibrotic and hyalinized, with calcified eggs (Fig. 35.5).

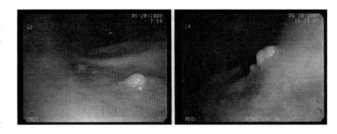

Fig. 35.1 Endoscopic photographs of multiple colonic pseudopolyps secondary to schistosomiasis. (Courtesy Dr. Becky Wheeler)

Fig. 35.2 An inflammatory infiltrate rich in eosinophils surrounds schistosome ova (**a**, courtesy Dr. George F. Gray, Jr.). Early granuloma with associated neutrophils. Embryos are visible in the ova, as they are not completely calcified (**b**, courtesy Dr. Joe Misdraji)

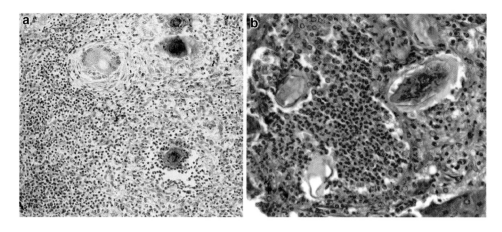

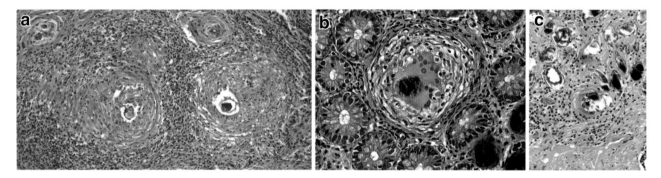

Fig. 35.3 Confluent schistosomal granulomas with fibrosis and a predominantly mononuclear cell infiltrate (**a**, courtesy Dr. Joe Misdraji). Colon biopsy showing granuloma with early fibrosis, eosinophils, and a multinucleate giant cell centered on an egg (**b**, courtesy Dr. Becky Wheeler). Sections of appendix show calcified ova and parts of ova with associated fibrosis, mononuclear cells, and rare eosinophils (**c**, courtesy Dr. Joe Misdraji)

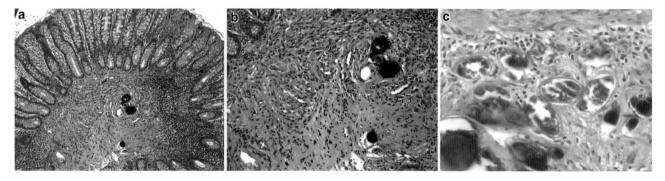

Fig. 35.4 Colon biopsy showing calcified ova in the submucosa, with associated fibrosis and rare inflammatory cells (**a** and **b**). High-power view of calcified ova in the submucosa, with associated fibrosis and rare mononuclear cells (**c**)

Schistosome eggs are variably acid-fast (Fig. 35.6); morphologic and staining characteristics of the eggs of the various species are given in Table 35.1. In H & E sections, the calcified eggs are generally dark blue or black and somewhat amorphous (Fig. 35.7). Decalcification may reveal partially preserved embryos (Fig. 35.8). The worms themselves are slender and elongated, measuring approximately 0.5–2.5 cm in length. Worms are occasionally found within veins in histologic sections (Fig. 35.9).

Differential diagnosis. The inflammatory reaction to the organism may mimic other infectious processes as well as chronic idiopathic inflammatory bowel disease. Schistosome eggs in tissue sections may be distinguished from the eggs of *Enterobius, Capillaria*, and trematodes by their spines

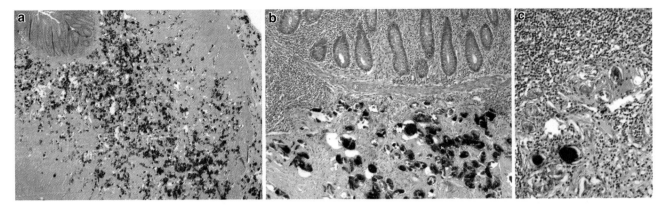

Fig. 35.5 Low-power view of appendix containing innumerable calcified ova, with associated fibrosis (**a**, courtesy Dr. Joe Misdraji). Higher power views showing calcified ova with associated fibrosis in the submucosa (**b**, courtesy Dr. Joe Misdraji; **c**, courtesy Dr. David Owen)

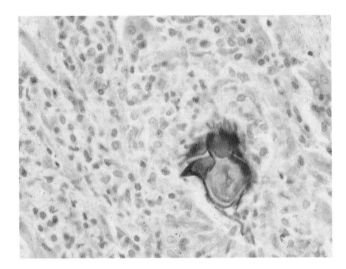

Fig. 35.6 Acid-fast shell and spine of a schistosome egg within a granuloma (Ziehl–Neelsen stain; courtesy Dr. George F. Gray, Jr.)

and the acid-fast properties of the eggs (see Table 35.1). Microscopic detection of eggs in stool or urine is the most reliable, cost-effective method of diagnosis, although multiple specimens may be required. Worms are occasionally retrieved from biliary lavage (Fig. 35.10). Serologic studies are also useful.

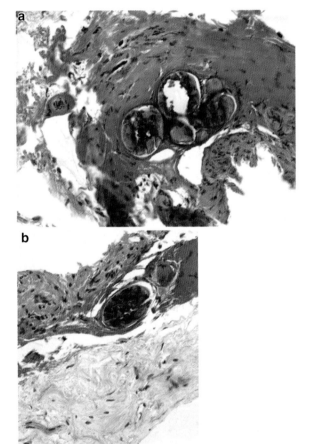

Fig. 35.7 Colon biopsies showing dark blue to black, amorphous calcified schistosome eggs (**a** and **b**). Note associated fibrosis and lack of inflammation in this remote infection

Selected References

1. Abdel-Moneim RI. Bilharziasis of the appendix. Int Surg 67:45–7, 1982.
2. Adebamowo CA, Akang EEU, Ladipo JK, et al. Schistosomiasis of the appendix. Br J Surg 78:1219-21,1991.
3. Cheever AW. Decalcification of schistosome eggs during staining of tissue sections: a potential source of diagnostic error. Am J Trop Med Hyg 35:959–61, 1986.
4. Davis A. Recent advances in schistosomiasis. Quart J Med 58:95–110, 1986.
5. Eldin OS, Nada N, Eldosoky I. Bilharzial lymphadenitis, a case report. Histopathol 52:655–6, 2008.
6. Elliott DE. Schistosomiasis: pathophysiology, diagnosis, and treatment. Gastroenterol Clin North Am 25(3):599–624,1996.
7. Gryseels B, Polman K, Clerinx J, Kestens L. Human schistosomiasis. Lancet 368(9541):1106–18, 2006.

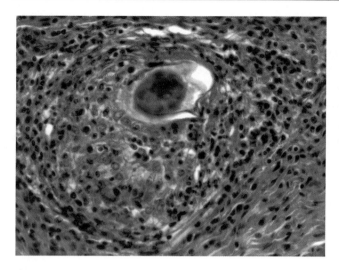

Fig. 35.8 Ova that are not yet calcified or that are subjected to histologic decalcification may reveal partially intact embryos

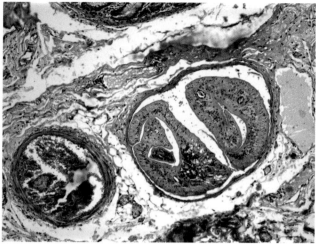

Fig. 35.9 Adult worms are occasionally seen within venules in the bowel. (Courtesy Dr. David Owen)

Table 35.1 Schistosome target organs, geographical distribution, and staining characteristics of schistosome eggs

Species	Egg shape	Staining properties	Target organs	Endemic areas
S. haematobium	Terminal spine	Acid-fast spine	Bladder, ureter, pelvis	Africa Southern Europe Western Asia
S. mansoni	Lateral spine	Acid-fast shell and spine	Gut, liver, lung	Africa Brazil West Indies Puerto Rico
S. japonicum	Small lateral spine	Acid-fast shell and spine	Gut, liver, lung	China Japan Philippines
S. intercalatum	Terminal spine	Acid-fast spine	Gut, liver	West Africa
S. mekongii	Small lateral spine	Acid-fast shell and spine	Gut, liver, lung	Laos Cambodia Thailand
S. malayi	Small lateral spine	Acid-fast shell and spine	Liver	Penang peninsula (Malaysia)

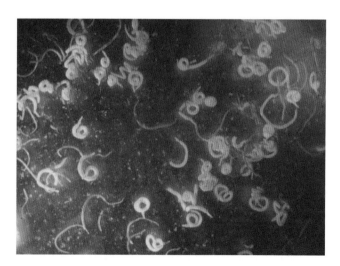

Fig. 35.10 Numerous schistosome worms retrieved via biliary lavage. (Courtesy Dr. George F. Gray, Jr)

8. Iyer HV, Abaci IF, Rehnke EC, Enquist IF. Intestinal obstruction due to schistosomiasis. Am J Surg 149:409–11, 1985.
9. Lamps LW. Appendicitis and infections of the appendix. Semin Diagn Pathol 21:86–97, 2004.
10. Satti MB, Tamimi DM, Al Sohaibani M, et al. Appendicular schistosomiasis: a cause of clinical acute appendicitis? J Clin Pathol 424–8, 1987.
11. Smith JH, Christie JD. The pathobiology of *Schistosoma haematobium* infection in humans. Hum Pathol 17:333–45, 1986.
12. Smith JH, Said MN, Kelada AS. Studies on schistosomal rectal and colonic polyposis. Am J Trop Med Hyg 26:80–4, 1977.
13. Strickland GT. Gastrointestinal manifestations of schistosomiasis. Gut 35:1334–7, 1994.
14. von Lichtenberg F. Schistosomiasis. In: Connor DH, Chandler FW, et al (eds): Pathology of Infectious Diseases, Stamford, CT: Appleton and Lange, 1997, pp. 1537–51.

Subject Index

L.W. Lamps, *Surgical Pathology of the Gastrointestinal System: Bacterial, Fungal, Viral, and Parasitic Infections*,
DOI 10.1007/978-1-4419-0861-2, © Springer Science+Business Media, LLC 2009

Printed in the United States of America